Forensic Learning Series

Sexually Transmitted Infection and Disease Assessment

for Health Care Providers and First Responders

Forensic Learning Series

STM **Learning,** Inc.

Leading Publisher of Scientific, Technical, and Medical Educational Resources
Saint Louis
www.stmlearning.com

Sexually Transmitted Infection and Disease Assessment

for Health Care Providers and First Responders

Forensic Learning Series

Patricia M. Speck, DNSc, CRNP, FNP-BC, DF-IAFN, FAAFS, DF-AFN, FAAN
Professor
Coordinator Advanced Forensic Nursing
Department of Family, Community, & Health Systems
The University of Alabama at Birmingham School of Nursing

Diana K. Faugno, MSN, RN, CPN, SANE-A, SANE-P, FAAFS, DF-IAFN, DF-AFN
Forensic Nurse
Founding Board Director
End Violence Against Women International
Past President
Academy of Forensic Nursing

Stacey Mitchell, DNP, MBA, RN, SANE-A, SANE-P, DF-AFN, FAAN
Clinical Associate Professor
College of Nursing
Texas A&M University

Rachell A. Ekroos, PhD, APRN-BC, AFN-BC, FAAN
Chief Executive Officer
Center for Forensic Nursing Excellence International (CFNEI)

Melanie Gibbons Hallman, DNP, CRNP, CEN, FNP-BC, ACNP-BC, ENP-C, TCRN, FAEN
Assistant Professor
Department of Family, Community, & Health Systems
The University of Alabama at Birmingham School of Nursing

STM **Learning,** Inc.

Leading Publisher of Scientific, Technical, and Medical Educational Resources
Saint Louis
www.stmlearning.com

Publishers: Glenn E. Whaley and Marianne V. Whaley
Graphic Design Director: Glenn E. Whaley
Acquisitions Editor: Glenn E. Whaley
Associate Editor: Marika Betker
Book Design/Page Layout: Jennifer M. Jones and G.W. Graphics
Print/Production Coordinator: Jennifer M. Jones and G.W. Graphics
Cover Design: Jennifer M. Jones and G.W. Graphics
Color Prepress Specialist: Kevin Tucker
Developmental Editor: Marika Betker
Copy Editor: Marika Betker
Proofreader: Samantha Koester

Printed in the United States of America.

Publisher:
STM Learning, Inc.
Saint Louis, Missouri 63033
Phone: (314) 434-2424
http://www.stmlearning.com orders@stmlearning.com

Library of Congress Control Number: 2019954902
ISBN 9781936590865 (ebook) | ISBN 9781936590858 (pbk. : alk. paper)

Contributors

Kathy Bell, MS, RN, SANE-A, SANE-P, DF-AFN
Forensic Nursing Administrator
Tulsa Police Department

Alice Springer Bristow, DNP, CRNP, FNP-BC, CWCN, CNE
Instructor
The University of Alabama at Birmingham School of Nursing
Nurse Practitioner
Cahaba Medical Care
Woodstock, Alabama

Pamela H. Bryant, DNP, CRNP, CPNP-AC/PC
Assistant Professor
Pediatric Primary Care Specialty Track Coordinator
Family/Community and Health Systems
The University of Alabama at Birmingham, School of Nursing

Elizabeth Coleman, MSN, CRNP, CPNP-PC
Nursing Instructor
The University of Alabama at Birmingham School of Nursing

William DeClue, DNP, FNP-BC, MHA
Assistant Professor
Goldfarb School of Nursing
Barnes-Jewish College

Nancy R. Downing, PhD, RN, SANE-A, SANE-P, FAAN
Associate Professor
Center of Excellence in Forensic Nursing
Texas A&M University

Angela Ellis, MSN, RN, SANE-A, SANE-P
Forensic Nurse Consultant
Anchorage, Alaska
Adjunct Professor
School of Nursing
The University of Alaska Anchorage
Medical-Forensic Expert
The Alaska Network on Domestic Violence and Sexual Assault

Ashley Feldman, BSN, RN
Clinical Forensic Registered Nurse
Nevada HealthRight

Amanda Flynn, DNP, MSN, RN, FNP-BC
Assistant Professor
Goldfarb School of Nursing
Barnes-Jewish College

Kathy Gill-Hopple, PhD, RN, SANE-A, SANE-P, DF-AFN
Adjunct Professor
Masters of Nursing Forensic Program
Fitchburg State University
Clinical Forensic Program Coordinator (retired)
Medical University of South Carolina

Kelsey Tucker Geer, MSN, FNP-C
Nurse Practitioner
Marshall Medical Center South
Boaz, Alabama

David T. House, DNP, CRNP, ENP-C, FNP-BC, CNS
Assistant Professor
Department of Family, Community, & Health Systems
The University of Alabama at Birmingham School of Nursing

Trinity Ingram-Jones, DNP, MSN, APRN, CPNP, PCNS, AFN-BC, SANE-A, SANE-P, DF-AFN
Owner
Ingram-Jones & Associates, LLC
Executive Director and Medical-Forensic Examiner
The Cottage, Richmond Hill

Katie Jett, DNP, FNP-BC, RN
Assistant Professor
Director, BSN Program Upper Division at West Campus
Director, Clinical Simulation Institute
Goldfarb School of Nursing
Barnes-Jewish College

Kelsey Kincaid, BA
Las Vegas, Nevada

April Love, MSN, RN, RNC-OB, CNE
Instructor
The University of Alabama at Birmingham School of Nursing

Nicole Marnell, DNP, APRN, CPNP-PC
Assistant Professor
School of Nursing
The University of Alaska Anchorage

Lauren Mays, DNP, CRNP, FNP-BC
Instructor
Nurse Practitioner
The University of Alabama at Birmingham School of Nursing

Elisabeth Pelt, MSN, APRN, WHNP-BC
Instructor
Family, Community, & Health Systems
The University of Alabama at Birmingham School of Nursing

Cheryl L. Pullium, DNP, APRN, RN, ACNS-BC
Clinical Assistant Professor
College of Nursing
Texas A&M University

Sallie Johnson Shipman, EdD, MSN, RN, CNL, NHDP-BC
Clinical Assistant Professor
Family, Community, and Health Systems Science
The University of Florida College of Nursing
Gainesville, Florida

Rebecca Suttle, DNP, CRNP, AGACNP-BC
Adult-Gero Acute Care Nurse Practitioner
The University of Alabama at Birmingham School of Nursing

Kathleen Thimsen, DNP, MSN, WOCN, FNS
Assistant Professor
Goldfarb School of Nursing
Barnes-Jewish College

Lauren Traveller, DNP, APRN, FNP-C
Assistant Director of Clinical Services
Clinical Forensic Specialist
Nevada HealthRight

Angelia Trujillo, DNP, MSN, WHNP-BC
Associate Professor
School of Nursing
The University of Alaska Anchorage

Robert Vargas, BS
Las Vegas, Nevada

Cindy Weston, DNP, APRN, CCRN, CNS-CC, FNP-BC
Assistant Professor
Associate Dean for Clinical and Outreach Affairs
College of Nursing
Texas A&M University

Foreword

The effective detection and management of sexually transmitted infections (STIs) is integral to health and overall well-being in our patient populations. Of concern are patients who have experienced sexual assault as they are at particular risk and require STI evaluation immediately following the assault, as well as during the recommended follow-up examination. The Centers for Disease Control and Prevention states, "Examinations of survivors of sexual assault should be conducted by an experienced clinician in a way that minimizes further trauma to the survivor."[1]

It is important that caregivers are competent and confident when caring for this vulnerable and complex patient population. *Sexually Transmitted Infection and Disease Assessment for Health Care Providers and First Responders* provides health care providers information in a succinct and comprehensive format which not only increases the reader's essential knowledge, but allows learners to synthesize, apply, and review essential information in practical case history exercises. The integration and practical application of this knowledge within the scenarios allows learners to synthesize key information to transform their practice at a self-directed pace. Authored by internationally recognized experts, readers are presented with case histories and corresponding exercises in STI evaluation, which are ideal for self-directed study or group instruction and will benefit novice and advanced practitioners alike.

Catherine H. Rossi, FNP-BC, RN, MSN, SANE-A, SANE-P, DF-AFN
President (2020)
Academy of Forensic Nursing
Program Manager
Cone Health Forensic Nursing
Greensboro, North Carolina

1. *2015 sexually transmitted diseases treatment guidelines: sexual assault and abuse and STDs. Centers for Disease Control and Prevention Web site. https://www.cdc.gov/std/tg2015/sexual-assault.htm. Updated June 4, 2015. Accessed September 21, 2019.*

Our Mission

To become the world leader in publishing and information services on child abuse, maltreatment, diseases, and domestic violence. We seek to heighten awareness of these issues and provide relevant information to professionals and consumers.

FOREWORD

In 2018, the Centers for Disease Control and Prevention reported 2 457 118 combined cases of sexually transmitted infections (STIs) in the United States.[1] Because many cases of common STIs such as syphilis, gonorrhea, *Chlamydia*, human papillomavirus, and herpes simplex are not identified or reported, the number of STIs may be considerably higher. *Sexually Transmitted Infection and Disease Assessment for Health Care Providers and First Responders* was written with the intent of creating an evidence-based, self-directed teaching tool and reference for providers across all disciplines who deal with patients of all ages at risk for STIs. The text, in both handbook and ebook format, provides clear and concise information with drawings and full-color photographs that are useful for the veteran forensic or nonforensic clinician as well as for the clinician just entering practice.

This all-new handbook is written by content experts in forensic nursing, advanced emergency nursing practice, and advanced outpatient nursing practice. A review of male and female anatomy, with drawings and full-color photographs, details normal anatomy as well as variants of normal anatomy. An overview of STIs is provided with photographs. Each chapter provides a section on Disease and Mimics which assists in the differential diagnosis of the suspected STI. Epidemiology and focused diagnostic methods are described along with the use of checklists and concise algorithms that provide a clear pathway to diagnosis. Critical thinking is reinforced through pediatric and adult/geriatric case studies that teach and refine diagnostic skills in STI identification, treatment protocols, and follow-up based on the current evidence-based recommendations. Importantly, the reader is reminded frequently that any child diagnosed with an STI should be referred to child protective services for investigation of potential sexual abuse. With increasing international travel, the risk of STIs increases.[2] This text reinforces the need for greater STI awareness and screening for all who are at risk for STIs.

Sexually Transmitted Infection and Disease Assessment for Health Care Providers and First Responders is a resource that all practitioners caring for patients at risk for STIs will want in their pocket.

William E. Somerall, Jr, MD, MAEd
Assistant Professor of Nursing
The University of Alabama at Birmingham School of Nursing
Birmingham, Alabama

1. *DC fact sheet: reported STDs in the United States, 2018. Centers for Disease Control and Prevention Web site. https://www.cdc.gov/nchhstp/newsroom/docs/factsheets/std-trends-508.pdf. Accessed November 13, 2019.*
2. *Memish ZA, Osoba AO. International travel and sexually transmitted diseases.* Travel Med Infect Dis. *2006;4(2):86-93.*

Preface

Understanding sexually transmitted infections (STIs) is a large part of medical forensic practices, whether it is registered nurses trained to recognize disease and refer the patient to experts, or advanced nurse practitioners and physicians charged with diagnosis and treatment. *Sexually Transmitted Infection and Disease Assessment* provides the latest information on STIs for medical practitioners at every level. Each chapter covers a different STI and includes information for a rapid check of presenting symptoms, current testing procedures, and treatment options according to the latest recommendations with updates from the Centers for Disease Control and Prevention. In addition, the book has patient education recommendations, as well as sexual health practices recommendations.

The case study review section helps the provider maintain skills with an assessment for differential diagnosis of the most commonly seen STIs and offers an opportunity for students to test their knowledge. Both the experienced and novice provider will benefit from the chance to review and refine their skills.

The authors want to thank the support of their employers and colleagues, and everyone who contributed to the important information included in this book. We believe health care providers will find this assessment to be an invaluable addition to their library and will keep this book on their desk, becoming their favorite frequent reference.

Patricia M. Speck, DNSc, CRNP, FNP-BC, DF-IAFN, FAAFS, DF-AFN, FAAN

Diana Faugno, MSN, RN, CPN, SANE-A, SANE-P, FAAFS, DF-IAFN, DF-AFN

Stacey Mitchell, DNP, MBA, RN, SANE-A, SANE-P, DF-AFN, FAAN

Rachell A. Ekroos, PhD, APRN-BC, AFN-BC, FAAN

Melanie Gibbons Hallman, DNP, CRNP, CEN, FNP-BC, ACNP-BC, ENP-C, TCRN, FAEN

Reviews

As a forensic nurse or first responder, we are the source that patients count on for answers. For this reason, we need powerful resources that are easy to use. Sexually Transmitted Infection and Disease Assessment for Health Care Providers and First Responders *delivers this in a big way—providing essential and plentiful detail in a naturally intuitive structure. This is the rare combination of breadth, depth, and simplicity. Breadth: covering both common and rare STIs and STDs; depth: providing definitions, pictures, and case examples; and simplicity: each chapter makes sense and provides the information you need, where you expect to find it.*

Whether you are an experienced practitioner or new to the field, this text provides evidence-based and current best practices including identification, modes of transmission, symptoms, and treatments of STIs or STDs. This book supports case reviews or serves as a quick reference during patient care. The user-friendly format delivers the information you need quickly and concisely. The value of a simple to use, accurate, and in-depth handbook like this cannot be overstated for the first responder. I recommend having this book readily available in all patient care scenarios.

Sarah Pederson,
BSN, RN, SANE-A, SANE-P
Atlanta, Georgia

The Sexually Transmitted Infection and Disease Assessment *is a very detailed explanation of sexually transmitted infections. It not only discusses prevalence, epidemiology, assessment, and treatment, but it provides great case studies and provides the reader with the ability to self-evaluate their understanding of the diseases. The tables give you quick references to immunization schedules and illustrations assist the provider in identifying diseases. This is the type of treatise that is so beneficial to front line providers to assist them in medical diagnosis and treatment. This is a "must purchase" for nurses who are pursuing degrees as advanced practice providers.*

Barbra A. Bachmeier,
JD, MSN, APRN, NP-C, DF-AFN,
FAEN
Advanced Practice Provider/Forensic Nurse
Indianapolis, Indiana

Sexually Transmitted Infection and Disease Assessment *is an exceptional guide, which offers health care professionals the opportunity to engage in a self-directed or group learning experience in the evaluation for sexually transmitted infections. The thoughtful range and breadth with which each chapter is written provides a comprehensive and detailed understanding of sexually transmitted infections. It affords readers the opportunity to assess case histories and identify treatment options with photographs for reference, demonstrating basic concepts as well as difficult issues. The evaluation exercises included enhance and strengthen abilities in sexually transmitted infection identification, treatment, and follow-up care. This book is an invaluable resource and clearly articulates the highest standards of care for professionals providing sexual health assessments and care to this population.*

Sinead Maher, MSc, RM, RNP, RGN
CNS Sexual Assault Forensic Examiner
Sexual Assault Treatment Unit
Cork, Ireland

Sexually Transmitted Infection and Disease Assessment *provides health care professionals with the tools necessary to deliver appropriate care for patients who may have been exposed to, or are exhibiting symptoms of, STIs. It is an exceptional resource for any health care provider, from physicians to forensic nurses, who interact with patients across the lifespan. Novice and experienced providers will find this resource to be an invaluable addition to their medical library.*

Beginning with clear and accurate definitions, diagrams, and labeled images, this text guides the learner through several STIs. Individualized case studies allow the learner to test their own knowledge of anatomical structures and work through case presentations from presentation to treatment. Each case study builds on the previous one and serves to provide a well-rounded description of many STIs. I highly recommend Sexually Transmitted Infection and Disease Assessment *for any health care professional who wishes to expand their knowledge-base.*

Laurie Charles, MSN, RN,
CA-CPSANE, SANE-A, SANE-P, CHSE
Clinical Assistant Professor
Texas A&M University College of Nursing
Center of Excellence in Forensic Nursing

Sexually Transmitted Infection and Disease Assessment *presents a complex and challenging health care topic for the various levels of health care professionals. This workbook promotes a practical, self-directed approach to an ever-challenging problem in today's society. The most common sexually transmitted infections are discussed through a variety of applicable learning activities. To refine and reinforce the content, anatomical reviews, case studies, special populations, treatment plans, and full color photographs are incorporated to enhance the reader's knowledge. A collaborative, trauma-informed approach provides an approach to prevention, assessment, identification, and treatment.*

Frankie Wallis,
DNP, NP-C, NEA-BC, COI
University of Alabama Hospital - UAB
Senior Director of Nursing
Emergency & Trauma Services
Birmingham, Alabama

Reviews

The Sexually Transmitted Infection and Disease Assessment *is a practical, clinically focused workbook designed to improve the diagnostic skills of health professionals at every level. This expertly authored text examines disease processes, contextual relevance, and clinical management for each topic using clear, concise delivery augmented by photographic exemplars and thoroughly supported with case studies. Whether used for reference or self-study, the authors' wealth of knowledge cultivated over many decades of patient care experience and curated in this well-organized volume will benefit novice first responders and experienced health care providers alike.*

Chelsea Hayman, BSN, RN, CEN
Doctor of Nursing Practice Student
The University of Alabama at Birmingham

This comprehensive guide on sexually transmitted infections (STIs) is a must-have for all medical professionals and frontline health care workers. This guide is insightful and practical in the layout of the pathophysiology and treatment of STIs which allows information to be incorporated in forensic practice. The use of detailed case studies and laboratory information increase the learner's knowledge about STIs. All health care workers need to access this guide to enhance their knowledge about infections to better manage the care of their patients. The authors use an excellent approach to capture the attention of its audience and brings to light a much-needed topic in the health care arena.

Beverly N. Brown, MSN, APRN, FNP-C
Student
The University of Alabama at Birmingham

The Sexually Transmitted Infection and Disease Assessment *is a beneficial educational exercise for clinicians providing care in a multitude of settings. The succinct and relevant review of pathophysiology, diagnostics, and management of STIs is enriched by case histories and application activities for the learner. The competency gained through completion of the educational exercises will empower care providers to address patient needs according to best practice guidelines.*

Jessica Griffith Sparks, RN-BSN
Candidate for Doctor of Nursing Practice
The University of Alabama at Birmingham

This assessment is an excellent resource for forensic medical professionals to review sexually transmitted infections and diseases. The case studies and photographs allow the medical professional to understand the diagnosis and treatment plan. It is a great addition to any medical professionals' library.

Elizabeth McCord,
MSN, FNP-C, SANE-A
Operations Manager
Bridge Forensic Clinic
Pearl, Mississippi

This comprehensive workbook serves as an insightful guide for students and teachers everywhere. The authors' vast knowledge is clearly visible and allows for this book to serve as a valuable resource. The special attention to detail in laboratory testing, treatments, and special considerations is key in diagnosis and treatment. The case studies provide a unique and realistic perspective into clinical practice and allow for updated information to be readily and easily available. This workbook is useful to all health care workers as a tool for educating others, as well as for self-education to be the best health care provider possible and promote patient safety.

Sameera A. Rajpari, BSN, RN
Candidate for Doctor of Nursing Practice
The University of Alabama at Birmingham

Contents in Brief

Contents in Detail

Sexually Transmitted Infection and Disease Assessment

for Health Care Providers and First Responders

Forensic Learning Series

STM **Learning,** Inc.

Leading Publisher of Scientific, Technical, and Medical Educational Resources

Saint Louis

www.stmlearning.com

Section I

Definitions and Anatomical Review

Objectives

After reviewing the figures presented in this section, the student will be able to:

1. Correctly identify oral, genital, and anal anatomy.

2. Accurately define structures of the oral, genital, and anal anatomy.

Instructions

Anatomical diagrams and photographs have been provided to assist the student with correctly identifying anatomical landmarks. These diagrams and photos should be used when documenting normal anatomy, injuries, and any other variant conditions or findings throughout the *Sexually Transmitted Infection and Disease Assessment.*

STI Definitions

— ***Abstinence:*** Not having sexual intercourse.

— ***Acquired immunodeficiency syndrome (AIDS):*** A disease of the human immune system caused by the human immunodeficiency virus (HIV). HIV/AIDS represents the entire range of diseases caused by the HIV virus from early infection to late stage symptoms.

— ***Anal intercourse:*** Sexual contact in which the penis enters the anus.

— ***Antibiotic:*** A medication that either kills or inhibits the growth of a bacteria.

— ***Antiviral:*** A medication that either kills or inhibits the growth of a virus.

— ***Atrophic:*** A thinning of tissue modified by the location. In epidermal atrophy, the epidermis becomes transparent with a loss of skin texture and cigarette paper–like wrinkling. In dermal atrophy, there is a loss of connective tissue and the lesion is depressed.

— ***Bacterial vaginosis (BV):*** A polymicrobial clinical syndrome resulting from replacement of the normal hydrogen peroxide producing *Lactobacillus* sp. in the vagina with high concentrations of anaerobic bacteria. A common symptom of BV is abnormal homogeneous, off-white, fishy-smelling vaginal discharge.

— ***Cervical motion tenderness (CMT):*** A sign found on pelvic examination suggestive of pelvic pathology; when movement of the cervix during the bimanual examination elicits pain.

— ***Cervix:*** The lower, cylindrical end of the uterus that forms a narrow canal connecting the upper (uterus) and lower (vagina) parts of a woman's reproductive tract.

— ***Chlamydia:*** The most common reported sexually transmitted bacterial infection in the United States, caused by the bacteria *Chlamydia trachomatis*. Often, no symptoms are present, especially in women. Untreated *Chlamydia* can cause sterility and pelvic inflammatory disease (PID) and increase the chances for life-threatening tubal pregnancies. *Chlamydia* is treated with antibiotics and can be prevented by avoiding sexual intercourse or by using protection (eg, a latex or polyurethane condom) with every sexual act and encounter.

— ***Condom (male):*** A device that covers the penis, worn during sex to prevent sexually transmitted infections (STIs) and pregnancy. Condoms can be made of animal skin, latex, or polyurethane, but only latex and polyurethane condoms protect against diseases.

— ***Condom (female):*** A device worn internally that lines the vagina during sexual intercourse as a barrier contraceptive to prevent exposure to ejaculated sperm and STIs. The female condom is a thin, soft, loose-fitting sheath with a flexible ring at each end made out of polyurethane or synthetic nitrile.

— ***Confidential:*** Private information that identifies a person and, by law, is required to be kept in a secured location with access restricted only to authorized personnel. For example, a confidential HIV test would be one where a person's file would be kept in a locked area where only authorized medical personnel (physician, nurse practitioner, or counselor) would have access.

— ***Cryotherapy:*** Freezing with liquid nitrogen or cryoprobe; one of the recommended provider-administered treatments for external genital warts.

— ***Dark field:*** A simple and reliable microscopic test for the direct detection of *Treponema pallidum*, the bacteria that causes syphilis. Exudates and fluids from genital lesions are examined as a wet mount using dark-field microscopy. Dark-field microscopy is most suitable when the lesions are located in the genital region, are moist, and the examination can be done immediately after specimen collection. Testing nongenital lesions, especially oral lesions, can result in false positives because of the presence of nonpathogenic spirochetes and is not recommended.

— ***Dental dam:*** A thin, rectangular sheet, usually latex rubber, used as a barrier to prevent the transmission of STIs during oral sex.

— ***Disease intervention specialist (DIS):*** A public health worker who investigates cases and contacts of reportable STIs. The DIS locates and counsels people with STIs and HIV to identify exposed individuals and ensure testing and treatment. A DIS provides recommendations to physicians and health departments on the testing and treatment of patients and facilitates rapid referrals to service and follow-up.

— ***Dyspareunia:*** Painful sexual intercourse.

— ***Dysuria:*** Difficult or painful urination.

— ***Enzyme-linked immunosorbent assay (ELISA):*** A screening test used to detect HIV infection by looking for antibodies to the virus in a patient's serum. If antibodies to HIV are present (positive), it is followed by confirmatory testing according to guidelines from the Centers for Disease Control and Prevention (CDC).

— ***Ectopic pregnancy:*** Also referred to as ***tubal pregnancy;*** a pregnancy in which the fertilized egg that grows into a fetus attaches itself to the fallopian tube instead of the walls of the uterus. Ectopic pregnancy can be life threatening. Rates of ectopic pregnancy increase significantly in women who have PID, an effect of untreated bacterial STIs such as *Chlamydia* and gonorrhea.

— ***Edematous:*** A condition marked by an excessive accumulation of watery fluid in cells and tissues.

— ***Expedited partner therapy (EPT):*** The clinical practice of treating the sex partners of patients diagnosed with *Chlamydia* or gonorrhea by providing prescriptions or medications to the patient to take to his or her partner without the health care provider first examining the partners. Although legality varies by state, the clinical practice is allowed by the majority of the United States. In these cases, the health care provider does not examine the partner but is required to provide treatment through state law.

— ***Fallopian tubes:*** Tubes on each side of the uterus through which an egg moves from the ovaries to the uterus.

— ***Fluorescent treponemal antibody (FTA) test:*** A blood serum test for syphilis that detects the presence or absence of specific antibodies directed against the organism *Treponema pallidum*. The FTA is a "treponemal test" used in the diagnosis of syphilis infection and detects the majority of, but not all, cases of infection. False negatives can occur in early syphilis infection, and false positives are relatively uncommon. The FTA should be used in conjunction with the rapid plasma reagin to properly diagnose syphilis infection.

— ***Genital warts:*** A viral infection caused by the nononcogenic or low-risk types of human papillomavirus (HPV), usually types 6 and 11. Genital warts are diagnosed by visual inspection and most commonly occur in the genital or anal areas of the body. They typically appear cauliflower-shaped and can be flesh-colored, pink, or hyperpigmented. Because genital warts are caused by a virus, there is no real cure—the warts themselves can be treated, but the virus still lives inside a person's body. HPV is passed through direct skin-to-skin contact, even if no symptoms are present.

— ***Gonorrhea:*** The second most commonly reported bacterial STI in the United States, caused by the bacteria *Neisseria gonorrhoeae*. Many people who are infected show no signs of the disease, particularly women. When symptoms are present, they usually appear 2 to 5 days after sexual contact with an infected partner. Gonorrhea can cause PID if left untreated. Gonorrhea is treated with antibiotics and can be prevented by avoiding sexual contact with infected individuals or by using protection (eg, a latex or polyurethane condom) with every sexual contact.

— ***Gynecologist:*** A physician or nurse practitioner who specializes in women's reproductive health.

— ***Hepatitis A:*** An acute viral infection of the liver caused by the hepatitis A virus (HAV). Hepatitis A is often asymptomatic and generally self-limiting. Symptoms may include nausea, vomiting, diarrhea, jaundice (yellowish discoloration of the skin), fever, and abdominal pain. Incubation period is 2 to 6 weeks. It rarely results in chronic infection, chronic liver disease, or acute liver failure. Transmission is primarily by the fecal-oral route via food or water contaminated with feces. The hepatitis A vaccine is available for the prevention of hepatitis A.

— ***Hepatitis B:*** An infectious illness of the liver caused by the hepatitis B virus (HBV). Acute illness causes liver inflammation, vomiting, jaundice, and, rarely, death. Chronic hepatitis B may eventually cause cirrhosis and liver cancer. It is transmitted by exposure to infectious blood or body fluids such as semen and vaginal fluid. There is no specific treatment for the acute infection. Treatment is recommended for some with chronic infection to suppress the virus and may include antiviral medications (eg, entecavir [Baraclude], tenofovir [Viread], lamivudine [Epivir], adefovir [Hepsera], telbivudine [Tyzeka]) which fight the virus, slowing down its ability to damage the liver. It is preventable with the hepatitis B vaccine series.

— ***Hepatitis C:*** An infectious disease affecting primarily the liver caused by the hepatitis C virus (HCV). Infection is often asymptomatic, but chronic infection can lead to scarring of the liver and ultimately to cirrhosis. Those with cirrhosis may go on to develop liver failure or liver cancer. Transmission occurs through blood-to-blood contact associated with intravenous drug use, poorly sterilized medical equipment, transfusions, and rarely through sexual transmission. Chronic infection can be treated with medication, and cure rates range from 50% to 80%. HCV is the leading reason for liver transplantation. No vaccine against hepatitis C is available.

- ***Human immunodeficiency virus (HIV):*** A retrovirus, causing AIDS. It is the best-known lentivirus (***lenti*** is Latin for "slow"), which is a genus of retroviruses that causes chronic and deadly disease, characterized by long incubation periods in humans. There is slow progressive failure of the immune system, which allows life-threatening opportunistic infections and cancers to thrive. HIV is transmitted via blood, semen, vaginal fluid, pre-ejaculate, and breast milk. The virus infects vital cells in the human immune system such as helper T cells, macrophages, and dendritic cells, leading to a loss of cell-mediated immunity. As a result, the body becomes progressively susceptible to opportunistic infections. HIV is highly treatable, but there is no cure or vaccine for prevention.

- ***Human papillomavirus (HPV):*** A DNA virus from the papillomavirus family that establishes infection in keratinocytes of the skin and mucous membranes. Most HPV infections are subclinical and will cause no physical symptoms; however, some subclinical infections may become clinical and cause benign papillomas (warts) or squamous cell papillomas (cancers). Approximately 30 to 40 types of HPV are typically transmitted through sexual contact and infect the anogenital region. HPV types 6 and 11 are commonly associated with genital warts and rarely progress to cancer. High-risk HPV types 16 and 18 are associated with progression to precancerous lesions and invasive cancer. The HPV vaccine prevents HPV types 16 and 18, the 2 types that cause 80% of cervical cancer. The vaccine is routinely recommended for girls and boys ages 11 or 12, although it can be given as early as age 9. It is ideal for girls and boys to receive the vaccine before they have sexual contact and are exposed to HPV.

- ***Herpes simplex virus (HSV):*** A chronic, lifelong viral infection spread when an infected person is producing and shedding the virus in an infected area of the skin. Two types of HSV have been identified, HSV-1 and HSV-2. Most cases of genital herpes are caused by HSV-2 and oral lesions are typically caused by HSV-1, but both types can be found in the genital and oral areas. A large majority of individuals with HSV are asymptomatic and unaware of their exposure. The infection is manageable and treatable with antiviral therapy, but there is no vaccine for prevention.

- ***Injection drug use:*** A term used to describe a method of injecting drugs using a needle.

- ***Long-acting bicillin (LAB):*** Also known as benzathine penicillin. The antibiotic recommended for the treatment of syphilis because of its prolonged, low-concentration, antibacterial action over 2 to 4 weeks after a single intramuscular dose.

- ***Loop electrosurgical excision procedure (LEEP):*** A procedure using a fine wire-loop diathermy for biopsy or excision for treatment of cervical intraepithelial neoplasia.

- ***Lymphogranuloma venereum (LGV):*** An STI caused by certain subtypes of *Chlamydia trachomatis*, specifically serovars L1, L2, L2a, and L3. LGV is primarily an infection of lymphatics and lymph nodes. Although there have been sporadic outbreaks among men who have sex with men in the United States, it is endemic in parts of Africa, India, Southeast Asia, South America, and the Caribbean. Incidence and hence, prevalence, is unknown as LGV has been nonreportable since 2003.

- ***Macerated:*** Softened or broken-down skin resulting from prolonged exposure to wetness that leads to whitening and thickening of the keratin, sometimes with redness, oozing, and scaling.

- ***Macule:*** A circumscribed flat discoloration (eg, a freckle, a small vitiligo spot).

— ***Men who have sex with men (MSM):*** A term used to describe a male person who has sex with men. The CDC now recommends *gay, bisexual,* and *other men who have sex with men* be collectively referred to as MSM.

— ***Men who have sex with women (MSW):*** A term used to describe a male person who has sex with women.

— ***Mucoid:*** An adjective used to describe secretions that are slippery and rich in glycoproteins and water.

— ***Mucopurulent cervicitis (MPC):*** Inflammation of the cervix characterized by purulent or mucopurulent endocervical exudate visible in the endocervical canal or on an endocervical swab specimen.

— ***Mycoplasma genitalium (Mgen):*** An emerging STI. The bacterium is sexually transmitted and can cause inflammation of the urinary and genital tracts in men and women. Mgen, like other STIs, can cause inflammation of delicate genital tissue. Although nucleic acid amplification tests detect the organism, they are not readily available at this writing.

— ***Nodule:*** A circumscribed, elevated solid lesion. A large nodule is a tumor (ie, wart, hemangioma).

— ***Nongonococcal urethritis (NGU):*** An inflammation of the urethra not caused by gonorrheal infection; characterized by urethral discharge, painful urination, or itching at the end of the urethra.

— ***Nucleic acid amplification test (NAAT):*** A molecular technique used to detect a virus or bacterium by detecting the genetic material of an infecting organism. NAATs are able to detect the presence of infection earlier after exposure than antigen or antibody tests; however, NAATs are not used for test of cure within 3 months as the detection of noninfective residual DNA may yield false positives long after treatment.

— ***OLDCARTS:*** Acronym (Onset, Location, Duration, Character, Aggravating/relieving, Radiation, Timing, Severity) used when subjective history is provided to ensure complete assessment.

— ***Oral sex (oral intercourse, oral copulation):*** Sex in which the mouth comes in contact with the genital or anal areas (penis, vagina, or anus).

— ***Ovaries:*** The pair of female reproductive glands in which the ova, or eggs, are formed. The ovaries are located in the lower abdomen, 1 on each side of the uterus.

— ***Papanicolaou test (Pap smear):*** A method of cervical screening used to detect potentially precancerous and cancerous cells in the endocervical canal. A speculum is used to open the vaginal canal and allow the collection of cells from the outer opening of the cervix and the endocervix. Cells are then examined for abnormalities.

— ***Papule:*** A small superficial bump that is elevated and less than 1 cm (ie, papular dermatitis).

— ***Partner notification:*** A process in which a person with an infection, such as an STI, lets his or her sexual partner(s) know about the infection so that testing and treatment can be sought. DISs in the health departments can assist with the notification process.

— ***Patch:*** A large macule equal to or greater than 1 cm across, commonly involving some type of subtle skin surface changes, such as scaling or wrinkling, though the lesion itself is not palpable.

— ***Patient-delivered partner therapy (PDPT):*** A form of EPT in which providers supply infected patients with treatment packets to deliver to their partners without requiring the partners to come into the clinic for a medical examination or testing.

— ***Pelvic inflammatory disease (PID):*** An inflammatory disorder of the upper female genital tract, including any combination of endometritis, salpingitis, tubo-ovarian abscess, and pelvic peritonitis. The infection (usually caused by sexually transmitted organisms) spreads from the vagina to the upper parts of a woman's reproductive tract in the pelvic cavity. It can be difficult to diagnose because of the wide variety of symptoms and signs, which can be mild and subtle in many women. If left untreated, PID can cause infertility and in severe cases may even spread to the liver and kidneys, causing dangerous internal bleeding, liver and lung failure, and death.

— ***Pelvis:*** The lower part of the abdomen between the hip bones. Organs in a female's pelvis include the uterus, vagina, ovaries, fallopian tubes, bladder, and rectum.

— ***People who inject drugs (PWID):*** Refers to those who currently inject drugs or have a history of injection drug use.

— ***Plaque:*** A broad papule, or confluence of papules, equal to or greater than 1 cm; an elevated, plateau-like lesion greater in its diameter than in its depth (ie, psoriasis).

— ***Polycystic ovarian syndrome/disease (PCOS/PCOD):*** A condition in which a woman's ovaries or adrenal glands produce more male hormones than normal, possibly resulting in the development of cysts (fluid-filled sacs) on the ovaries. Women who are obese are more likely to have PCOS. Women with PCOS are at increased risk of developing diabetes and heart disease.

— ***Postexposure prophylaxis (PEP):*** A preventative medical treatment started immediately after a high-risk exposure to a pathogen such as HIV to prevent infection and development of the disease. To be effective, PEP for HIV must be taken within 72 hours of exposure; it consists of 2 to 3 antiretroviral medications taken for 28 days.

— ***Pre-exposure prophylaxis (PrEP):*** A preventative medical treatment used before exposure to a disease-causing agent to prevent rather than treat or cure a disease. PrEP most commonly refers to an HIV-prevention strategy that uses antiretroviral medications to protect high-risk HIV-negative people from acquiring HIV.

— ***Pruritus:*** Sensation that causes the desire or reflex to scratch; itchiness.

— ***Pubic lice:*** The crab louse *(Pthirus pubis)*, also known as the pubic louse. A tiny insect that is an obligate ectoparasite of humans. They are typically found in the pubic hair but may also live on other areas of coarse hair, including the eyelashes. They cannot jump, and they feed exclusively on blood. They are spread through sexual contact as well as through sharing of infested bed sheets, clothing, or towels. Females lay 3 eggs a day, and the eggs take 6 to 8 days to hatch. Itching is the main symptom of pubic lice. Skin may be irritated, and a rash may develop from extensive scratching and digging. Pubic lice can be treated with a medicated shampoo.

— ***Purulent:*** Producing or containing pus.

— ***Pustule:*** A small circumscribed elevation on the skin containing pus.

— ***Rapid plasma reagin (RPR):*** A macroscopic serological test that looks for nonspecific antibodies in the blood of a patient that may be infected with *Treponema pallidum*, the bacteria that causes syphilis. The test does not look for antibodies against the actual organism but rather for antibodies against substances released by cells when they are damaged by *T. pallidum*. The RPR is used to screen for syphilis and a RPR level (also called a ***titer***) can be used to track the progress of the disease over time and the patient's response to therapy. Because it is a nonspecific test, false positives can be seen as a result of a variety of different circumstances and conditions. The RPR is the test of choice by most laboratories across the United States and has largely replaced the Venereal Disease Research Laboratory, a similar nontreponemal syphilis test. There has been an increase in the adoption of automated treponemal tests by laboratories as the initial screening test for *T. pallidum*, followed by a nontreponemal test. While this algorithm is timelier and more cost-effective, it does have a 14% to 40% false-positive rate, with a second treponemal test often being used to help determine what clinical action should be taken.

— ***Reporting:*** The process of notifying the federal, state, regional, or local authorities of a new case of a reportable disease. Individual states have reporting laws on which diseases are required to be reported and who is required to submit the report (laboratory, clinic, or both).

— ***Scabies:*** A contagious skin infection caused by the mite *Sarcoptes scabiei*. The mite is tiny and not directly visible. The parasite burrows under the host's skin, causing intense itching. The mite may be transmitted by direct skin-to-skin contact and from infested bed sheets, towels, or clothes. Extensive scratching can also cause a rash. Like pubic lice, scabies can be cured with a medicated shampoo.

— ***Semen:*** The fluid from a man's penis that contains sperm.

— ***Sensitivity:*** A statistical measurement of the performance of a test that measures the proportion of actual positives that are correctly identified. The ability of a test to be positive in the presence of disease (also known as the ***true positive rate***).

— ***Sexually transmitted infection (STI):*** An infection that is passed during oral, anal, or genital/vaginal sexual contact. STIs include *Chlamydia*, gonorrhea, syphilis, genital herpes, HIV, genital warts, and trichomoniasis.

— ***SOAP:*** Acronym (Subjective history, Objective findings, Assessment, Plan of care) used when diagnosising STIs.

— ***Specificity:*** A statistical measurement of the performance of a test that identifies the proportion of negatives that are correctly identified. The ability of a test to be negative in the absence of disease (also known as the ***true negative rate***).

— ***Spermatozoa (sperm):*** The male reproductive cells. In mammals, they develop in the testicles and are released from the penis. Sperm cannot divide and have a limited life span of 3 to 5 days within the female genital tract. A sperm joins an ovum (female egg cell) during fertilization to form a zygote and contributes half of the nuclear genetic information. In mammals, the sex of the offspring is determined by the sperm cell.

— ***Spermicide:*** An agent that kills spermatozoa. Spermicide can be found in some condoms. Frequent use of spermicides containing nonoxynol-9 has been associated with disruption of the genital epithelium and is therefore not recommended for STI or HIV prevention.

— ***Squamous:*** Related to or covered with scales.

— ***Sterility:*** The inability to get pregnant, or to get someone pregnant; often caused by the effects of untreated bacterial infections such as *Chlamydia* or gonorrhea.

— ***Symptom:*** Any noticeable change in the body or its functions that indicates disease or infection; a physical sign that disease is present.

— ***Syphilis:*** A bacterial infection caused by the spirochete *Treponema pallidum*. The primary route of transmission is through sexual contact, but it may also be transmitted from mother to fetus during pregnancy or at birth, resulting in congenital syphilis. Signs and symptoms vary depending on which of the 4 stages it presents (primary, secondary, latent, and tertiary). Diagnosis is usually made using blood tests and an enzyme immunoassay test. This blood test checks for syphilis antibodies. Other tests include fluorescent treponemal antibody absorption test, *Treponema pallidum* particle agglutination assay, dark-field microscopy, and microhemagglutination assay. Syphilis can be effectively treated with antibiotics, specifically the preferred intramuscular penicillin G.

— ***Transmission:*** The spread of disease from 1 person to another.

— ***Trichomoniasis:*** Also referred to as "trich," it is an infection of the urogenital tract caused by the single-celled protozoan *Trichomonas vaginalis*. The most common sites of infection in women are the urethra and the vagina. Symptoms in women can include vaginal discharge, "fishy" odor, burning, and itching. Men rarely experience symptoms but can carry, and therefore transmit, the parasite through intercourse. It can be effectively treated with oral antibiotics.

— ***Ulcer:*** An open lesion on the surface of the skin or a mucosal surface caused by superficial loss of tissue, usually with inflammation.

— ***Urethra:*** The tube in the penis that carries both urine and semen.

— ***Urethritis:*** Inflammation (swelling) of the urethra. The most common symptom is painful or difficult urination. Urethral discharge is also commonly present. STIs (eg, gonorrhea, *Chlamydia*, *Mycoplasma genitalium* infection) often cause urethritis in men.

— ***Urinalysis:*** A laboratory test in which urine is examined microscopically for normal and abnormal elements to assist in diagnosing infections of the urinary tract.

— ***Uterus:*** The small, hollow, pear-shaped organ in a woman's pelvis. The organ in which the fetus develops during gestation; also called the ***womb.***

— ***Vaginal intercourse:*** Sexual contact in which the penis is inserted inside the vagina.

— ***Vaginal fluid:*** The natural liquids produced inside a woman's vagina. In an infected person, STIs can be passed when vaginal fluids come in contact with the genital area of a woman's sex partner.

— ***Vaginitis:*** Inflammation (swelling) of the vagina associated with symptoms of vaginal discharge, itching, pain, and irritation or infection of the vulva. The 3 main causes of vaginitis are BV, vulvovaginal candidiasis (VVC or ***yeast***), and trichomoniasis.

— ***Venereal disease research laboratory (VDRL):*** A microscopic serological test that looks for nonspecific antibodies in the blood of a patient that may be infected with *Treponema pallidum*, the bacteria that causes syphilis. The test does not look for antibodies against the actual organism but rather antibodies against substances released by cells when they are damaged by *T. pallidum*. The VDRL is used to screen for syphilis, and a VDRL level (also called a ***titer***) can be used to track the progress of the disease over time and the patient's response to therapy. Because it is a nonspecific test, false positives can be seen as a result of a variety of different circumstances and conditions. The VDRL has largely been replaced by the RPR as the nontreponemal syphilis test of choice by most laboratories in the United States.

— ***Vesicle:*** A small, fluid-filled bubble, usually superficial, and less than 0.5 cm.

— ***Vulvovaginal candidiasis (VVC):*** A vaginal infection typically caused by excessive growth of *Candida albicans*, a fungal species normally present in the vagina in small numbers and usually harmless. VVC is occasionally caused by other *Candida* species. Symptoms include pruritus, vaginal soreness, dyspareunia, external dysuria, and abnormal vaginal discharge. Treatment is an antifungal medication, either topical or oral. An estimated 75% of women will have at least 1 episode of VVC in their lifetime.

— ***Western blot:*** A confirmatory test used to detect specific anti-HIV antibodies in a human serum sample using a gel electrophoresis technique. The Western blot has been the traditional confirmatory test for HIV after 2 positive ELISA tests.

— *Wet prep:* A microscopic laboratory procedure used for the diagnosis of vaginal infections, primarily yeast, trichomoniasis, and BV. A sample of vaginal discharge is put in a saline suspension and viewed under the microscope. Reported abnormal findings should include whether the test is positive or negative for clue cells (must be 20%), yeast pseudohyphae, motile trichomonads, and increased white blood cells.

— *Zygote:* A single cell with a complete set of chromosomes that normally develops into an embryo.

Additional Definitions

The student may find reviewing the following definitions useful in completing the activities within this book. Terminology for indicators of direction when documenting findings during a medical forensic examination include ***anterior, posterior, inferior, superior, medial, lateral, proximal,*** and ***distal.***

— ***Abrasions:*** Superficial injuries representing the removal of the outermost layers of the skin; usually caused by lateral rubbing, sliding, or compressive forces.

— ***Anterior:*** Situated toward the front of the body.

— ***Avulsion:*** A forceful separation or detachment that may occur traumatically or surgically; tearing away of a body part or structure.

— ***Bruises (contusions):*** Injuries that lie below the intact epidermis and result from extravascular collection of blood that has leaked from ruptured capillaries or blood vessels after sufficient force has been applied to distort the soft tissues and tear 1 or more vessels.

— ***Cut:*** An opening in the skin that occurs when a sharp object comes into contact with skin or tissue with enough pressure to divide it; cuts have even, regular edges.

— ***Drug-facilitated sexual assault (DFSA):*** Term for all types of sexual assault when drugs, alcohol, or other intoxicants are deliberately given to the victim by the perpetrator.

— ***Distal:*** Farther away; situated away from the center of the body or from the point of attachment.

— ***Inferior:*** Low; situated lower in position.

— ***Lacerations:*** Injuries that occur when the continuity of the skin is broken and disrupted by blunt force such as tearing, ripping, crushing, overstretching, pulling apart, over bending, or shearing of tissue.

— ***Lateral:*** Situated toward the one side.

— ***Incapacitated rape:*** Self-induced intoxication creating vulnerability and lack of legal consent before rape.

— ***Medial:*** Middle; situated in the middle or inside.

— ***Petechiae:*** Multiple hemorrhagic spots; pinpoint to pinhead in size.

— ***Posterior:*** Behind; situated toward the back of the body.

— ***Proximal:*** Near; situated nearer to the center of the body or the point of attachment.

— ***Superior:*** Above; situated above another structure.

Oral Cavity

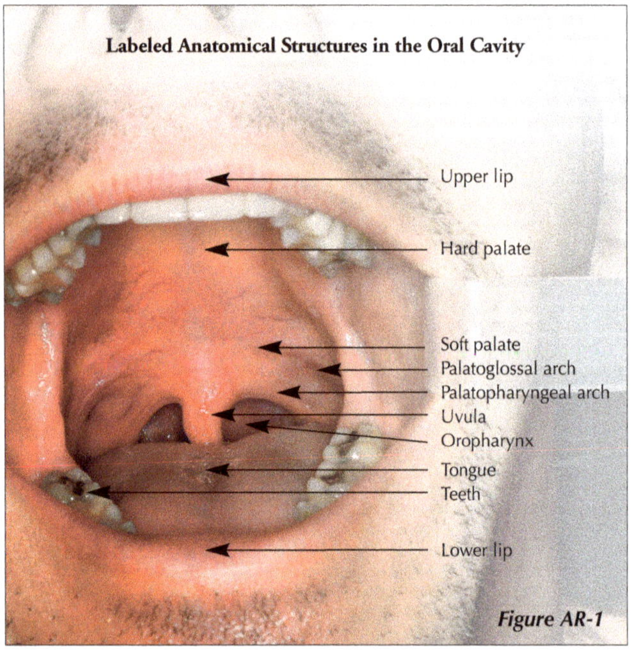

Figure AR-1

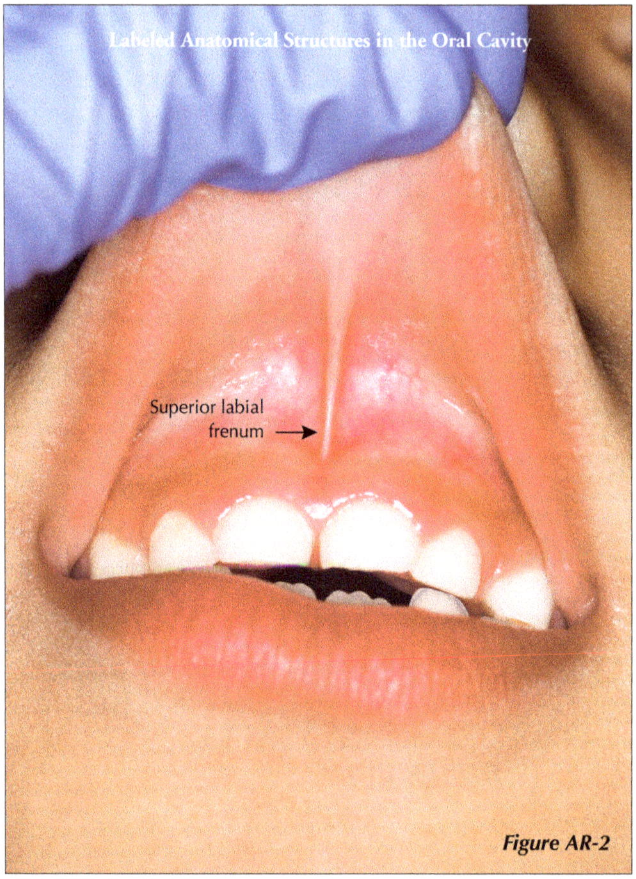

Figure AR-2

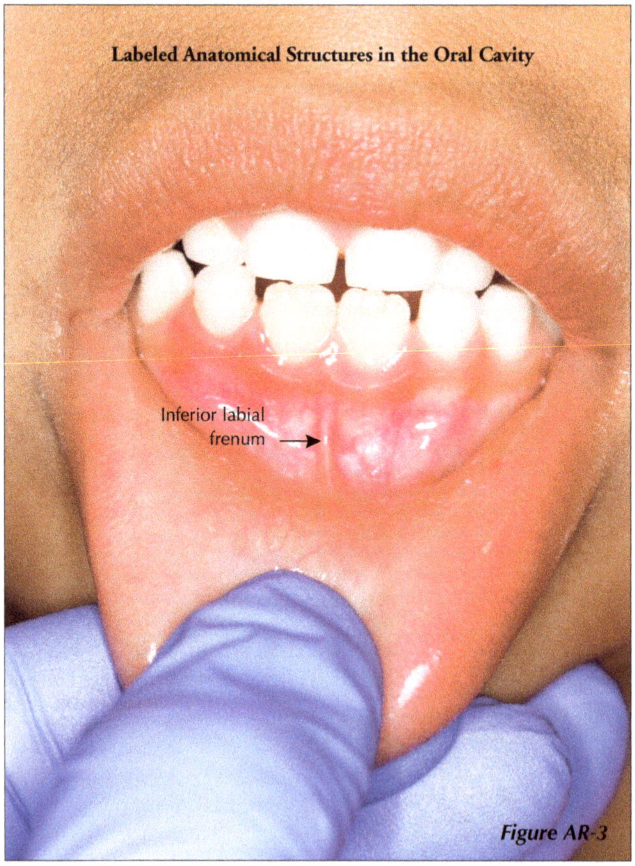

Figure AR-3

Definitions

— ***Fordyce spots:*** Enlarged ectopic sebaceous glands in the mucosa of the mouth and genitals, appearing as small yellow spots.

— ***Frenum*** (original term: frenulum): A small fold of mucous membrane that limits the movements of an organ or anatomical structure (eg, lingual frenum, maxillary labial frenum, mandibular labial frenum).

— ***Gingiva:*** The soft tissue overlying the crowns of unerupted teeth and encircling the necks of those that have erupted. Wisdom teeth are the last set of molars to erupt, usually at age 18 to 25 years.

— ***Hard palate:*** The anterior part of the palate, covered above by the mucous membrane of the nose and below by the mucoperiosteum of the roof of the mouth.

— ***Lips:*** The soft external structures that form the boundaries of the mouth; the opening to the oral cavity.

— ***Oropharynx:*** The area of the pharynx between the soft palate and the upper aspect of the epiglottis; area of the throat in the back of the mouth.

— ***Palatine raphe:*** A ridge or line along the median line of the palate that sometimes turns into a slight groove at its posterior end.

Labeled Anatomical Structures in the Oral Cavity

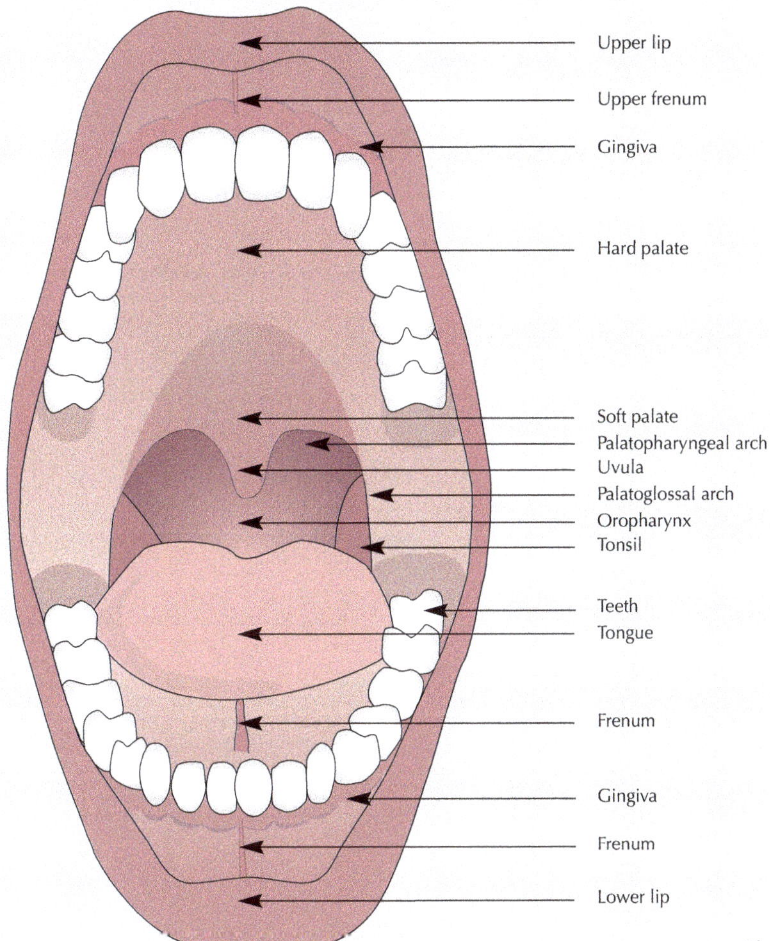

Figure AR-4

— ***Palatoglossal arch:*** The anterior of the 2 folds of mucous membrane on either side of the oropharynx, enclosing the palatoglossal muscle.

— ***Palatopharyngeal arch:*** The posterior of the 2 folds of mucous membrane on either side of the oropharynx, enclosing the palatopharyngeal muscle.

— ***Soft palate:*** A movable fold consisting of muscular fibers enclosed in mucous membrane. The soft palate is suspended from the rear of the hard palate and separates the nasal cavity from the oral cavity during swallowing or sucking.

— ***Teeth:*** The hardest bone in the body. Deciduous teeth are commonly called baby teeth or primary teeth; the first set usually consists of 20 teeth. For most, there are a total of 32 permanent, or adult, teeth.

— ***Tongue:*** A mobile mass of muscular tissue that is covered with mucous membrane; occupies much of the cavity of the mouth; forms part of its floor; is the organ of taste; and assists in chewing, swallowing, and speech.

— ***Tonsil:*** A small oral mass of lymphoid tissue, especially either of 2 such masses embedded in the lateral walls of the opening between the mouth and the pharynx. Also called faucial tonsil or palatine tonsil.

— ***Uvula:*** A small, soft structure hanging from the free edge of the soft palate in the midline above the root of the tongue. The uvula is composed of muscle, connective tissue, and mucous membrane.

MALE GENITALIA

Labeled Anatomical Structures in the Male

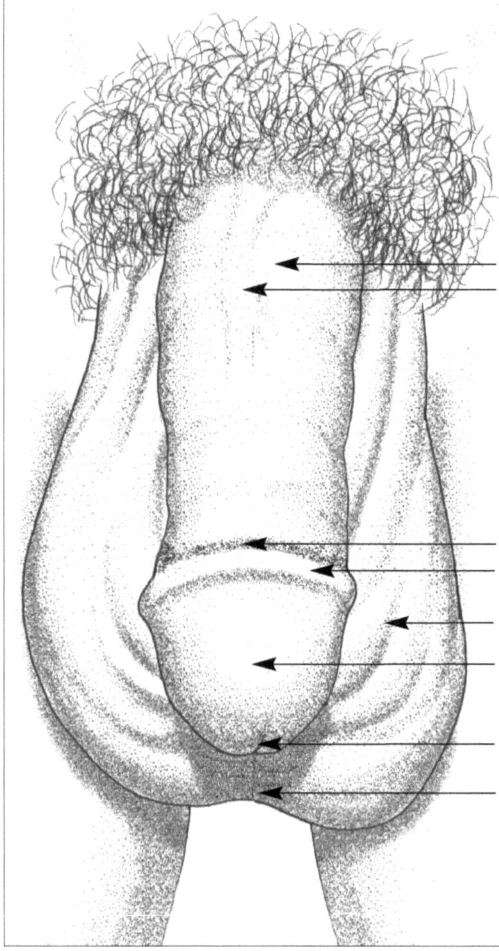

Figure AR-5

Labeled Anatomical Structures in the Prepubescent Male (Circumcised)

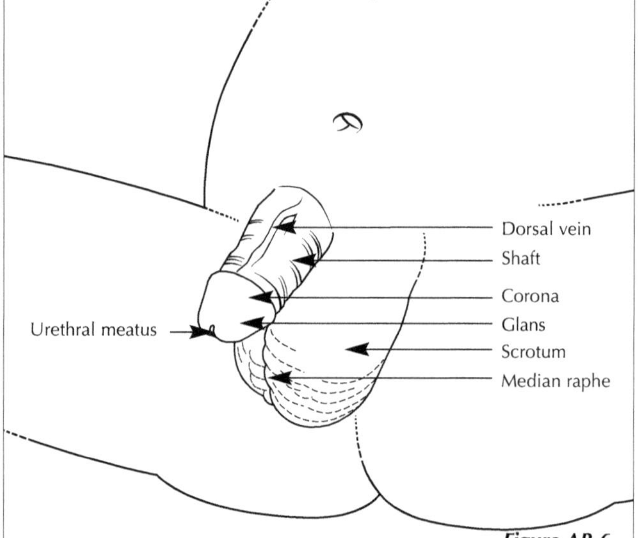

Figure AR-6

Labeled Anatomical Structures in the Prepubescent Male (Uncircumcised)

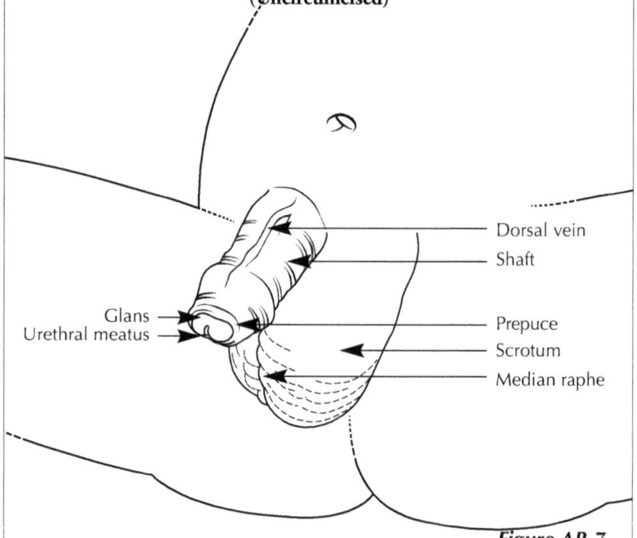

Figure AR-7

DEFINITIONS

— ***Corona of glans penis:*** The rounded, prominent border of the glans on the distal portion of the penile shaft.

— ***Coronal sulcus:*** The rounded border of the glans penis, curving under before the shaft, separated from the corpora cavernosa penis by the neck of the glans.

— ***Corpus spongiosum:*** A column of spongy tissue that runs through the shaft (body) and glans (head) of the penis. Surrounds the urethra (the tube through which urine and sperm pass from the body) and contains blood vessels that fill with blood to help make an erection and keep the urethra open during the erection.

— ***Dorsal vein:*** Tributaries spanning the dorsal surface of the penile shaft.

— ***Fordyce spots:*** Enlarged ectopic sebaceous glands in the mucosa of the mouth and genitals, appearing as small yellow spots.

— ***Glans (also called glans penis or balanus):*** The cap-shaped expansion of corpus spongiosum at the distal end of the penis, which is covered by loose skin (foreskin or prepuce), enabling it to expand during an erection.

— ***Median raphe:*** A visible line of tissue extending from the anus to the perineum. The median raphe is located between the scrotum and the anus in the male and the vestibule and the anus in the female.

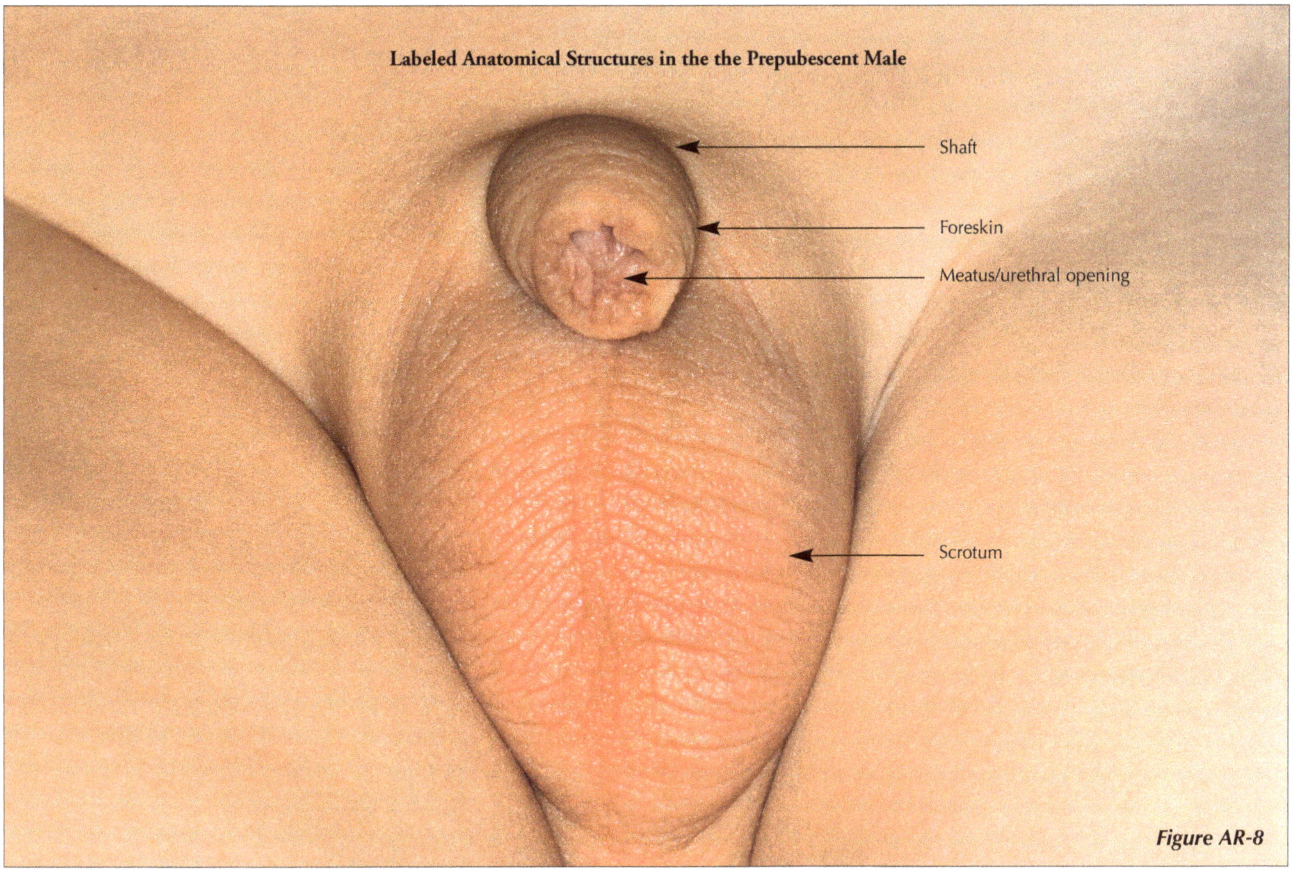

Labeled Anatomical Structures in the the Prepubescent Male

Figure AR-8

— ***Perineum:*** The external surface or base of the perineal body, lying between the scrotum and anus. This network of muscles, located between and around the scrotum and anus, supports the pelvic cavity and maintains the structure of the pelvic floor by keeping the organs in place.

— ***Scrotum:*** The pouch containing the testicles and their accessory organs. The scrotum is located inferiorly to the penis and is covered with hair in males of reproductive age.

— ***Shaft:*** The part of the penis between the glans and the body.

— ***Urethral meatus:*** A slit-like opening located at the tip of the glans. Urine and seminal products, including spermatozoa, exit the body through the urethral meatus.

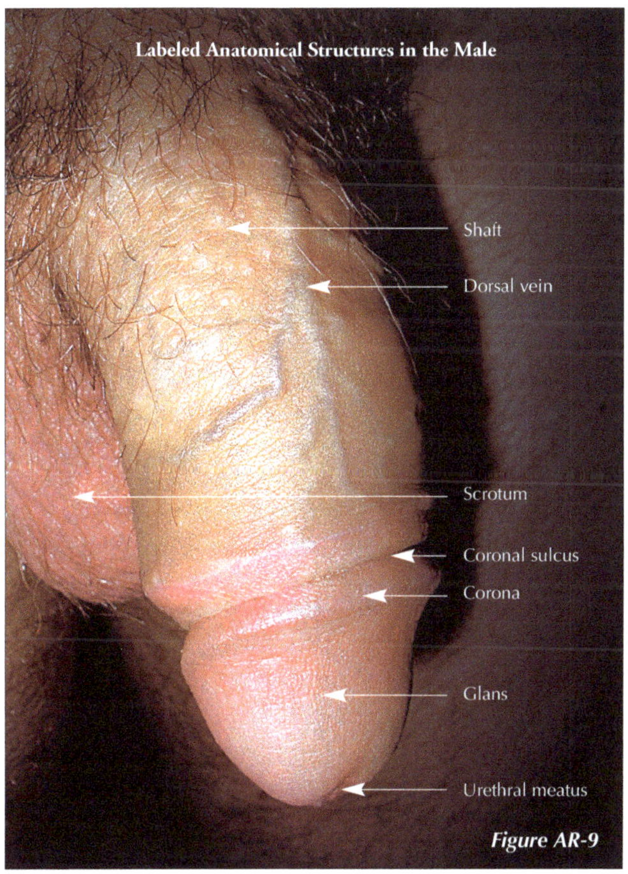

Labeled Anatomical Structures in the Male

Figure AR-9

Female Genitalia

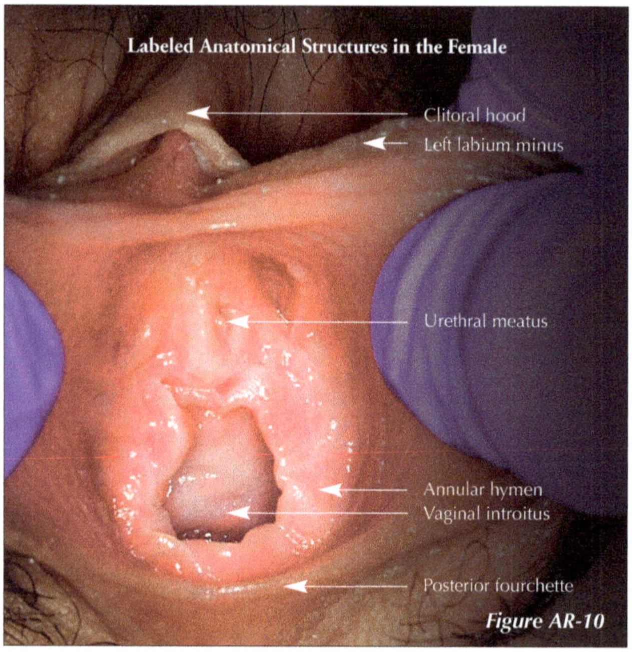

Figure AR-10

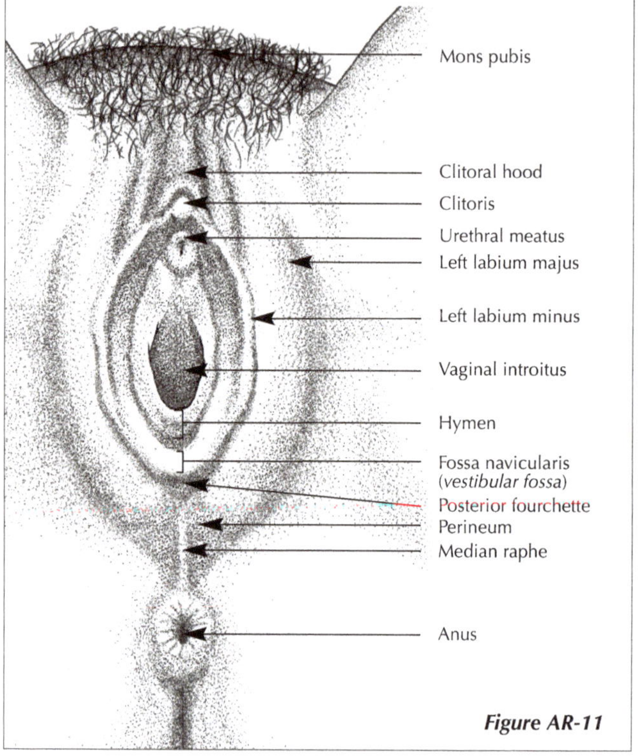

Figure AR-11

Definitions

— ***Cervical os:*** The opening in the cervix that leads to the endometrial cavity of the uterus. This area consists of unstratified columnar epithelium cells.

— ***Cervix:*** The portion of the uterus between the isthmus and the vagina.

— ***Posterior fornix:*** Vault-like recess inferior to the cervix; it is created from the protrusion of the cervix into the upper vagina.

— ***Clitoral hood:*** A fold of skin covering the clitoris.

— ***Clitoris:*** An erectile structure, homologous to the male penis, formed by 2 corpora cavernosa and the glans, covered by the prepuce. The clitoris is connected to the mons pubis and pubic symphysis by the suspensory ligament. Only a fifth (or less) is visible (glans) positioned under the prepuce, which is a hooded flap of integument. The glans is exposed, representing the most innervated part of the clitoris. The hidden part of the clitoris is covered by muscle, reaching up to 7 cm or more in length.

— ***Fordyce spots:*** Enlarged ectopic sebaceous glands in the mucosa of the mouth and genitals, appearing as small yellow spots.

— ***Fossa navicularis:*** The cupping or concavity of the lower part of the vestibule, limited by the vestibular corona adjacent to the hymen attachment and the posterior fourchette, 2 to 4 cm distal to the vestibular corona, and approximately 4 to 8 o'clock. The vestibular corona color represents larger capillaries in the dermis, and the color of the integument varies from red to pink, dependent on estrogen influence, thickness of the vestibular tissues, and BMI (folding), but not race since all have varying shades of pink with macules or papules (some pathological, requiring referral to specialist) if in the fossa navicularis.

— ***Hymen:*** A collar or semicollar of tissue surrounding the vaginal orifice. Normal variations in appearance of the hymen include:

— ***Annular:*** Hymenal tissue present all around the vaginal opening, including at the 12 o'clock location.

— ***Crescentic hymen:*** Hymenal tissue is absent at some point above the 3 to 9 o'clock locations.

— ***Imperforate hymen:*** Hymen with no opening.

— ***Microperforate hymen:*** Hymen with 1 or more small openings.

— ***Redundant hymen:*** Hymen with multiple flaps folding over each other.

— ***Septate hymen:*** Hymen with 1 or more septa across the opening.

Labeled Anatomical Structures in the Prepubescent Female

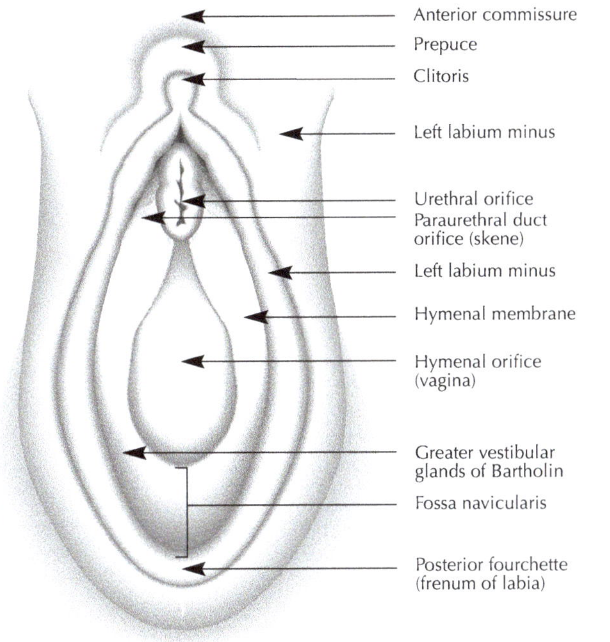

Figure AR-12

— ***Hymenal mound (bump):*** Round and thickened tissue at any location on the rim of the hymen.

— ***Hymenal notch (cleft):*** A V-shaped indentation on the rim of the hymen. A superficial notch (cleft) above the 3 o'clock and 9 o'clock locations is normal. Any partial notch or cleft below the 3 o'clock and 9 o'clock locations is also considered a normal variant. Notches between the 3 o'clock and 9 o'clock locations that extend through the hymenal corona (hymenal attachment in the vestibule and vaginal tube) are considered penetrating injury.

— ***Interlabial sulci:*** Grooves between the labia majora and the labia minora.

— ***Labia majora:*** Two folds of skin on either side of the labia minora. This area usually is covered with hair that appears during puberty.

— ***Labia minora:*** The longitudinal thin folds of nonkeratinized skin medial to the labia majora. The labia minora are hairless but have many sensory nerve endings that engorge when stimulated.

— ***Median raphe:*** A visible line of tissue extending from the anus to the perineum. It is located between the vestibule and the anus in the female and the scrotum and the anus in the male.

Labeled Anatomical Structures in the Prepubescent Female

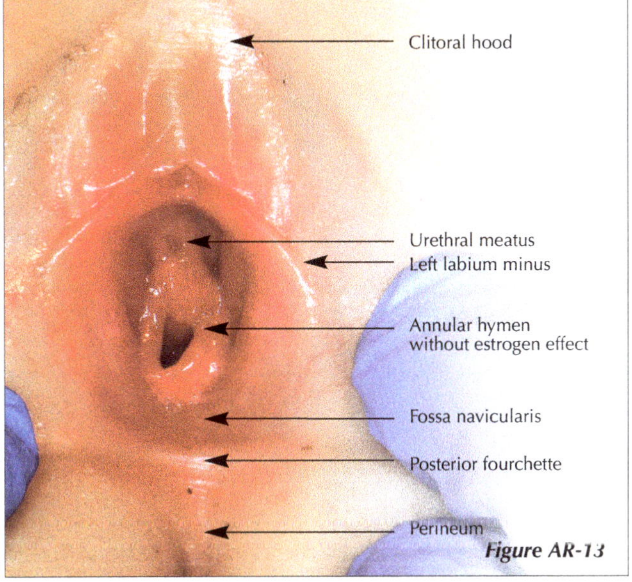

Figure AR-13

— ***Mons pubis:*** The rounded fleshy prominence created by adipose tissue overlying the pubic symphysis bone.

— ***Perineum:*** The external surface or base of the perineal body, lying between the vulva and anus. This network of muscles, located between and around the vagina and anus, supports the pelvic cavity and maintains the structure of the pelvic floor by keeping the organs in place.

— ***Periurethral bands*** (also called vestibular bands or urethral ligaments): Structures that support the urethra and the pelvic floor and are often confused with adhesive scarring. When seen, these bands are usually symmetrical, found in pairs, and attached to the pubic symphysis area.

— ***Posterior fornix:*** Vault-like recess inferior to the cervix; it is created from the protrusion of the cervix into the upper vagina.

— ***Posterior fourchette*** (also called Hart's line or the posterior commissure): An area where the 2 labia meet posteriorly.

Female Genitalia

Annular Hymen Orifice

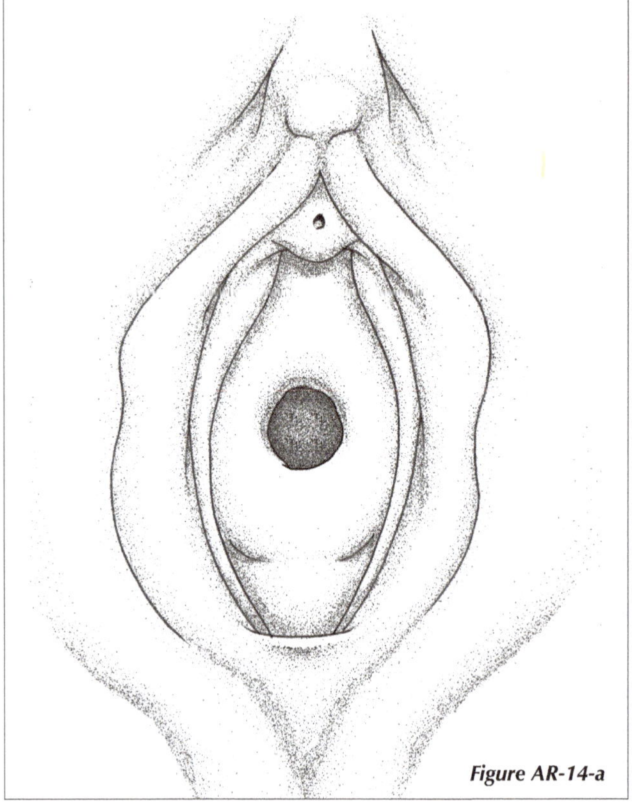

Figure AR-14-a

Annular Hymen Orifice

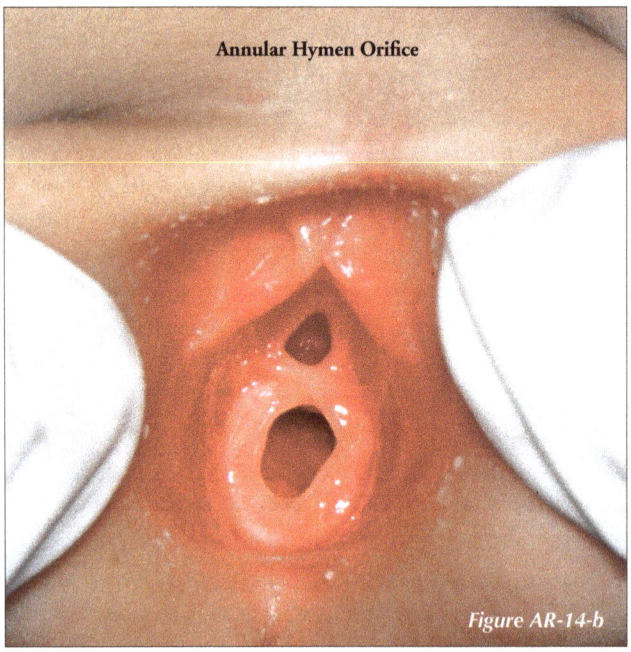

Figure AR-14-b

Crescentic Hymen Orifice

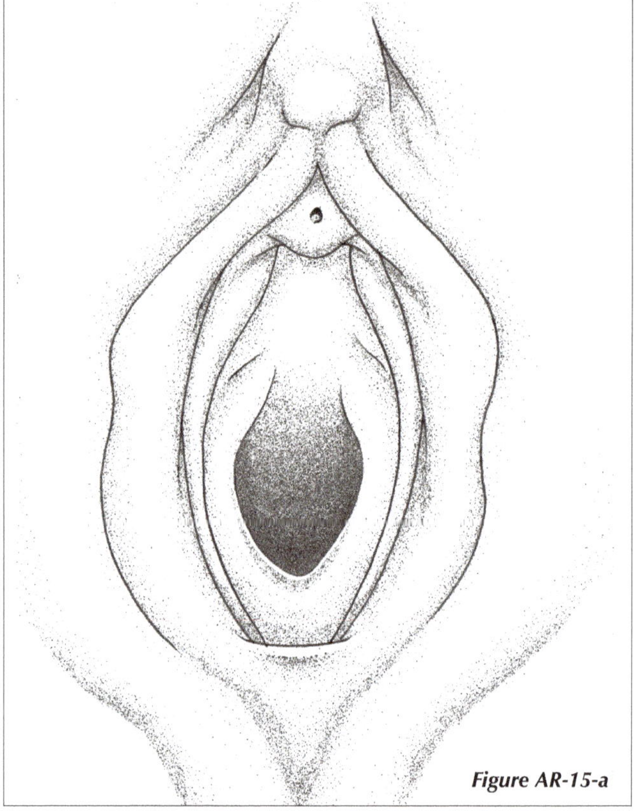

Figure AR-15-a

Crescentic Hymen Orifice

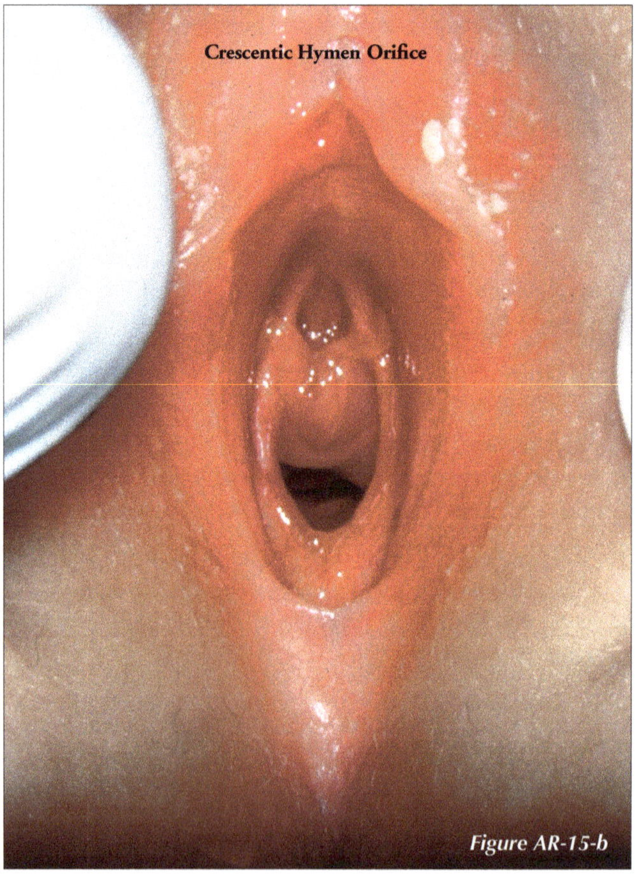

Figure AR-15-b

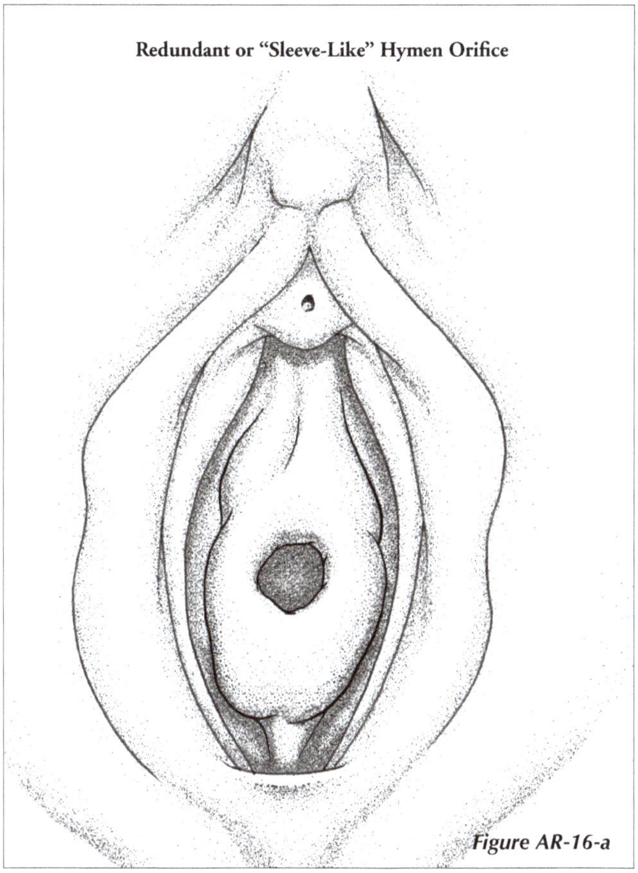

Redundant or "Sleeve-Like" Hymen Orifice

Figure AR-16-a

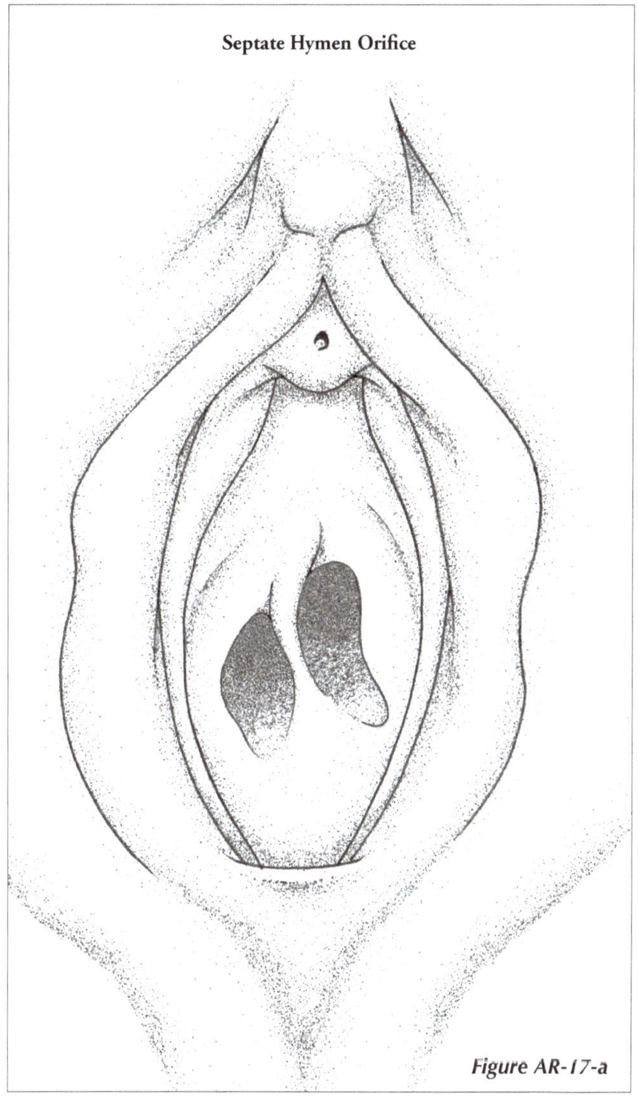

Septate Hymen Orifice

Figure AR-17-a

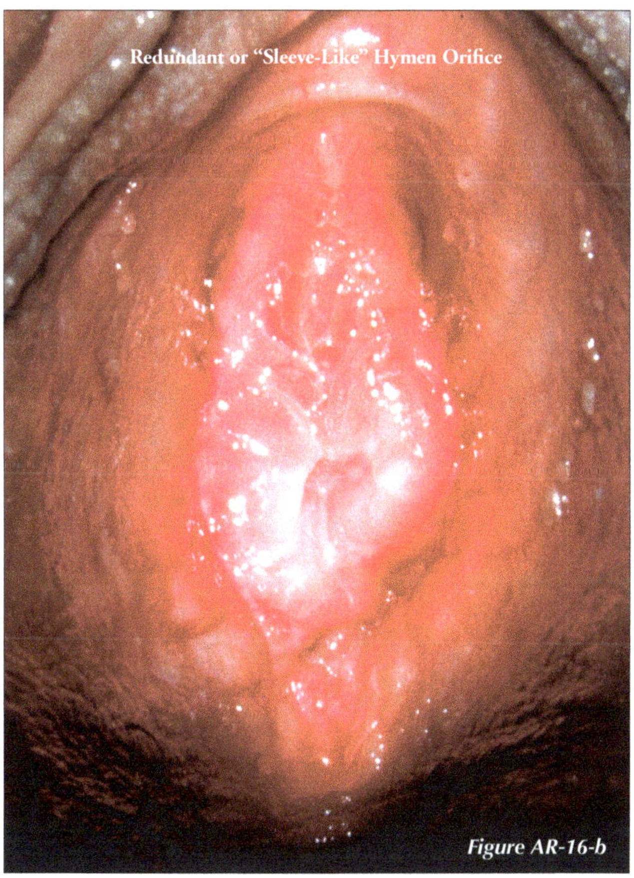

Redundant or "Sleeve-Like" Hymen Orifice

Figure AR-16-b

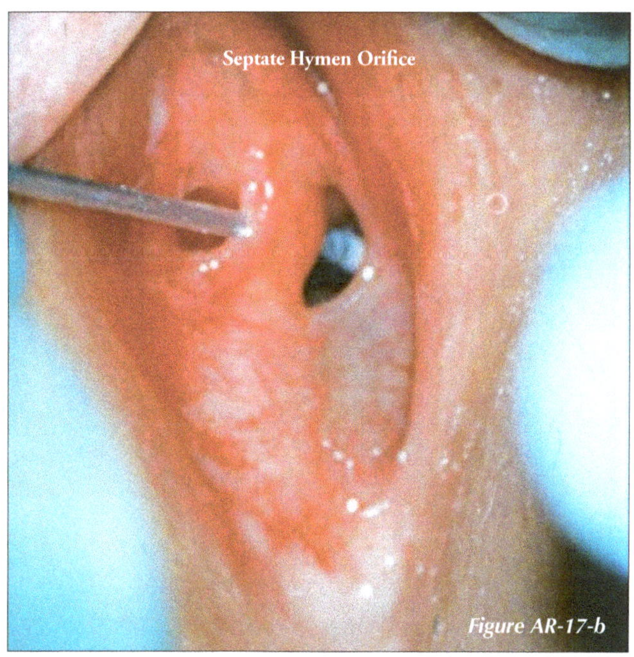

Septate Hymen Orifice

Figure AR-17-b

Female Genitalia

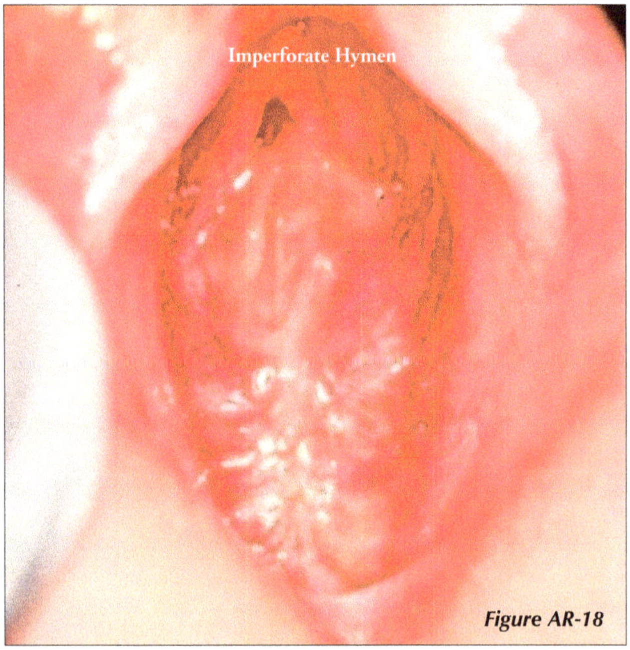

Figure AR-18

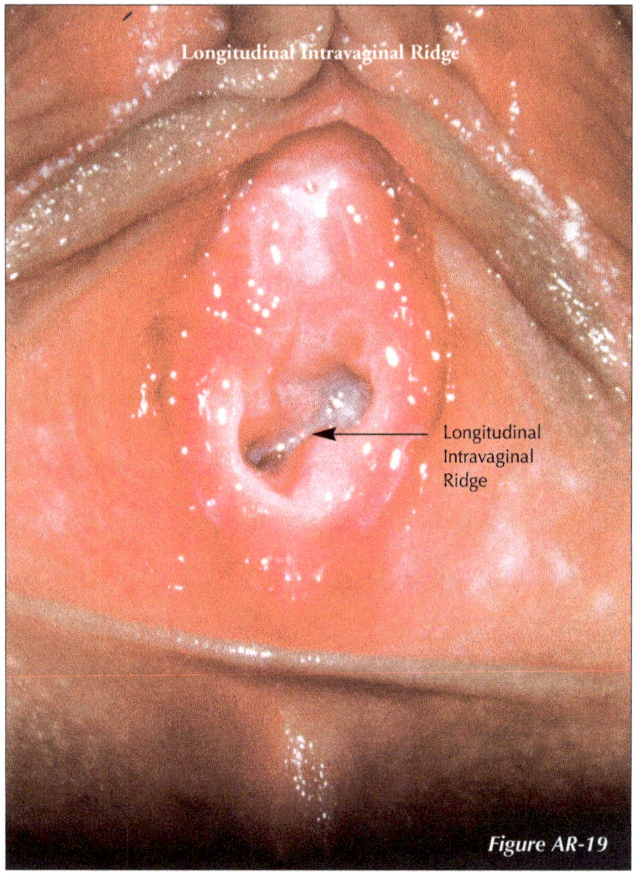

Figure AR-19

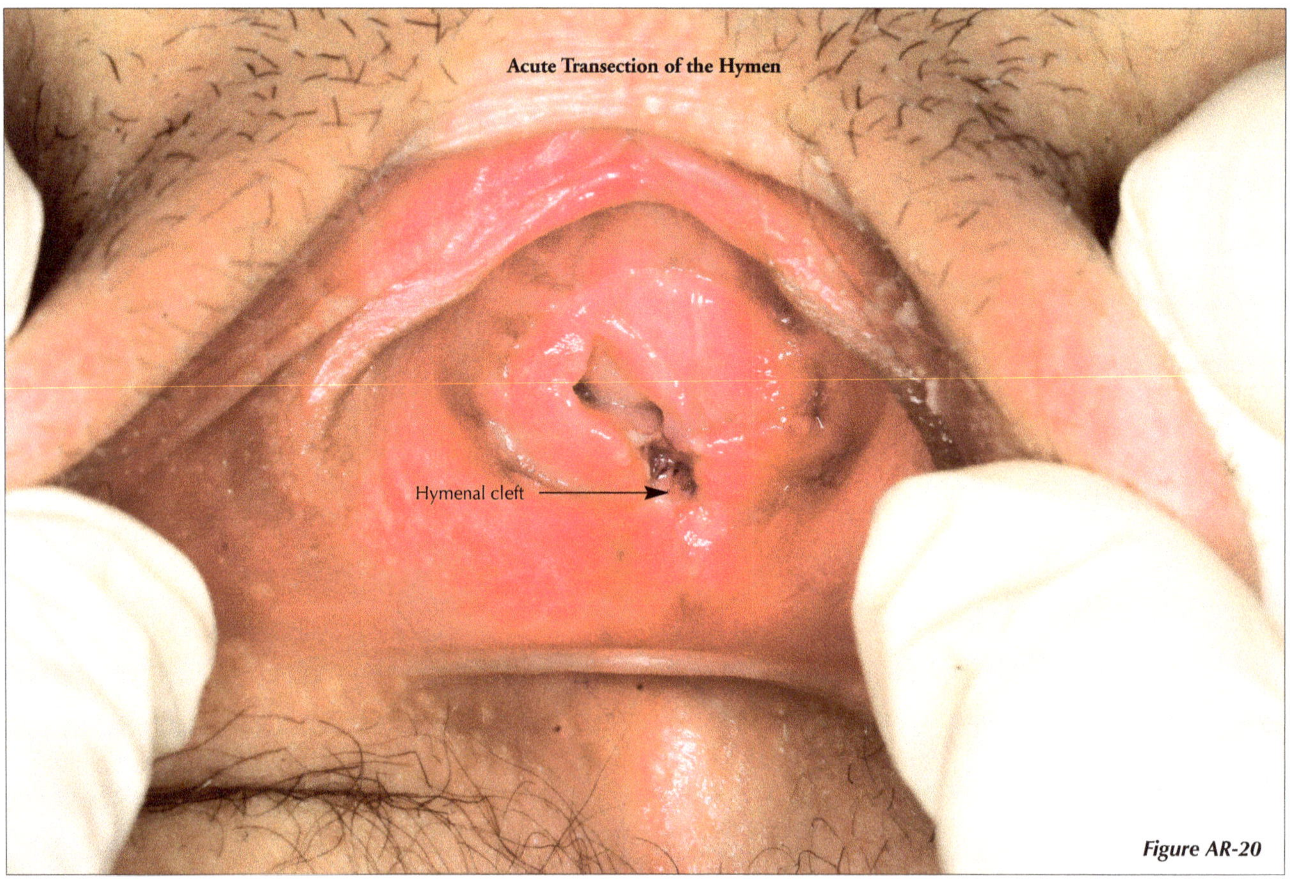

Figure AR-20

Speculum Examination

Labeled Anatomical Structures in the Female During Examination

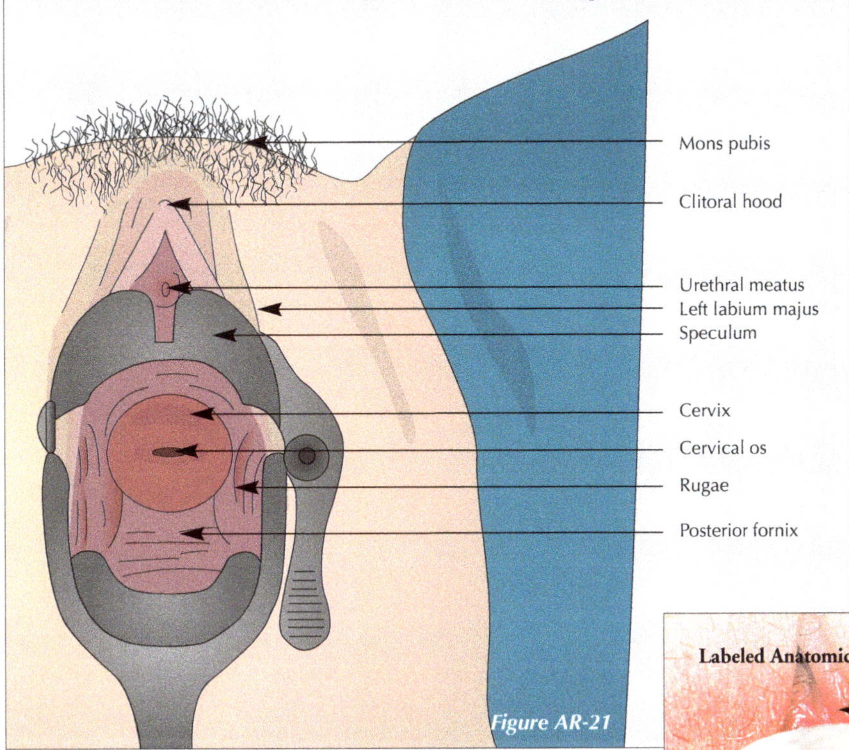

Figure AR-21

Labeled Anatomical Structures in the Female During Examination

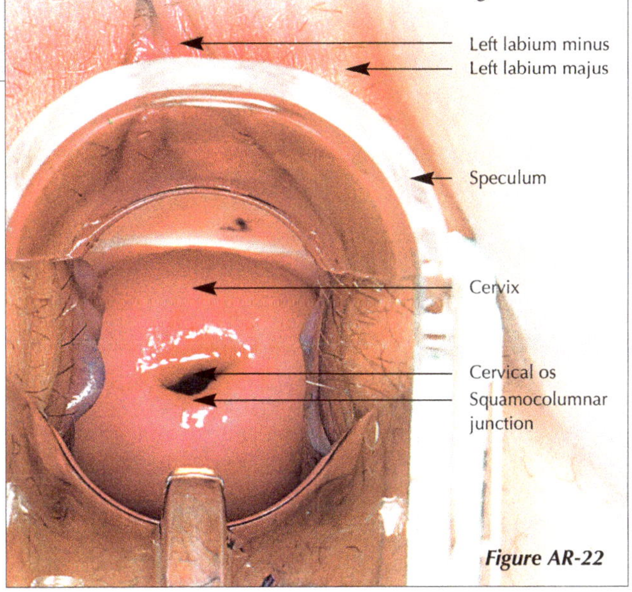

Figure AR-22

Definitions

— ***Rugae:*** Normal folds of epithelium that run circumferentially from the vaginal columns in the vagina. They are not present when there is no estrogen or estrogen effect.

— ***Speculum:*** An instrument for opening or distending an orifice to permit visual inspection.

— ***Squamocolumnar junction:*** A clinically visible line demarcating nonkeratinized squamous epithelia from simple columnar cells in the cervical canal.

— ***Urethral meatus:*** A location on the urethra that encircles the lumen of the external opening of the urethral tube. The urethra connects the urinary bladder to the urethral meatus for the purpose of releasing urine.

— ***Vagina:*** The muscular canal, usually 6 to 7 inches in length, extending from the cervix to the hymen. Its walls are lined with squamous cells, creating a mucous membrane with a pH range of 3.8 to 4.5.

— ***Vaginal fornix:*** The protrusion of the cervix into the upper vagina creating vault-like recesses known as the anterior fornix and posterior fornix.

— ***Vaginal introitus:*** Opening of the vagina.

— ***Vaginal vault:*** The enlargement of the internal end of the vagina.

— ***Vaginal vestibule:*** An anatomical area containing the openings of the vagina, urethra, and Bartholin's glands. Anatomical boundaries include the clitoris anteriorly, the labia laterally, and the posterior fourchette posteriorly.

— ***Vestibular papillae:*** Multiple, tiny, filiform, rosy papules symmetrically distributed on the inner sides of the vestibular tissue.

— ***Vulva:*** An area of the female genitalia lying posterior to the mons pubis that includes the labia majora, labia minora, clitoris, vaginal vestibule, vaginal introitus, and Bartholin's glands.

ANORECTAL ANATOMY

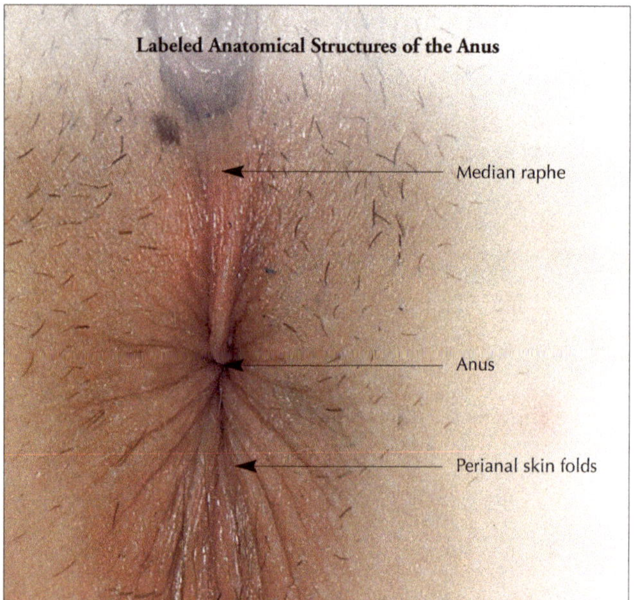

Figure AR-23

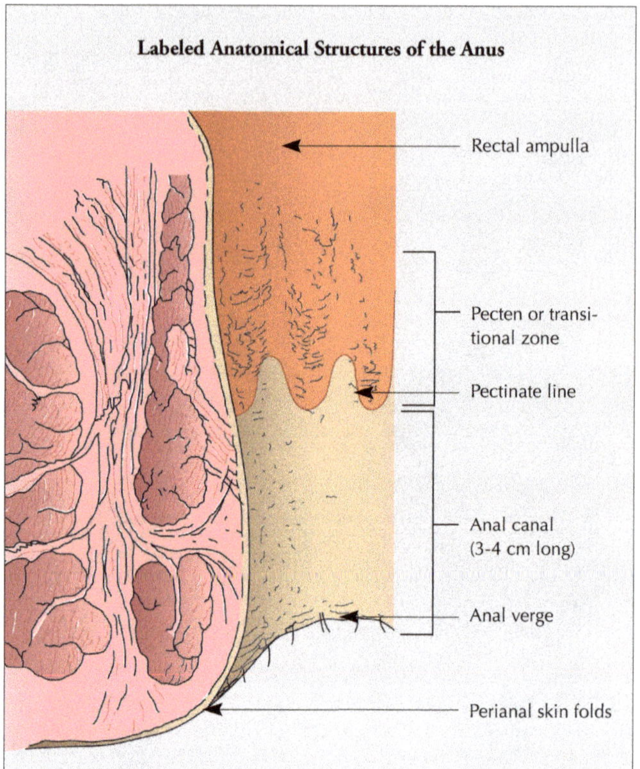

Figure AR-24

DEFINITIONS

— ***Anal canal:*** Terminal part of the large intestine, 3 to 4 cm in length, sensitive to pain, surrounded by sphincter muscles, and without lubricating glands.

— ***Anal verge:*** The distal end of the anal canal; overlies the subcutaneous tissue of the external anal sphincter and extends exteriorly to the margin of anal skin.

— ***Anus:*** The opening of the anal canal, lying between the buttocks, viewed as a linear, slit-like opening, visible with retraction of the buttocks.

— ***Median raphe:*** A visible line of tissue extending from the anus to the perineum. The median raphe is located between the vestibule and the anus in the female and the scrotum and the anus in the male.

— ***Pectinate line*** (also called the ***dentate line***): The saw-toothed line of demarcation between the lower portion of the anal verge and the pectin, a smooth zone of stratified squamous epithelium extending to the anal verge.

— ***Perianal skin folds:*** Wrinkles of perianal skin created by the contraction of the anal sphincter.

— ***Perianal venous engorgement:*** The pooling of venous blood in the circumferential veins of the anus, marked by a bulging of the veins and flat, purple discoloration of the perianal tissues.

— ***Rectal ampulla:*** The proximal portion of the rectum that dilates when the anus opens.

— ***Rectum:*** The distal portion of the large intestine, beginning anterior to the third sacral vertebra.

Examination Techniques

Supine Frog-Leg Position

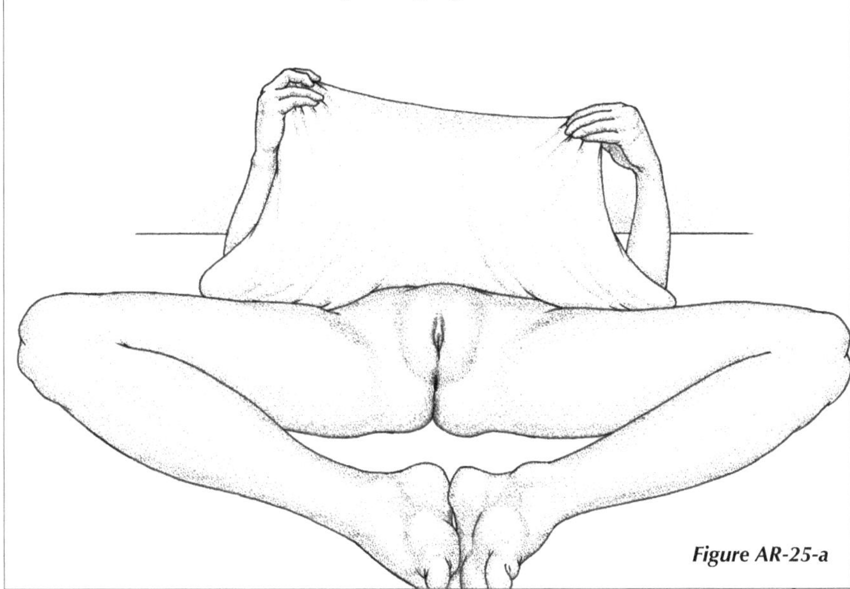

Figure AR-25-a

Supine Frog-Leg Position

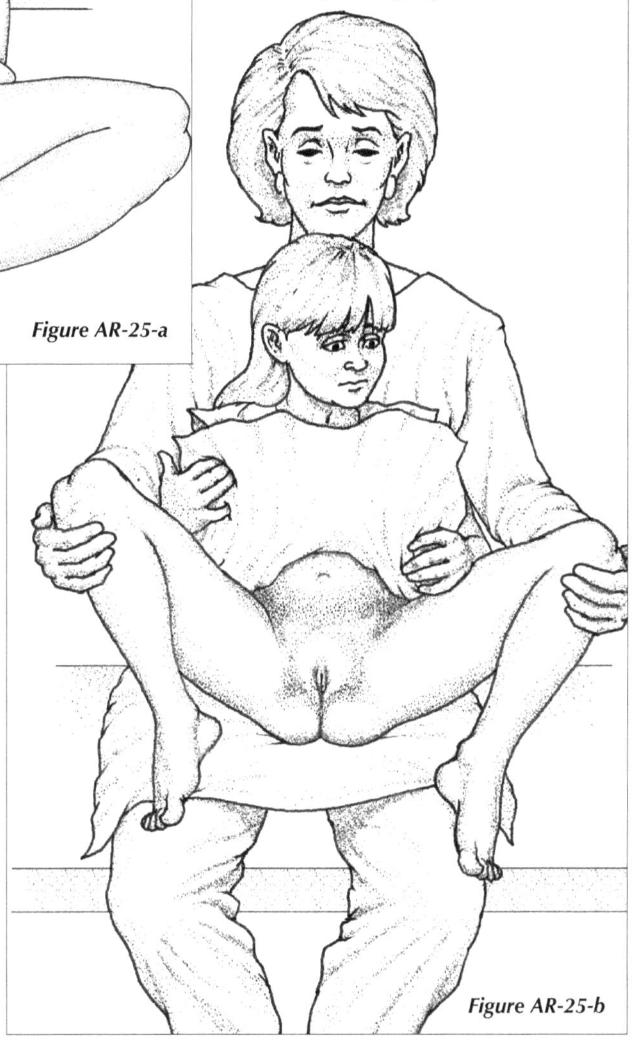

Figure AR-25-b

Prone Knee-Chest Position

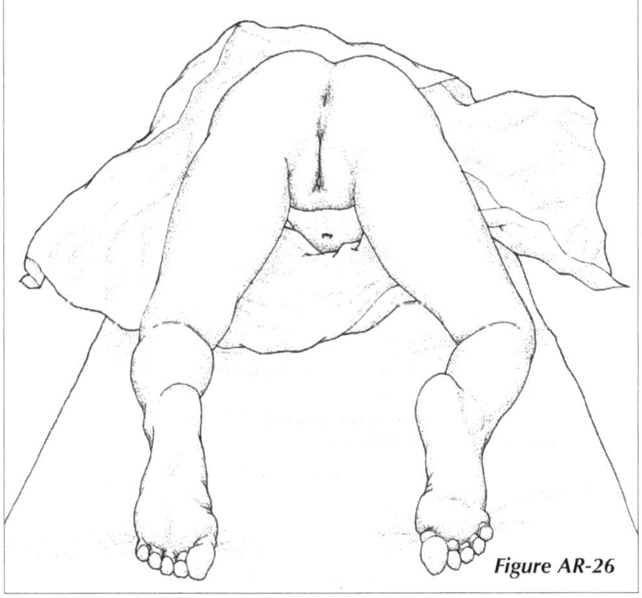

Figure AR-26

Definitions

— ***Examination positions:*** There are 5 positions that may be helpful during the medical examination. Most examinations require only 2 of these positions—either the supine frog-leg position or the supine lithotomy position (depending on the child's age and size) and the prone knee-chest position. For males, the genitalia may be examined while the patient is lying supine on the examination table. Although the legs need to be parted during the testicular examination, a frog-leg position often hides the anal orifice. The prone knee-chest position is still recommended for males, as this position provides the best visualization of the perianal structures.

— ***Lateral decubitus position:*** This position can be used for all age groups to examine the anus. The knees should be together and drawn up on the chest such that the anus can be visualized with minimal gluteal separation or distortion of the tissue.

— ***Prone knee-chest position:*** This position provides a different view of the vestibule and hymen in females and is the best view of the perianal area in both biological sexes. The child's shoulders, elbows, and forearms are placed on the table in order to make the lower back lordotic and to extend the hips upward. The knees are placed about 18 inches apart. The angle of the knee should be approximately 90 degrees.

Examination Techniques

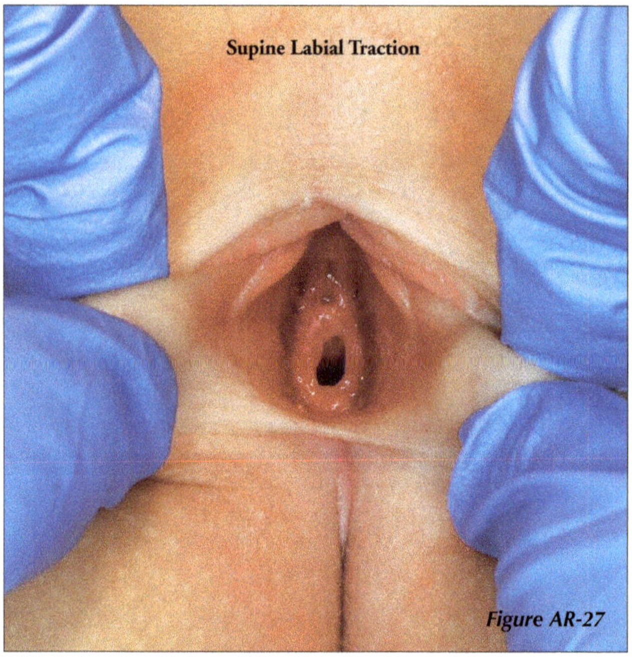

Supine Labial Traction

Figure AR-27

— ***Supine frog-leg position:*** This position is used for smaller prepubertal female children. The child places the soles of the feet together with knees flexed laterally. Some clinicians allow the child to adopt a modified version of this position while sitting in the guardian's lap.

— ***Supine knee-chest position:*** This position is generally used to examine the anus of infants and small toddlers. The knees are drawn up onto the chest to visualize perianal structures.

— ***Supine lithotomy position:*** This position is used for larger female prepubertal children and all female adolescents. The feet are first placed in the examination table stirrups. The child then moves or slides the hips and buttocks to the end of the table and flexes the knees outward.

— ***Labial separation:*** Separation of the labia majora is accomplished with gentle outward pressure using the palmar side of fingers.

— ***Labial traction:*** Visualization of the hymen and possibly the vaginal introitus can be accomplished by gently, yet firmly, grasping the labia majora between the index finger and thumb and carefully pulling outward (toward the examiner).

— ***Prone knee-chest labial traction and separation:*** With the child prone, have her bring her knees up under her, leaving her trunk/head down toward the examination table. Firmly grasp the buttocks and gently lift upward and slightly apart.

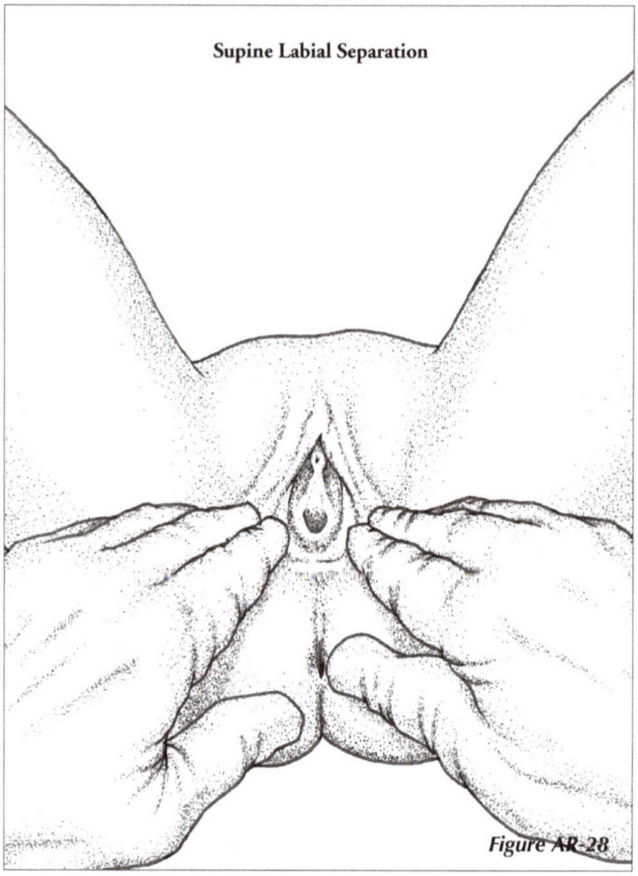

Supine Labial Separation

Figure AR-28

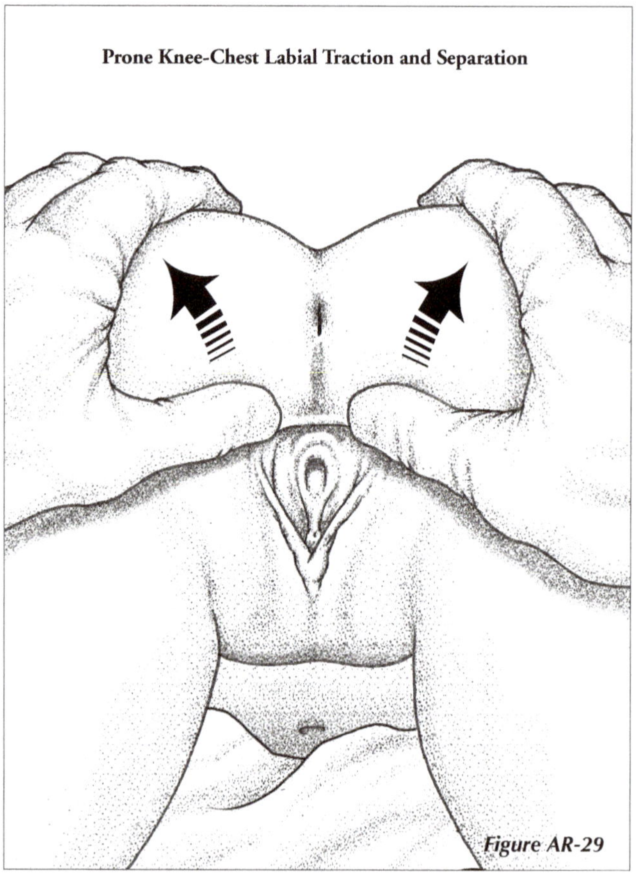

Prone Knee-Chest Labial Traction and Separation

Figure AR-29

Section II

Bacterial Infections

Chapter 1

Bacterial Vaginosis

Cheryl L. Pullium, DNP, APRN, RN, ACNS-BC

Disease and Mimics

— Bacterial vaginosis (BV) is the most prevalent cause of vaginal infection in women ages 14 to 49 years.

— Pregnant women with BV have increased risk of preterm delivery and low-birthweight babies.

— Children diagnosed with BV warrant evaluation for sexual abuse, but BV alone does not prove sexual abuse; conversely, screening for BV is indicated when screening children for sexual victimization (**Figure 1-1**).[1]

— Sexual activity is a risk factor for BV, especially new sexual contact, multiple sexual partners, nonuse of condoms, and women who have sex with women (WSW).

— BV is not only a risk factor for acquiring herpes simplex virus (HSV), gonorrhea, *Chlamydia*, and trichomoniasis, there is also an increased prevalence of BV in women with sexually transmitted infections (STIs).

— ***Differentiating BV from trichomoniasis:*** Similarities in the presentation of BV and trichomoniasis include prolonged, malodorous vaginal discharge and elevated vaginal pH. However, trichomoniasis discharge is purulent and accompanied by symptoms of burning, pruritus, dysuria, frequent urination, dyspareunia, and lower abdominal pain. Untreated, trichomoniasis infection can lead to cystitis or urethritis.

— BV is a risk factor for acquiring, as well as transmitting, human immunodeficiency virus (HIV).

— Treatment of a male sexual partner does not prevent reinfection of the female partner.

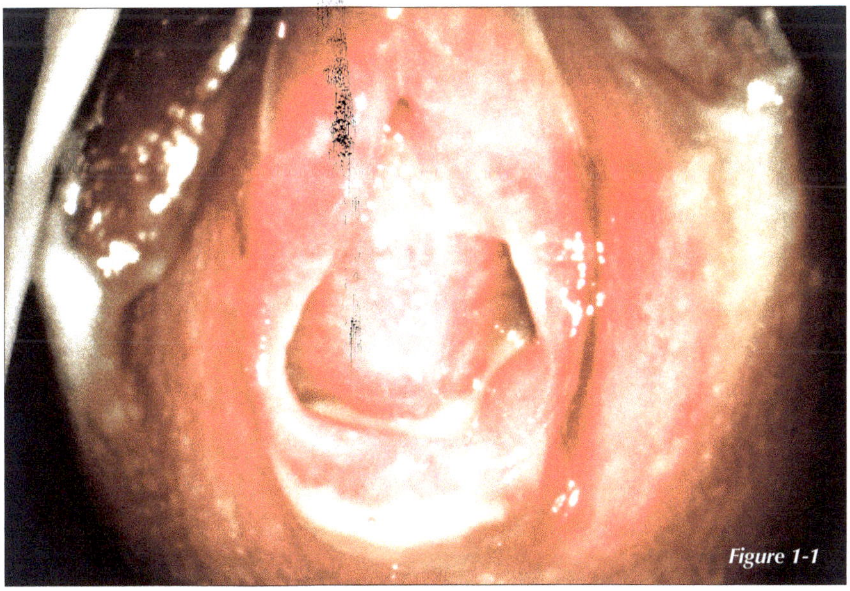

Figure 1-1. *Profuse, thin, gray malodorous discharge in a 7-year-old girl with BV.*

Epidemiology

BV is a noninflammatory condition and occurs as a result of disrupted vaginal flora. Women with BV have a decrease in the normally dominant, hydrogen peroxide–producing *Lactobacillus*, which allows for an increase in opportunistic organisms that exist at low levels in the vaginal environment. The majority of women with BV are asymptomatic and do not require treatment. Women with symptomatic BV present with a thin vaginal discharge that is off-white in color and has a noticeable "fishy" odor (**Figure 1-2** and **1-3**).

BV can be diagnosed using clinical criteria (ie, Amsel's Diagnostic Criteria) or Gram stain. A Gram stain, which is considered the gold standard laboratory method for diagnosing BV, is used to determine the relative concentration of lactobacilli (ie, long Gram-positive rods), Gram-negative and Gram-variable rods and cocci (ie, *G. vaginalis*, *Prevotella*, *Porphyromonas*, peptostreptococci), and curved Gram-negative rods (ie, *Mobiluncus*) characteristic of BV.[2] In the clinical setting, where microscopy is available, BV is based on the Amsel criteria. The Amsel criteria requires the presence of at least 3 of the following points for a diagnosis of BV:

— Thin, off-white discharge that coats the vaginal walls

Vaginal pH is greater than 4.5

— Positive whiff-amine test (presence of a fishy odor when 1 drop of 10% potassium hydroxide [KOH] is added to a sample of the vaginal discharge)

— Clue cells on saline wet mount (if an experienced technician is available to evaluate)

Using the Amsel criterial to diagnose BV has been correlated with results by Gram stain. Other tests, including Affirm VP III (Becton Dickinson, Sparks, MD) and the OSOM BV Blue test (Sekisui Diagnostics, Framingham, MA), have acceptable performance characteristics compared with Gram stain. Although a proline aminopeptidase test card is available for the detection of elevated pH and trimethylamine, it has low

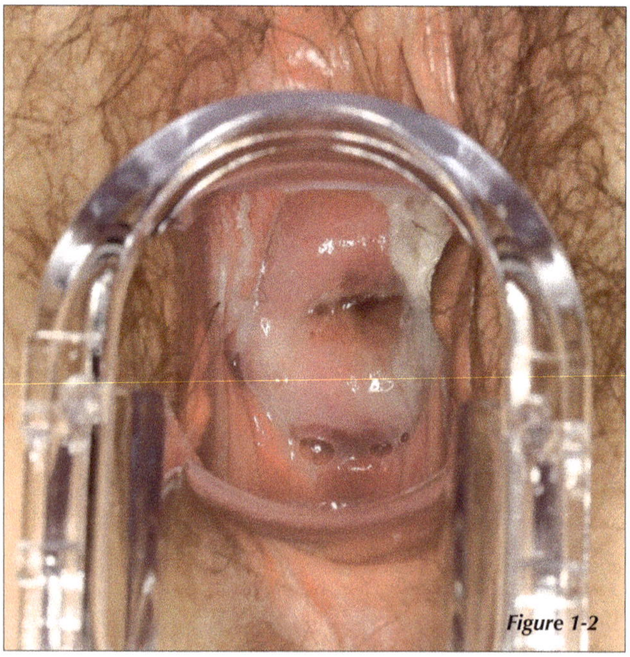

Figure 1-2. *Thin vaginal discharge that is off-white in color and has a noticeable "fishy" odor. (Courtesy of Diana Faugno, MSN, RN, CPN, SANE-A, SANE-P, FAAFS, DF-IAFN, DF-AFN)*

Figure 1-3. *Thin, off-white vaginal discharge indicative of symptomatic BV. (Courtesy of Diana Faugno, MSN, RN, CPN, SANE-A, SANE-P, FAAFS, DF-IAFN, DF-AFN)*

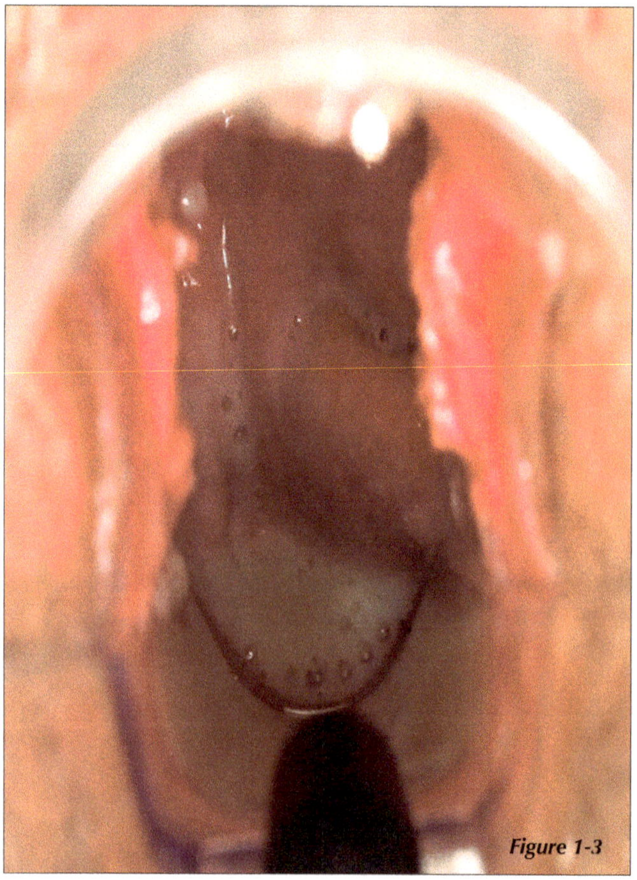

sensitivity and specificity and therefore is not recommended. PCR have been used in research settings for the detection of a variety of organisms associated with BV, but evaluation of its clinical utility is still underway.[2]

Treatment Guidelines

Treatment of asymptomatic BV is not recommended because improvement typically occurs spontaneously in 2 to 3 months. Condom use is recommended for the next 3 months. Treatment is recommended for women with symptoms. The benefits of therapy in nonpregnant women are relieved vaginal symptoms and signs of infection and reduced risk of acquiring *C. trachomatis*, *N. gonorrhoeae*, *T. vaginalis*, HIV, and herpes simplex type 2.[2]

The recommended guidelines for the treatment of BV in symptomatic, nonpregnant women are as follows:

— Metronidazole 500 mg orally twice daily for 7 days ***OR***

— Metronidazole 0.75% gel 5 g (1 applicator full) intravaginally once daily for 5 days ***OR***

— Clindamycin 2% cream 5 g (1 applicator full) intravaginally once daily for 7 days

Alternative treatments for symptomatic nonpregnant women include the following:

— Tinidazole 2 g orally once daily for 2 days ***OR***

— Tinidazole 1 g orally once daily for 5 days ***OR***

— Clindamycin 300 mg orally twice daily for 7 days ***OR***

— Clindamycin ovules 100 mg intravaginally once daily for 3 days

Recommended guidelines for treatment of pregnant women with symptomatic BV include the following:

— Metronidazole 250 mg orally 3 times daily for 7 days ***OR***

— Metronidazole 500 mg orally twice daily for 7 days ***OR***

— Clindamycin 300 mg orally twice daily for 7 days

Treatment of asymptomatic BV among pregnant women who are at high-risk for preterm delivery (ie, those with a previous preterm birth) has been evaluated by several studies, which have yielded mixed results.[2] Current recommendations do not support routine treatment of pregnant women with asymptomatic BV.

Recommended guidelines for treatment of BV in children are as follows:

— Metronidazole 15 to 25 mg/kg per day, taken orally in 3 divided doses (maximum 2 g per day) for 7 days[1]

Special Considerations

— ***Alcohol:*** Alcohol consumption should be avoided during treatment with nitroimidazoles. To reduce the possibility of a disulfiram-like reaction, abstinence from alcohol use should continue for 72 hours after completion of tinidazole.[2]

— ***Recurrence:*** More than half of women treated for symptomatic BV have a recurrence within 12 months. Follow-up visits are unnecessary if symptoms resolve. Persistent or recurrent BV is common, so women should be advised to return for evaluation if symptoms recur.[2] Reinfection, failure of treatment to eradicate the organism (antimicrobial resistance), and failure to restore the normal vaginal flora have been linked to recurrence. Using a different recommended treatment regimen can be considered for women who have a recurrence; however, retreatment with the same recommended regimen is an acceptable approach for treating persistent or recurrent BV after the first occurrence.[2] In women with multiple recurrences despite completion of the recommended course of treatment, consideration should be given to 0.75% metronidazole gel twice a week for 4 to 6 months. This has been shown to reduce recurrences, but this benefit might not persist when suppressive therapy is discontinued.[2]

— ***Coinfection:*** All women with BV should be tested for HIV and other STIs.[2]

Case Studies

Adult Case Study 1-1

A 20-year-old female university student presents to the student health center with a complaint of foul-smelling vaginal discharge after "lots of sex" over a 3-day beach vacation with her current boyfriend. She reports she had sex multiple times daily for the 3 days they were at the beach. She has been monogamous with this same sexual partner for the past 2 months but had multiple sexual partners, both male and female, over the past 2 years. She uses oral contraceptives to prevent pregnancy; however, she does not use any type of barrier protection because she "always forgets." She denies dysuria, cloudy urine, frequent urination, pruritus, dyspareunia, burning sensation, and vaginal erythema or edema. When asked to describe the vaginal discharge, she states that it is constant, white in color, fishy smelling, and has a thin consistency. She reports that she did not notice the discharge before her beach weekend, but now it is worrisome because of the amount of discharge and the odor, which is very noticeable.

Examination

The patient's discharge is off-white and thin with a "fishy" odor.

Laboratory Testing

Patient has a positive whiff test and a vaginal pH of 5.1. Urine pregnancy test is negative.

Treatment

Based on the patient's description of the discharge and the lack of any other symptoms, BV is the most obvious diagnosis. Definitive diagnosis is made in this case by meeting 3 of the 4 Amsel Criteria: (1) characteristic discharge; (2) positive whiff test; and (3) vaginal pH greater than 4.5. A prescription for metronidazole 500 mg twice daily for 7 days was provided to the patient.

Child Case Study 1-2

A 15-year-old girl presents to her primary care provider with a complaint of vaginal discharge for 3 days. She is not sexually active. When asked to describe her symptoms, she complains of a vaginal discharge that "smells funny."

Examination

Speculum exam reveals off-white discharge on the cervix and in the vaginal vault.

Laboratory Testing

Urinalysis is negative. Vaginal pH is 4.9.

Treatment

Based on the physical assessment and laboratory testing, the provider diagnoses the patient with BV. Vaginal pH is greater than 4.5. There is no bladder infection. Vaginal discharge is off-white and has a "fishy" smell. A prescription for metronidazole 500 mg twice daily for 7 days is provided to the patient.

References

1. American Academy of Pediatrics. STIs in children. In: Kimberlin DW, Brady, TB, Jackson, MA, eds. *Red Book: 2018 Report of the Committee on Infectious Diseases.* 31st ed. Elk Grove, IL: American Academy of Pediatrics; 2018:168-176.
2. 2015 sexually transmitted diseases treatment guidelines: bacterial vaginosis. Centers for Disease Control and Prevention Web site. https://www.cdc.gov/std/tg2015/bv.htm. Updated June 4, 2015. Accessed March 30, 2020.

Additional References

Khan Z, Bhargava A, Mittal P, et al. Evaluation of reliability of self-collected vaginal swabs over physician-collected samples for diagnosis of bacterial vaginosis, candidiasis and trichomoniasis, in a resource-limited setting: a cross-sectional study in India. *BMJ Open.* 2019;9(8):e025013.

Sobel JD. Bacterial vaginosis: clinical manifestations and diagnosis. UpToDate Web site. https://www.uptodate.com/contents/bacterial-vaginosis-clinical-manifestations-and-diagnosis. Updated February 11, 2019. Accessed August 1, 2019.

Chapter 2

Chancroid

Kathleen Thimsen, DNP, MSN, WOCN, FNS
Katie Jett, DNP, FNP-BC, RN

Disease and Mimics

- Chancroid is an acute ulcerative infection of the genital skin or mucous membrane caused by bacterial transmission of *Haemophilus ducreyi*.
- Characteristics of the presenting signs and symptoms include a history of acute onset of painful skin lesions.
- Chancroid is suspected in patients who have unexplained genital ulcers or buboes (which may be mistaken for an abscess) and have been in an endemic region (**Figure 2-1**).
- Lesions of the disease typically occur on the genital or anogenital area and are associated with inguinal lymphadenopathy.[1]
- Chancroid was once a highly prevalent condition in many areas of the world, but with global efforts directed to increasing social awareness and related sexual behavior changes, along with improved diagnostic and treatment options, chancroid is not often seen in industrialized nations.[1]
- Chancroid is now recognized for its ability to amplify the transmission of human immunodeficiency virus (HIV) infection.[3,4]
- Chancroid is an important cofactor for HIV transmission, and up to 10% of patients with chancroid are coinfected with syphilis or herpes simplex virus (HSV).[1,4]

Epidemiology

Chancroid has declined in incidence since 2000[2] but was once considered endemic to developing regions of Africa, Asia, and the Caribbean. Although very few cases are seen in the United States, periodic outbreaks of chancroid have occurred.[1] The outbreaks are usually among minority populations and in urban settings. The proportion of chancroid among genital ulcerative diseases decreased from 69% to 15% worldwide.

Figure 2-1. *Chancroid, male. Regional adenopathy. (Courtesy of CDC, Atlanta, GA.)*

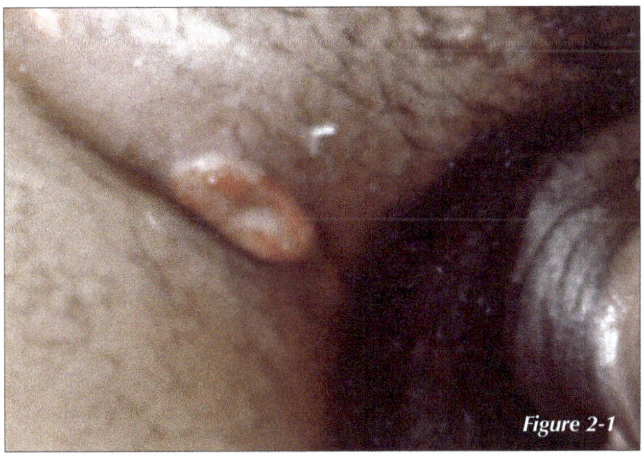

If available, a sample of purulent drainage from a bubo or exudate from the edge of a lesion should be sent to the laboratory for analysis to identify the specific causative organism. In cases of chancroid, diagnosis is usually based on clinical findings alone given that bacterial culture is often difficult as a result of multiple organisms being found in the ulcer. Few institutions have the available highly sensitive, certified tests specific to *H. ducreyi*.

Serology for syphilis, HIV, and HSV should be ordered to exclude other causes of genital lesions. Caution should be taken because interpretation of test results may be complicated as a result of the common issue of coinfected lesions.

Infection and symptoms appear after an incubation period of 3 to 7 days. Small, painful papules appear and rapidly break down into shallow, soft, painful ulcers with ragged, undermined edges (ie, with overhanging tissue) and a red border. Ulcers vary in size and often coalesce. Deeper erosion occasionally leads to marked tissue destruction.

Patients with chancroid present with painful genital ulcers with inguinal adenopathy. Inguinal lymph nodes are tender, enlarged, and often matted together, forming a pus-filled abscess (bubo). The skin stretched over the abscess is red, warm-hot, shiny, and hard with palpation. The skin may be friable over the abscess itself and may open with minimal pressure. Often, the openings to the ulcerations may expose sinus tracts. The spread of the infection to other areas of the skin may occur and cause new ulcers or lesions. Phimosis, urethral stricture, and urethral fistula may also occur from chancroid.

Symptoms in women are less noticeable because complaints are typically related to painful urination or defecation, painful intercourse, rectal bleeding, or vaginal discharge. Diagnostic testing includes identification on specific culture media.[2] Polymerase chain reaction (PCR) assays provide specific diagnosis, but the testing is not available in most laboratories. There is no Food and Drug Administration approved PCR test for *H. ducreyi* available in the United States, though clinical laboratories have developed their own PCR test and have used Clinical Laboratory Improvement Amendments verification studies in specimens.[3] Diagnosis should include a thorough history of sexual activity and information regarding the formation of painful ulcers and lymphadenopathy.[1]

Treatment Guidelines

Patients who are diagnosed with chancroid should be educated that it is a bacterial infection, most likely transmitted sexually (depending on ulcer location), and can be treated with an antibiotic. Patients should also be educated about the cofactor relationship between chancroid and HIV transmission, as well as genital herpes and syphilis.[2]

After the initiation of antimicrobial therapy, symptoms should resolve within 1 to 2 weeks. It is important that patients abstain from all sexual contact until they and their sexual partner have completed the full course of antibiotic treatment.[2] Because of the nature of coinfection and the difficulty in distinguishing the infections based on clinical presentation, testing for HSV and syphilis should also be conducted in patients presenting with chancroid.[2]

Successful treatment for chancroid cures the infection, resolves the clinical symptoms, and prevents transmission to others. In advanced cases, scarring can result despite successful therapy.

Recommended Regimens

— Azithromycin 1 g orally in a single dose ***OR***

— Ceftriaxone 250 mg intramuscularly in a single dose ***OR***

— Ciprofloxacin 500 mg orally twice a day for 3 days ***OR***

— Erythromycin 500 mg orally 3 times a day for 7 days

Azithromycin and ceftriaxone offer the advantage of single-dose therapy. Worldwide, several isolates with intermediate resistance to either ciprofloxacin or erythromycin have been reported. However, because cultures are not routinely performed, data are limited regarding the current prevalence of antimicrobial resistance.

Antibiotic resistance has been reported for beta-lactamase–producing strains of *H. ducreyi* as well as plasmid-mediated resistance to tetracycline, sulfonamides, chloramphenicol, and aminoglycosides; this resistance has led to reports of treatment failure.[2] The most active drugs against *H. ducreyi* are azithromycin, ceftriaxone, ciprofloxacin, and erythromycin; however, antibiotic therapy should be decided based on local resistance and susceptibility patterns.[2]

Follow-Up

Patients should return for a follow-up examination 3 to 7 days after the start of antimicrobial therapy. Patients should have symptom improvement within that time frame. If symptoms or ulcer appearance is not improved, additional consideration regarding diagnosis, antimicrobial treatment, and medication compliance should be explored. Larger ulcers may take longer than 2 weeks to improve.[3] Healing may also be slower in uncircumcised men with ulcers located underneath the foreskin. Lymphadenopathy resolution will likely take longer than ulcer healing and, when fluctuance persists, may require needle aspiration or incision and drainage.[3]

Sexual partners, regardless of symptom presence, should be examined and, when indicated, treated if they participated in sexual contact with the infected partner during the 10 days preceding the infected partner's onset of symptoms.[3]

Because of the difficulties in definitively diagnosing chancroid, the Centers for Disease Control and Prevention guidelines for the diagnosis of chancroid state that a probable diagnosis can be made if all of the following criteria have been met[3]:

1. The patient has 1 or more painful ulcer(s).
2. The clinical presentation, appearance of the genital ulcer(s), and, if present, the lymphadenopathy are what is typically seen with chancroid.
3. The patient does not demonstrate any evidence of *Treponema pallidum* infection by dark-field examination of the exudate from the ulcer(s) or by a serological test for syphilis that was performed at least 7 days after the onset of the ulcer(s).
4. A negative HSV PCR test or negative HSV culture from exudate.

Special Considerations

Children can be treated with ceftriaxone. Ciprofloxacin is contraindicated for pregnant and lactating women as well as children and adolescents younger than 18 years of age.[2,3]

Men who are uncircumcised and patients with HIV infection do not respond as well to treatment as persons who are circumcised or HIV-negative. Patients should be tested for HIV infection at the time chancroid is diagnosed. If the initial test results were negative, a serologic test for syphilis and HIV infection should be performed 3 months after the diagnosis of chancroid.

Case Studies

Adult Case Study 2-1

A 21-year-old man presents to an outpatient sexually transmitted infection (STI) testing clinic with reports of a 7-day history of red, painful "spots" on his penis. He denies fever, chills, nausea, vomiting, dysuria, urethral discharge, and testicular pain. He reports a regular female sex partner as well as an additional female sexual contact 9 days before the onset of his symptoms. He denies condom use with either partner.

Examination

On examination the patient has 3 2-cm tender, erythematous, penile lesions on his glans penis and coronal sulcus. He has 2 palpable inguinal lymph nodes. There is no urethral discharge, and the remainder of the genitourinary examination is unremarkable.

Laboratory Testing

Specimens are collected for gonorrhea and *Chlamydia*, including first-catch urine for nucleic acid amplification test. Samples for serological testing for syphilis, HSV, and HIV are collected.

Treatment

All tests came back negative, and the patient returns to the clinic 7 days later for reevaluation. On examination, the lesions are ulcerated and remain painful. He has fluctuant lymphadenopathy to the inguinal area. Based on the negative laboratory tests and clinical presentation, a probable diagnosis of *H. ducreyi* is made, and the patient is given a stat dose of azithromycin 1 g. Sexual contacts are notified and treated with azithromycin 1 g.

Child Case Study 2-2

A 15-year-old girl presents to the emergency department (ED) with reports of burning and pain on urination for 2 days. She denies fever, chills, abdominal pain, frequent urination, and discharge. The child seems uncomfortable answering questions in front of her mother, who presents with the child for evaluation. When questioned separately from the mother, the child reports that she has been sexually active (vaginal penetration) with a 15-year-old boy for 1 month.

Examination

Examination reveals a single 2-cm ulceration to the left labia that is painful and erythematous. Speculum examination is unremarkable, and there is no cervical tenderness. No discharge is noted during examination. Three small lymph node enlargements are noted in left inguinal area.

Laboratory Testing

Cultures for gonorrhea and *Chlamydia* specimens are collected from the cervix. A swab of the ulcer for HSV PCR is also obtained. A culture is obtained for testing for *H. ducreyi*. Samples for serological testing for syphilis and HIV are also considered.

Treatment

Azithromycin 1 g was given orally while in the ED for probable *H. ducreyi* infection. Follow-up with the local STI clinic in 3 to 7 days is established to make sure the symptoms and ulcer appearance are resolving. Safe sexual practices are discussed. Testing results are sent to the patient's personal cellular device to maintain patient privacy. All other specimens are negative.

References

1. Mohammed TT, Olumide YM. Chancroid and human immunodeficiency virus infection—a review. *Int J Dermatol.* 2008;47(1):1-8.
2. Lautenschlager S, Kemp M, Christensen JJ, Mayans MV, Moi H. 2017 European guideline for the management of chancroid. *Int J STD AIDS.* 2017;28(4):324-329.
3. 2015 sexually transmitted disease treatment guidelines: chancroid. Centers for Disease Control and Prevention Web site. https://www.cdc.gov/std/tg2015/chancroid.htm. Updated June 4, 2015. Accessed October 21, 2019.
4. Morse SA, Trees DL, Htun Y, et al. Comparison of clinical diagnosis and standard laboratory and molecular methods for the diagnosis of genital ulcer disease in Lesotho: association with human immunodeficiency virus infection. *J Infect Dis.* 1997;175(3):583-589.

Chapter 3

Lymphogranuloma Venereum

Kathleen Thimsen, DNP, MSN, WOCN, FNS
Amanda Flynn, DNP, MSN, RN, FNP-BC

Disease and Mimics

- Lymphogranuloma venereum (LGV) is an ulcerative disease of the genital area caused by the gram-negative bacteria *Chlamydia trachomatis*.
- LGV primarily affects the lymphatic system. LGV is caused by L1, L2, and L3 serovars of *C. trachomatis* and most recently L_2b (***LGV biovar***).[1]
- The most common clinical manifestation of LGV among heterosexuals is tender inguinal or femoral lymphadenopathy that is typically unilateral.
- A self-limited ulcer or papule sometimes occurs at the site of inoculation, but by the time patients seek care, lesions have often disappeared.[2]
- Rectal exposure in women or in men who have sex with men (MSM) can result in proctocolitis mimicking inflammatory bowel disease. Clinical findings may include mucoid or hemorrhagic rectal discharge, anal pain, constipation, fever, or tenesmus. Rectal LGV can be asymptomatic.[2]
- If it is not treated early, LGV proctocolitis can lead to chronic colorectal fistulas and strictures.[2]
- LGV is common in the tropical and subtropical regions around the world but is rare in the United States.[3]

Epidemiology

LGV most likely affects both sexes equally, although it is more commonly reported in men because early symptom manifestations of LGV are more apparent in men. Men typically present with the acute form of the disease, whereas women often present when they develop complications from later stages of the disease. LGV may appear at any age, but the highest incidence is between ages 15 and 40 years (sexually active population). Most cases in Europe and North America have been identified among white MSM patients presenting with proctitis who are also often positive for human immunodeficiency virus (HIV).[4] Since 2003, there has been a series of LGV outbreaks reported across Europe.[5,6] This is a major public health concern because enhanced shedding of HIV during clinical proctitis could increase the risk of HIV transmission to uninfected men.[7] Before the outbreaks in MSM, LGV was primarily endemic in heterosexuals in areas of East and West Africa, India, parts of Southeast Asia, and the Caribbean, where it is manifested as the classic form of the disease with genital ulcers and lymphadenopathy (without proctitis).

Complications usually occur when the disease is left untreated and include necrosis and rupture of the lymph nodes, anogenital fibrosis and strictures, and anal fistula. Elephantiasis of the genital organs can also occur in some cases. Systemic complications like pneumonia and hepatitis also have been reported.[8]

Diagnosis is based on clinical suspicion, epidemiologic information, and the exclusion of other causes for proctocolitis, inguinal lymphadenopathy, or genital or rectal ulcers. Genital lesions, rectal specimens, and lymph node specimens can be tested for *C. trachomatis* by culture, direct immunofluorescence, or nucleic acid detection. MSM presenting with proctocolitis should be tested for *Chlamydia*.[2]

LGV infection has 3 phases. The first phase (primary stage) starts with a painless papule or ulcer at the site of inoculation. The second phase (secondary stage) of the infection is the invasion of regional lymph nodes, which can result in an inguinal or rectal syndrome. The third phase of LGV infection (tertiary stage) is the irreversible destruction of lymph tissue.[8]

Unlike other serovars of *C. trachomatis*, which cause mucosal infections by infecting columnar epithelial cells, the serovars L1, L2, and L3 cause systemic disease by infecting monocytes and macrophages and then invading submucosal sites and regional lymph nodes.[8]

Primary: Although often unnoticed by patients, about 3 to 30 days after inoculation localized inflammation manifests at the site of exposure (often genital or rectal, but it can be oropharyngeal).[9] Classically, this lesion is a transient papule that is about 1 to 6 mm in size, but it can be a pustule or ulcer. The lesions resolve or heal spontaneously after a few days.[2] Direct rectal inoculation, as in the outbreaks of LGV among MSM, can result in proctitis with symptoms of rectal pain, anorectal bleeding, mucoid or hemopurulent rectal discharge, tenesmus, and constipation.[9]

Secondary: About 2 to 6 weeks after the primary lesion appears, regional tissue invasion occurs and can be accompanied by constitutional symptoms (eg, fever, chills, malaise, myalgia, arthralgia).[10] Advancing systemic complications such as pneumonia and hepatitis have been reported.[2] Although symptoms depend on the site of inoculation, some individuals might be asymptomatic during this stage.[11] With penile, urethral, or vulvar inoculation, the main presentation is an inguinal syndrome.[9] In such cases, LGV induces often unilateral, painful, firm, inguinal or femoral lymphadenopathy known as ***buboes***. These lymph nodes can suppurate, ulcerate, and possibly lead to purulent discharge through cutaneous fistulas.[11] Concurrent inguinal and femoral lymphadenopathy can create the ***groove sign***, which is present in 10% to 20% of cases.[12,13] Cervical lymphadenopathy can occur with the onset of the oral syndrome of LGV.[2] Rectal inoculation results in proctitis and lower abdominal or low-back pain as a result of involvement of the pelvic and retroperitoneal lymph nodes.[12] In these cases lymphadenopathy is not evident on physical examination but can often be identified through imaging (eg, computed tomography, magnetic resonance imaging).[9]

Tertiary: If untreated, LGV can lead to irreversible tissue destruction and scarring.[10] In particular, the chronic lymphangitis and subsequent lymphatic obstruction caused by LGV can lead to regional lymphedema and genital elephantiasis. In severe cases, necrosis and rupture of the lymph nodes have been reported.[14] In cases of rectal involvement, perirectal abscesses, anal fistulas, and strictures are possible.[8]

Treatment Guidelines

Currently there is no vaccination against LGV. The treatment of choice (supported by more than 50 years of clinical experience) is doxycycline. The Centers for Disease Control and Prevention's (CDC's) Sexually Transmitted Disease (STD) Treatment Guidelines recommend doxycycline 100 mg orally twice daily for 21 days and an alternative regimen of erythromycin 500 mg orally 4 times a day for 21 days. Although clinical data are lacking, azithromycin 1 g orally once weekly for 3 weeks is probably effective based on its chlamydial antimicrobial activity.[2] Fluoroquinolone-based treatments also might be effective, but the optimal duration of treatment has not been evaluated.[2] Doxycycline is not recommended for use in pregnant women. Pregnant and lactating women should be treated with erythromycin. Azithromycin may prove useful for treatment of LGV in pregnancy, but no published data are available regarding its safety and efficacy.[2] Patients should abstain from sex until treatment is complete and symptoms have resolved. Sexual partners of a probable or confirmed LGV case should be tested for *Chlamydia* infection and presumptively treated with doxycycline 100 mg orally twice daily for 7 days.[2] Patients should be monitored until symptoms and signs of the disease have resolved, which may occur within 3 to 6 weeks. Tests of cure should be performed approximately 3 to 4 weeks after effective treatment is completed. All guidelines also recommend ongoing follow-up until signs and symptoms are resolved.[8] **Table 3-1** outlines possible treatment regimens for LGV.

Table 3-1. Lymphogranuloma Venereum Treatment Regimens[4]

Drug	Regimen	Mechanism/Possible Side Effects	Comments
Doxycycline	100 mg PO twice daily for 21 days	— Inhibits protein synthesis by binding to 30S ribosomal subunits of susceptible bacteria — Dyspepsia; nausea; diarrhea; photosensitivity; darkening of skin, nails, eyes, teeth, gums, or scars; esophageal ulceration; Fanconi syndrome (nephrotoxicity); steatosis (hepatotoxicity); headache and vision problems (secondary intracranial hypertension–pseudotumor cerebri)	— First choice; recommended by CDC — Contraindicated in pregnancy and breastfeeding — Antacids that contain aluminum, calcium, or magnesium or any product that contains iron, such as vitamin or mineral supplements, should not be taken
Erythromycin	500 mg PO 4 times daily for 21 days	— Inhibits bacterial growth by blocking dissociation of peptidyl transfer RNA from ribosomes — Diarrhea, stomach pain, nausea, vomiting	Second choice; recommended by CDC
Azithromycin	1 g PO stat, then 1 g PO weekly for 3 weeks	— Inhibits bacterial protein synthesis by binding to the 50S ribosomal subunit of the bacterial 70S ribosome — The same as for erythromycin	Should be considered as second choice, but evidence is lacking to recommend this drug
Tetracycline	500 mg PO 4 times daily for 21 days	— The same as for doxycycline — The same side effects listed for doxycycline	The same as for doxycycline
Minocycline	300 mg loading dose, followed by 200 mg PO twice daily for 21 days	— The same as for doxycycline — Vertigo, dizziness, ataxia, tinnitus, and the side effects listed for doxycycline	The same as for doxycycline
Moxifloxacin	400 mg PO once daily for 21 days	— Blocks DNA gyrase enzyme (responsible for production and repair of bacterial DNA), leading to bacteria death — Nausea, dizziness, diarrhea, QT prolongation, and photosensitivity	— Administration should be separated from aluminum- and magnesium-containing antacids, sucralfate, and multivitamins because they can lower absorption of moxifloxacin and reduce its effectiveness — Should be used with caution with warfarin (increases risk for bleeding) and sotalol (abnormal heart rhythm)

For more information on treatment, see the CDC's sexually transmitted diseases guidelines at https://www.cdc.gov/std/tg2015/lgv.htm.[2]
Modified from Ceovic R, Gulin SJ. Lymphogranuloma venereum: diagnostic and treatment challenges. Infect Drug Resist. 2015;8:39-47.

Diagnosis

Evaluation should involve a thorough history, including a sexual history. Diagnosis is based on clinical suspicion, epidemiological information, and the exclusion of other causes for proctocolitis, inguinal lymphadenopathy, or genital or rectal ulcers.[2-4] Genital lesions, rectal specimens, and lymph node specimens (ie, lesion swab, bubo aspirate) can be tested for *C. trachomatis* by culture, direct immunofluorescence, or nucleic acid detection. Nucleic acid amplification tests (NAATs) for *C. trachomatis* perform well on rectal specimens but are not approved by the Food and Drug Administration for this purpose.[2] However, MSM presenting with proctocolitis should be tested for *Chlamydia*, and NAAT performed on rectal specimens is the preferred approach to testing.[2-4] Sex partners from within the last 60 days of a patient with probable or confirmed LGV should be tested for *Chlamydia* and empirically treated with doxycycline 100 mg orally twice daily for 7 days.[2] Patients should have an appropriate sexually transmitted infection (STI) evaluation per the CDC's STD Treatment Guidelines for HIV, syphilis, herpes simplex virus, gonorrhea, or chancroid, and treatment or linkage to care should be provided as needed. As required by state law, these cases should be reported to the health department.[2]

Special Considerations

HIV infection: Persons with both LGV and HIV infection should receive the same regimens as those who are HIV negative. Prolonged therapy might be required, and there may be a delay in the resolution of symptoms.[2]

Recently there have been outbreaks of LGV among HIV-positive MSM. Symptoms include proctocolitis, inguinal lymphadenopathy, and penile lesions.[15]

Pregnancy: Pregnant and lactating women should be treated with erythromycin. Doxycycline should be avoided in the second and third trimester of pregnancy because of risk for discoloration of teeth and bones; however, it is compatible with breastfeeding.[2]

Case Studies

Adult Case Study 3-1

A 31-year-old man presents to an outpatient STI testing clinic. He reports a 2-week history of a painful, red, swollen ulcer on his penis. He denies fever, chills, night sweats, rashes, genital lesions, dysuria, urethral discharge, testicular pain, proctitis, rectal discharge, tenesmus, and diarrhea. He reports previous unprotected receptive and penetrative oral and anal sexual contacts with male partners.

Examination

Examination reveals a 3 cm, tender, erythematous, penile lesion free of discharge and ulceration. There is no visible groove sign (ie, inflammation of the inguinal nodes above and femoral nodes below the inguinal ligament). The genitourinary examination is otherwise unremarkable, as is the examination of his cervical lymph nodes and oropharynx.

Laboratory Testing

Specimens are collected to test for gonorrhea and *Chlamydia*, including first-void urine for NAAT and pharyngeal and rectal swabs for culture. LGV genotyping is requested for all specimens that have positive test results for *Chlamydia*. Samples for serological testing for syphilis, HIV, and *Chlamydia* serovar L are also sent.

Treatment

Based on a presumptive clinical diagnosis of LGV, the patient is prescribed 100 mg doxycycline orally twice daily for 21 days. Follow-up in 2 to 3 weeks is requested. The subsequent follow-up shows complete resolution of symptoms. Serological testing for *Chlamydia* serovar L has positive results, with a titer of 1:512

by microimmunofluorescence. The HIV test results are negative. All other results are negative and, because titer *Chlamydia* is not detected in the urine, pharyngeal, and rectal specimens, the laboratory does not perform LGV genotyping. No public health reporting or follow-up occurs. The patient is encouraged to refrain from sexual activity until 7 days after he has completed his treatment and to inform all sexual partners from the previous 60 days to present for testing and empiric treatment.

Child Case Study 3-2

AC is a 13-year-old boy who is brought to the emergency department by his mother and maternal grandmother with concerns of abdominal pain, constipation, and bleeding from the rectum. The child has been away at camp for the last 2 weeks. The child seems withdrawn and avoids eye contact.

Examination

The child is observed guarding his abdomen. The abdomen is hard without rebound tenderness. Visual inspection of the genital and perianal areas for genital discharge, odor, bleeding, irritation, warts, and ulcerative lesions is completed. The child has some anorectal bleeding with a small pustule approximately 4 mm in circumference.

Laboratory Testing

Culture is completed for *Neisseria gonorrhoeae* from specimens collected from the pharynx and anus. Culture for *C. trachomatis* is completed from specimens collected from the anus. Only standard culture systems for the isolation of *C. trachomatis* should be used. The isolation of *C. trachomatis* is confirmed by microscopic identification of inclusions by staining with fluorescein-conjugated monoclonal antibody specific for *C. trachomatis*. Isolates are preserved for additional testing. Nonculture tests for *Chlamydia* are not specific enough for use in cases of possible child abuse or assault. Serological testing for HIV infection is also considered.

Treatment

Treatment based on height, weight, and age is recommended. Doxycycline is generally avoided in children younger than 8 years because of the possibility of teeth staining. This child is 13 years old and currently weighs 125 lb. Current guidelines recommend ceftriaxone 250 mg intramuscularly in a single dose with azithromycin 1 g orally in a single dose plus metronidazole 2 g orally in a single dose. Follow-up in 2 to 3 weeks with AC's primary care physician to confirm the resolving of symptoms is recommended. A report to the local authorities about possible sexual abuse is made. A serum sample is collected for evaluation of HIV, hepatitis B, and syphilis infections. The HIV test results are negative. All other results are negative, and *Chlamydia* is not detected in the urine, pharyngeal, and rectal specimens.

References

1. Saxon C, Hughes G, Ison C; UK LGV Case-Finding Group. Asymptomatic lymphogranuloma venereum in men who have sex with men, United Kingdom. *Emerg Infect Dis*. 2016;22(1):112-116.
2. 2015 sexually transmitted diseases treatment guidelines: lymphogranuloma venereum (LGV). Centers for Disease Control and Prevention Web site. https://www.cdc.gov/std/tg2015/lgv.htm. Updated June 4, 2014. Accessed July 15, 2019.
3. Rawla P, Limaiem F. *Lymphogranuloma Venereum*. Treasure Island, FL: StatPearls Publishing; 2019.
4. Ceovic R, Gulin SJ. Lymphogranuloma venereum: diagnostic and treatment challenges. *Infect Drug Resist*. 2015;8:39-47.
5. Ward H, Alexander S, Carder C, et al. The prevalence of lymphogranuloma venereum infection in men who have sex with men: results of a multicentre case finding study. *Sex Transm Infect*. 2009;85(3):173-175.

6. Savage EJ, van de Laar MJ, Gallay A, et al; European Surveillance of Sexually Transmitted Infections (ESSTI) network. Lymphogranuloma venereum in Europe, 2003-2008. *Euro Surveill.* 2009;14(48):19428.

7. Ward H, Martin I, Macdonald N, et al. Lymphogranuloma venereum in the United Kingdom. *Clin Infect Dis.* 2007;44(1):26-32.

8. O'Byrne P, MacPherson P, DeLaplante S, Metz G, Bourgault A. Approach to lymphogranuloma venereum. *Can Fam Physician.* 2016;62(7):554-558.

9. de Vrieze NH, de Vries HJ. Lymphogranuloma venereum among men who have sex with men. An epidemiological and clinical review. *Expert Rev Anti Infect Ther.* 2014;12(6):697-704.

10. Stamm WE. Lymphogranuloma venereum. In: Holmes KK, Sparling PF, Stamm WE, et al, eds. *Sexually Transmitted Diseases*, 4th ed. New York, NY: McGraw-Hill; 2008:595-605.

11. White J, O'Farrell N, Daniels D; British Association for Sexual Health and HIV. 2013 UK National Guideline for the management of lymphogranuloma venereum: Clinical Effectiveness Group of the British Association for Sexual Health and HIV (CEG/BASHH) guideline development group. *Int J STD AIDS.* 2013;24(8):593-601.

12. de Vrieze NH, van Rooijen M, Schim van der Loeff MF, de Vries HJ. Anorectal and inguinal lymphogranuloma venereum among men who have sex with men in Amsterdam, The Netherlands: trends over time, symptomatology and concurrent infections. *Sex Transm Infect.* 2013;89(7):548-552.

13. de Vrieze NH, van Rooijen M, Sperksnijder AG, de Vries HJ. Urethral lymphogranuloma venereum infections in men with anorectal lymphogranuloma venereum and their partners: the missing link in the current epidemic? *Sex Transm Dis.* 2013;40(8):607-608.

14. Workowski KA, Bolan GA; Centers for Disease Control and Prevention. Sexually transmitted diseases treatment guidelines, 2015. *MMWR Recomm Rep.* 2015;64(RR-03):1-137.

15. Health alert template for LGV. Centers for Disease Control and Prevention Web site. https://www.cdc.gov/std/program/outbreakresources/HANtemplate-lgv.htm. Updated May 13, 2019. Accessed December 3, 2019.

Chapter 4

Granuloma Inguinale (Donovanosis)

William DeClue, DNP, FNP-BC, MHA
Kathleen Thimsen, DNP, MSN, WOCN, FNS

Disease and Mimics

- Granuloma inguinale is a genital ulcerative disease caused by the intracellular gram-negative bacterium *Klebsiella granulomatis*.[1]
- It occurs rarely in the United States but is endemic in some tropical and developing areas.[1]
- Granuloma inguinale is commonly characterized by painless, slowly progressive ulcerative lesions on the genitals or perineum *without* regional lymphadenopathy (**Figure 4-1**). Lesions are highly vascular and bleed easily.[1] Lesions can also appear in the oral cavity.[2]
- Granuloma inguinale is contracted by having unprotected vaginal or anal intercourse with an infected partner. A person may contract it through oral sex, but this is rare.[2]
- The signs and symptoms of granuloma inguinale have a slow onset. The usual progression of the infectious process can take up to 5 to 7 days, and it can take up to 12 weeks for symptoms of the disease to progress to their peak state.[2]

Epidemiology

The causative organism of granuloma inguinale is difficult to culture, and diagnosis requires visualization of dark-staining Donovan bodies on tissue crush preparation or biopsy. No Food and Drug Administration–approved molecular tests for the detection of *K. granulomatis* DNA exist.[1] If a person has a history of recent travel and sexual contact in an endemically infected area, a diagnosis of granuloma inguinale should be considered.[2]

Treatment Guidelines

Treatment for adults is azithromycin 1 g orally once per week or 500 mg daily for at least 3 weeks and until lesions have completely healed; ciprofloxacin 750 mg orally twice daily for at least 3 weeks and until all lesions have completely healed; or erythromycin base 500 mg orally 4 times daily for at least 3 weeks and until all lesions have completely healed. Single-dose, directly observed therapy is preferred. For more information on treatment, see the Centers for Disease Control and Prevention's sexually transmitted disease guidelines at https://www.cdc.gov/std/tg2015/donovanosis.htm.

Doxycycline (Vibramycin) may be used, but the health care provider must be aware of special considerations for administration and dosing. If doxycycline is being used, the dose is 100 mg orally twice a day for a minimum of 3 weeks and continued until all lesions have completely healed.[2]

Figure 4-1. *Granuloma inguinale, male. (Courtesy of CDC, Atlanta, GA.)*

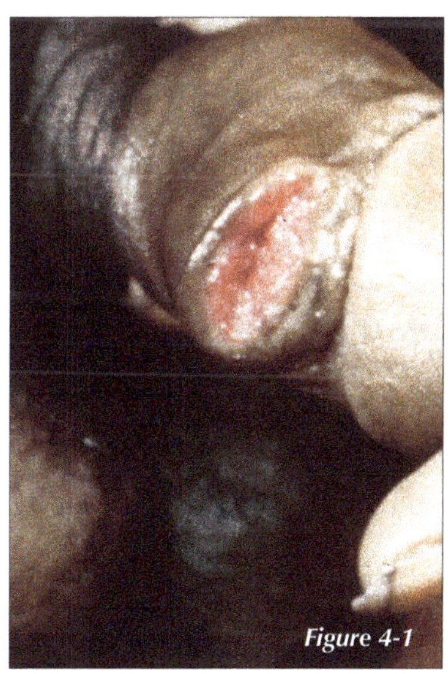

Special Considerations

Early treatment is optimal to prevent scarring and swelling in the genital, anal, or inguinal areas. The infected person has the responsibility to let sex partners know that he or she has the infection.[2]

- ***Pregnancy:*** Doxycycline should be avoided in the second and third trimester of pregnancy because of the risk for discoloration of teeth and bones of the developing fetus. Ciprofloxacin presents a low risk to the developing fetus during pregnancy. Sulfonamides are associated with rare but serious kernicterus in those with G6PD deficiency and should be avoided in the third trimester of pregnancy and during breastfeeding.[1]

— ***HIV infection:*** Persons with granuloma inguinale and human immunodeficiency virus (HIV) infection should receive the same regimens as those who do not have HIV infection.[1]

Case Studies

Adult Case Study 4-1

A 42-year-old woman comes into the sexually transmitted infection (STI) outpatient department with a complaint of an ulcer over the right labium majus for a month. She reports itching but is nontender, and no pain is noted. When questioned about sexual contact, the patient states she had unprotected sex with 2 people recently. The patient has type 2 diabetes and is taking metformin 1000 mg twice daily.

Examination

The clinical picture of the ulcer closely resembles a granuloma inguinale. The base of the ulcer is raised above the surrounding skin and consists of large, coarse, pale red, warty granulation tissue that gives the surface a buckled appearance. Further clinical examination of the ulcer reveals 2 cm peri-ulcer margins, but it is not indurated.

Laboratory Testing

A smear taken from the base of the lesion is sent to the laboratory for testing. Diagnosis occurs when the pathologist stains the tissue with Wright stain and Donovan bodies turn dark purple.

Treatment

The patient is treated with doxycycline 100 mg twice a day for 2 weeks until the ulcer heals. The patient is educated on self-care and protection when having sexual intercourse to prevent the recurrence of the disease process.[3]

Child Case Study 4-2

A 16-year-old boy presents to the pediatrician with a "sore" on his penis. The pediatrician completes subjective and objective assessments on the patient. The patient reports having unprotected sexual intercourse approximately 8 weeks prior. The patient reports having 2 sexual experiences with the same person.

Examination

The pediatrician assesses the penile lesion, noting a 2 cm x 2 cm, beefy-red, velvety, raised ulcer with irregular margins that has gradually increased in size. The patient states that it "hurts a little."

Laboratory Testing

A smear taken from the base of the lesion is sent to the laboratory for testing. Diagnosis occurs when the pathologist stains the tissue with Wright stain and Donovan bodies turn dark purple.

Treatment

The treatment plan is azithromycin 1 g orally in a single dose. The pediatrician educates the patient on how to protect himself to avoid STIs. This includes the use of condoms and abstinence.[4]

References

1. 2015 sexually transmitted diseases guidelines: granuloma inguinale (donovanosis). Centers for Disease Control and Prevention Web site. https://www.cdc.gov/std/tg2015/donovanosis.htm. Updated June 4, 2015. Accessed August 27, 2019.
2. Santiago-Wickey JN, Crosby B. *Granuloma Inguinale (Donovanosis)*. Treasure Island, FL: StatPearls Publishing; 2019.
3. Deivam S, Kuruvilla PC, Balasubramanian N, et al. A case report of Donovanosis: granuloma inguinale. *British Biomedical Bulletin*. 2014;2(3):472-476.
4. Ballard R. Klebsiella granulomatis (Donovanosis, Granuloma Inguinale). Oncohema Key Web site. https://oncohemakey.com/klebsiella-granulomatis-donovanosis-granuloma-inguinale/. Published July 1, 2017. Accessed August 27, 2019.

Chapter 5

Mycoplasma Genitalium

Angelia Trujillo, DNP, MSN, WHNP-BC
Nicole Marnell, DNP, APRN, CPNP-PC
Angela Ellis, MSN, RN, SANE-A, SANE-P

Disease and Mimics

— *Mycoplasma genitalium* (Mgen) is a sexually transmitted bacterium that lives on skin cells of the urinary and genital tracts in humans. It was first identified in the 1980s and causes signs and symptoms similar to those that occur with *Chlamydia*.[1,2] However, Mgen is less common than *Chlamydia* and is not as easily transmitted.[3]

— Mgen is recognized as a cause of male urethritis. It is responsible for 15% to 20% of nongonococcal urethritis cases, 20% to 25% of nonchlamydial urethritis cases, and approximately 30% of persistent or recurrent urethritis cases.[4] The pathogenic role of Mgen is less definitive in women than it is in men. In women, Mgen can be found in the vagina, cervix, and endometrium. The infection is commonly asymptomatic.[4]

— Mgen can be detected in 10% to 30% of women with clinical cervicitis, and most studies have found that Mgen is more common among women with cervicitis than those without. It is also found more often in the cervix or endometrium of women with pelvic inflammatory disease (PID) than in women without PID.[4]

Epidemiology

Mgen is difficult to diagnose via Gram stain and microscopy because it does not have a cell wall and is difficult to diagnose via culture because of its slow growth rate (6 months).[4-6] Diagnosis via nucleic acid amplification tests (NAATs) is possible but has only recently been approved by the Food and Drug Administration (FDA) in the United States.[4] Hologic laboratories, located in San Diego, is the first to receive FDA approval for Mgen testing. Roche received approval in May 2019 and, at the time of printing, SpeeDx is seeking approval.[7] NAATs are only available at a limited number of medical centers and commercial laboratories and are for research purposes only.[4,8] Specimen types for NAATs include urine, vaginal, endocervical, endometrial, urethral, penile-meatal, and rectal. For transgender and non-binary persons, the type of sexual activity will determine the most suitable swabs to collect. Oropharyngeal swabs are rarely collected because of low detection from the oropharynx.[4,6]

Screening in asymptomatic patients is not currently recommended.[4,8] In persistent or recurrent urethritis, cervicitis, or PID, Mgen should be suspected, tested for, and treated.[3,7] Mgen mimics other genital infections such as *Chlamydia trachomatis*, trichomoniasis, and bacterial vaginosis (BV).[4,8] Those who test positive for Mgen should discuss testing and treatment with current sex partners.[3]

As a result of the lack of knowledge and difficulty in diagnosis, estimates of the prevalence of Mgen vary. More common than *Neisseria gonorrhoeae*, but less common than *Chlamydia trachomatis*,[4-6] the prevalence of Mgen throughout the United States and Europe is estimated to be 1% to 4% among low-risk patients[2,4,6] and as high as 33% in high-risk populations.[5,6] The highest prevalence of infections are among adolescents and young adults (>24%) as well as African American men (27.9%) and women (23.2%).[6] Mgen infections are also associated with other sexually transmitted infections (STIs), such as those caused by *Chlamydia trachomatis* and *Neisseria gonorrhoeae,* making it easy to overlook.[8,10] Mgen can be found in the male urethra, rectum, and epididymis.[4,5] In female patients, Mgen has been detected in the vagina, cervix, endometrium, and fallopian tubes.[5]

Symptomology and Long-Term Sequelae

As with other STIs, Mgen is often asymptomatic in many patients. Clinical presentation may include dysuria, vaginal pruritus, mucopurulent discharge from the cervix, cervical friability, irregular bleeding, painful intercourse, increased leukocytes, and PID symptoms in females.[7] Males may experience dysuria, urethral discharge, and pruritus, as well as rectal symptoms and prostatitis. Other complaints can include painful ejaculation, watery or cloudy discharge from the tip of the penis, and inflammation of the foreskin of the penis.[3] Detection of Mgen in the anal canal ranges from 2% to 12%, with males having a higher rate of infection than females (12% versus 8.1%).[6] Because of the presence of these symptoms in other infections, clinical diagnosis is unfeasible by symptoms alone.[4] If left untreated, Mgen infections may lead to PID, sexually acquired reactive arthritis, preterm delivery, spontaneous abortion, and infertility.[6,8]

Treatment Guidelines

Mgen does not have a cell wall, so antibiotics targeting cell-wall biosynthesis are not effective against this organism. Mgen is not susceptible to cell wall synthesis-inhibiting medications such as penicillins and cephalosporins.[5] Treatment usually occurs in the context of syndromic management for urethritis, cervicitis, and PID.[4]

Mgen should be suspected and treated presumptively in cases of persistent or recurrent urethritis, cervicitis, and PID. For patients presenting with urethritis, cervicitis, or PID, treatment with a single, 1 g dose of azithromycin or a 7-day dose of doxycycline 100 mg is recommended, with azithromycin having been found to be more effective.[5] For persistent infections, treatment may be increased to a 5-day dose of azithromycin. If symptoms do not respond to treatment with azithromycin within 7 to 10 days or the patient tests positive with NAAT, moxifloxacin 400 mg daily for 7, 10, or 14 days is recommended.[4,8,10]

Moxifloxacin has been successfully used to treat Mgen in patients with previous treatment failures caused by resistant Mgen. If a patient fails treatment with moxifloxacin, baseline fluoroquinolone resistance may be suspected. In these cases, pristinamycin 1 g 4 times daily for 10 days may be effective, but it is currently only available in European countries.[10] As with all STIs, sexual partners should also be treated. Patients should be instructed to refrain from sexual intercourse until the patient and any sexual partners have completely finished all treatment. Women with PID should refrain from intercourse until 14 days after the start of treatment or 14 days after signs and symptoms have resolved, whichever occurs later. Male and female condom use provides a high level of protection against Mgen by reducing direct contact with genital tissues.[3]

Special considerations

Because of a lack of testing facilities, most patients with Mgen are not diagnosed. In addition, a test of cure typically is not performed after therapy despite high rates of ineffective treatment.[6] Therefore, patient assessment and follow-up are important, as well as supporting availability of testing and development of evidence-based screening guidelines.

— ***HIV:*** Patients with human immunodeficiency virus (HIV) are at a high risk for contracting Mgen and for transmitting HIV and Mgen to sexual partners. The release of cytokines and resulting inflammation caused by an Mgen infection make patients more susceptible to contracting HIV.[8]

— ***Children:*** Children who test positive for STIs after age 2 years should be evaluated for child sexual abuse (CSA), because STIs are a marker for the diagnosis of CSA outside of the neonatal period.[10] Children with recurrent genital infections or infections not responding to treatment should be evaluated for Mgen and CSA.

— ***Men who have sex with men:*** As a result of the colonization of Mgen in the rectum, men who have sex with men are at a higher risk for urethral infections.[5,12] Circumcision can reduce the risk of infection by 50%, suggesting foreskin as an additional site for colonization.[5]

— ***Other STIs:*** Mgen is often associated with other STIs such as *Chlamydia*, gonorrhea, trichomoniasis, BV, and HIV.[6,9]

Case Studies

Adult Case Study 5-1

MB is a 23-year-old female office worker who presents to the clinic with a request for a vaginal examination. She reports yellowish discharge and pelvic pain during intercourse. She reports no new partners in the last 3 months.

Examination

Patient is found to have cervical motion tenderness; copious yellow, thick discharge; and vaginal inflammation.

Laboratory Testing

Routine cultures for *Chlamydia trachomatis* and *Neisseria gonorrhoeae* are obtained, and patient is presumptively treated with azythromycin 1 g orally and ceftriazone (Rocephin) 250 mg via intramuscular (IM) injection. On follow-up, the patient continues to have pelvic pain and discharge. NAAT for *Chlamydia trachomatis* and *Neisseria gonorrhoeae* are negative. NAAT for *Mycoplasma genitalium* is positive. (This NAAT is sent to a local research laboratory.)

Treatment

The patient and her partner were treated with a 14-day course of moxifloxacin 400 mg daily, which resolved the infection.

Child Case Study 5-2

JB is a 4-year-old boy (weight: 19 kg [42 pounds]) seen for a routine well child check with his primary pediatrician.

Examination

On examination of his genitals, he is noted to have discharge from his penis.

Laboratory Testing

NAAT returns negative results for *Chlamydia trachomatis* and *Neisseria gonorrhoeae.*

Treatment

For *Chlamydia*, children younger than 8 years who weigh less than 45 kg (99 pounds) should be given azithromycin 20 mg/kg to treat *Chlamydia trachomatis* (maximum dose 1 g). For *Neisseria gonorrhoeae*, children who weigh less than 45 kg should be treated with 25 to 50 mg/kg once IM (maximum dose 125 mg). This patient is treated with azithromycin 380 mg orally and ceftriazone (Rocephin) 125 mg IM. On follow-up, patient continues to have discharge and has developed pain during urination. A NAAT for Mgen is sent to a local research laboratory and returns with positive results. A report is made to child protective services. An investigation leads to the child disclosing sexual abuse by his father's girlfriend, who also tests positive for Mgen.

NOTE: The recommended treatment for Mgen in adults when azithromycin therapy fails is moxifloxacin 400 mg once daily for 14 days.[10,13] There is no documented information on pediatric treatment when azithromyacin fails and when NAAT confirms Mgen. The recommendation would be to consult with a pediatric infectious disease specialist. Moxifloxacin use in children is noted primarily for anthrax, community-acquired pneumonia, and multidrug-resistant tuberculosis.[10] Moxifloxacin dosage for children ages 2 to 5 years is 5 mg/kg per dose every 12 hours (maximum dose 200 mg per dose). Limited data are available for optimal treatment length.

References

1. *Mycoplasma genitalium* infections. Centers for Disease Control and Prevention Web site. https://www2c.cdc.gov/podcasts/media/pdf/EID_11-17_M_Genitalium Infections.pdf. Published November 2017. Accessed August 11, 2019.
2. Tully JG, Taylor-Robinson D, Cole RM, Rose DL. A newly discovered mycoplasma in the human urogenital tract. *Lancet.* 1981;1(8233):1288-1291.
3. Lowth M. Mycoplasma genitalium. Patient Web site. https://patient.info/sexual-health/sexually-transmitted-infections-leaflet/mycoplasma-genitalium-mgen. Updated October 5, 2018. Accessed March 30, 2020.
4. 2015 sexually transmitted diseases treatment guidelines: emerging issues. Centers for Disease Control and Prevention Web site. https://www.cdc.gov/std/tg2015/emerging.htm. Updated June 4, 2015. Accessed July 18, 2019.
5. Manhart LE. *Mycoplasma genitalium:* an emergent sexually transmitted disease? *Infect Dis Clin North Am.* 2013;27(4):779-792.
6. Manhart LE, Trent M. *Mycoplasma genitalium:* a review of current issues and challenges. Semantic Scholar Web site. https://pdfs.semanticscholar.org/b4d5/2b00be8a1ef99e2a5bae88c8bcfa46b51c8a.pdf. Published July 2017. Accessed August 1, 2019.
7. Sisson P. New test is first in US to help detect new STD threat. Medical Xpress Web site. https://medicalxpress.com/news/2019-08-std-threat.html. Published August 5, 2019. Accessed September 5, 2019.
8. Heavey E. *Mycoplasma genitalium.* Nursing2019. 2017;47(7):61-62.
9. Seña A, Lee JY, Schwebke J, et al. A silent epidemic: the prevalence, incidence and persistence of *Mycoplasma genitalium* among young, asymptomatic high-risk women in the United States. *Clin Infect Dis.* 2018;67(1):73-79.
10. Mobley V, Seña A. *Mycoplasma genitalium* infection in men and women. UpToDate Web site. https://www.uptodate.com/contents/mycoplasma-genitalium-infection-in-men-and-women. Updated February 15, 2019. Accessed August 9, 2019.
11. Rogstad KE, Wilkinson D, Robinson A. Sexually transmitted infections in children as a marker of child sexual abuse and directions of future. *Curr Opin Infect Dis.* 2016;29(1):41-44.
12. Read TRH, Murray GL, Danielewski JA, et al. Symptoms, sites, and significance of Mycoplasma genitalium in men who have sex with men. *Emerg Infect Dis.* 2019;25(4):719-727.
13. Jensen JS, Cusini M, Gomberg M, Moi H. 2016 European guideline on Mycoplasma genitalium infections. *J Eur Acad Dermatol Venereol.* 2016;30(10):1650-1656.

Chapter 6

CHLAMYDIA

Lauren Traveller, DNP, APRN, FNP-C
Ashley Feldman, BSN, RN
Rachell A. Ekroos, PhD, APRN-BC, AFN-BC, FAAN

DISEASE AND MIMICS

— *Chlamydia* is the most common reportable disease and most prevalent sexually transmitted disease (STD) in the United States.[1]

— *Chlamydia*, an infection caused by *Chlamydia trachomatis* (*C. trachomatis*), is spread through contact with the mouth, vagina, penis, or anus of an infected individual. *Chlamydia* can be transmitted during penile sexual contact without ejaculation occuring.[2]

— An infected and untreated mother can infect the infant during the birthing process, resulting in neonatal conjunctivitis or pneumonia.[3]

— A positive *Chlamydia* infection in a prepubertal child beyond the neonatal period requires further assessment, including screening for sexual abuse.[2]

— Patients who have a *Chlamydia* infection are often asymptomatic and no abnormal findings are observed during the physical examination.[2]

— The most common symptoms among symptomatic persons with a genitourinary *Chlamydia* diagnosis include cervicitis, urethritis, dysuria, and mucopurulent or watery discharge (**Figure 6-1**).[2]

— In the female genitalia, an ascending *Chlamydia* infection can spread from the cervix into the upper reproductive tract, resulting in pelvic inflammatory disease (PID).[2]

— Rectal *Chlamydia* infections can occur through direct contact or, in patients with vaginal infection, through transmission from the reproductive tract.[4] Rectal *Chlamydia* may cause proctitis (rectal inflammation that may be accompanied by pain, discharge, and bleeding).[5]

— Contact with infected genital secretions can cause chlamydial conjunctivitis in persons regardless of age.[6]

— Oral contact with an infected individual (via oral, penile, vaginal, or anal contact) may result in oropharyngeal *Chlamydia*. A *Chlamydia* infection in the throat is not typically associated with pharyngitis.[7]

— Untreated *Chlamydia* increases the risk for contracting human immunodeficiency virus (HIV), if exposed.[8]

Figure 6-1. *Vaginitis with purulent discharge caused by* Chlamydia trachomatis *in a prepubertal girl with no disclosure of sexual abuse.*

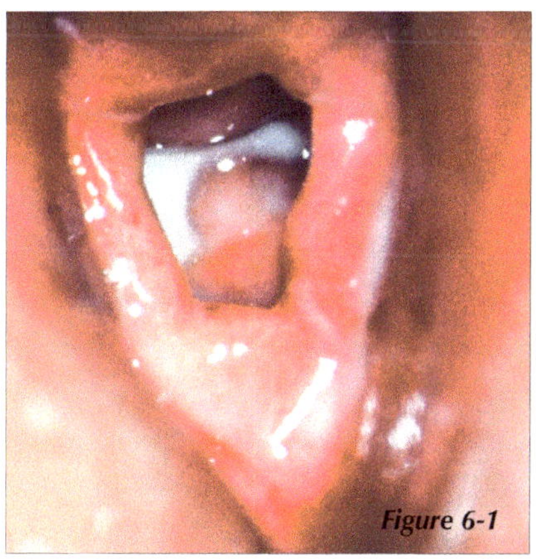

EPIDEMIOLOGY

The most recent report on chlamydial infections in the United States indicated 528.8 cases per 100 000 persons. Nearly two-thirds of chlamydial infections are among individuals between the ages of 15 to 24 years.[1] *Chlamydia* is more common in women, and an estimated 1 in 20 sexually active persons are infected.[8] Reported case rates of chlamydial infection are highest among black persons, with a 5.6 times greater likelihood of becoming infected than white persons.[1] Ejaculation is not needed to spread the infection; transmission of *Chlamydia* can occur when there is contact with infected secretions of the mouth, vagina, penis, or anus.[2] Avoiding direct contact with infected secretions through correct barrier use during sexual contact (eg, condoms, dental dams), as well as maintaining a mutually monogamous relationship with a partner who has tested negative for STDs, reduces the risk of transmitting or acquiring a chlamydial infection.[2]

Approximately 10% of men and 5% to 30% of women with laboratory-confirmed chlamydial infections develop symptoms.[9,10] The incubation period for *Chlamydia* is not well defined. However, because of the slow replication cycle of the organism, symptoms do not often appear until several weeks after exposure, if at all. Individuals with female genitalia who are symptomatic may report vaginal discharge, pyuria, dysuria, and frequent urination.[2] The infection can ascend from the cervix through the reproductive tract leading to PID. PID resulting from chlamydial infection may remain asymptomatic (or "subclinical"). It is estimated that 10% to 15% of women with untreated chlamydial infections present with classic signs and symptoms of acute PID, such as abdominal or pelvic pain, cervical motion tenderness, adnexal tenderness, and uterine tenderness. Regardless of presentation, untreated PID can cause permanent damage to the female reproductive tract, resulting in complications ranging from infertility and ectopic pregnancy to perihepatitis or reactive arthritis.[11-16] Men with urogenital symptoms may report urethral discharge and dysuria. Less common symptoms may include unilateral testicular pain, swelling, or tenderness, indicating possible epididymitis.[17]

Patients engaging in activities resulting in multiple site exposure risks (eg, genital, oral, anal) should receive screening for each point of contact. When screening is limited to urogenital testing (ie, urine), a negative result does not mean the person is free of infection. Despite a negative urine screen, a patient may have oropharyngeal infection, rectal infection, or both. Limiting screening to routine urine collection rather than contact history increases the risk of continued transmission because of untreated exposure, particularly when the infection is asymptomatic.

In adults, nucleic acid amplification tests (NAATs) are the most sensitive for detecting *Chlamydia* across multiple specimens and are therefore the gold standard for diagnosing *Chlamydia*. Urine, cervical swab, and vaginal swab specimens (**Figure 6-2**) can all be used to diagnose urogenital *Chlamydia* in women. Specimens can be collected by a health care provider or nurse or self-collected by the patient, particularly in cases where a pelvic examination is not indicated. Similarly, urine or urethral swab specimens can be used to diagnose urogenital *Chlamydia* in men.[18-21]

Figure 6-2. *Intracellular bodies of* Chlamydia *seen on Giemsa stain before fluorescein antibody staining.*

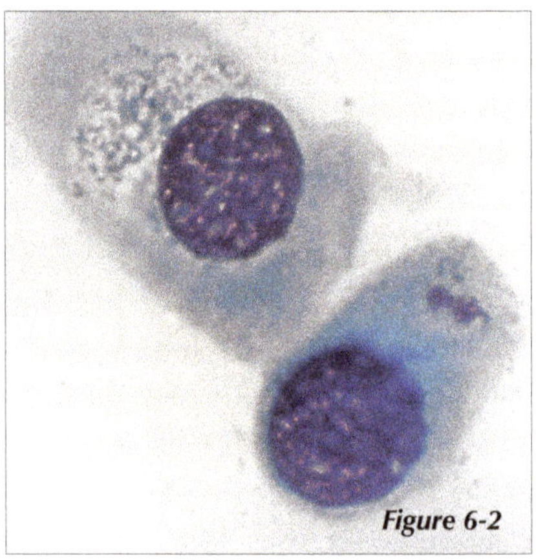

Rectal and pharyngeal swab specimens and NAATs have demonstrated increased sensitivity and specificity in detecting Chlamydia compared with cultures. In March 2019, the Food and Drug Administration approved the first diagnostic tests for extragenital testing for *Chlamydia*.[2,22-25]

Prepubertal children with chlamydial infections should receive further assessment for sexual abuse. There have been reports of perinatally transmitted chlamydial infections up to the age of 3 years, although most cases of perinatal acquired rectal or genital *Chlamydia* do not persist longer than 1 year.[3]

Treatment Guidelines

Antibiotics are used to treat *Chlamydia*. Azithromycin and doxycycline are recommended by the Centers for Disease Control and Prevention (CDC) to treat *Chlamydia* in those who are 8 years and older. For children younger than 8 years, treatment is weight-based with either erythromycin or azithromycin.[18] **Table 6-1** provides a summary of treatment guidelines.

Table 6-1. Summary of Treatment Guidelines for *Chlamydia*[18]

Infection	Population	Recommended Treatment	Alternative Treatment
Urogenital, oropharyngeal, anorectal	Adults	Azithromycin 1 g orally in a single dose ***OR*** Doxycycline 100 mg orally twice daily for 7 days	Erythromycin base 500 mg orally 4 times a day for 7 days ***OR*** Erythromycin ethylsuccinate 800 mg orally 4 times a day for 7 days ***OR*** Levofloxacin 500 mg orally once daily for 7 days ***OR*** Ofloxacin 300 mg orally twice a day for 7 days
	Adolescents and children ≥ 8 years old	Azithromycin 1 g orally in a single dose ***OR*** Doxycycline 100 mg orally twice daily for 7 days	
	Children < 8 years old and ≥ 45 kg	Azithromycin 1 g orally in a single dose	
	Children < 45 kg	Erythromycin base or ethylsuccinate 50 mg/kg/day orally divided into 4 doses daily for 14 days	
	Pregnant	Azithromycin 1 g orally in a single dose	Amoxicillin 500 mg orally 3 times a day for 7 days ***OR*** Erythromycin base 500 mg orally 4 times a day for 7 days ***OR*** Erythromycin base 250 mg orally 4 times a day for 14 days ***OR*** Erythromycin ethylsuccinate 800 mg orally 4 times a day for 7 days ***OR*** Erythromycin ethylsuccinate 400 mg orally 4 times a day for 14 days
	HIV positive	Same regimen as those without HIV infection	Same regimen as those without HIV infection
Ophthalmia neonatorum (chlamydial conjunctivitis)	Neonates (0-30 days)	Erythromycin or ethylsuccinate 50 mg/kg/day orally divided into 4 doses daily for 14 days	Azithromycin suspension, 20 mg/kg/day orally, 1 dose daily for 3 days
Pneumonia (chlamydial)	Infants (1-3 months)	Erythromycin base or ethylsuccinate 50 mg/kg/day orally divided into 4 doses daily for 14 days	Azithromycin 20 mg/kg/day orally, 1 dose daily for 3 days

For more information on treatment, see the CDC's sexually transmitted disease guidelines at validated https://www.cdc.gov/std/chlamydia/treatment.htm. For additional treatment guidance and medical management, refer to the CDC 2015 guidelines.[18]

Patients receiving treatment for *Chlamydia* should be informed to abstain from sexual contact for 7 days after treatment (eg, for 7 days after single-dose therapy, until completion of a 7-day regimen) and symptoms are no longer present, if applicable. Follow-up or repeat testing after treatment completion (also known as test of cure) is not routinely recommended except in pregnant patients and when there are questions regarding treatment adherence, continued symptoms, or concern for reinfection.[18]

Special Considerations

— ***Pregnancy:*** Screening all pregnant women for *Chlamydia* will help to prevent neonatal complications.[2,26] A single oral dose of azithromycin is recommended to treat pregnant women infected with *Chlamydia*. Amoxicillin and erythromycin are alternative treatments. Second- and third-trimester pregnancy is a contraindication for treatment with doxycycline. A test of cure is recommended 3 to 4 weeks after treatment and again in 3 months after treatment.[18]

— ***HIV infection:*** The treatment regimen used for patients who are HIV positive is the same as that used for patients who are HIV negative.[18]

— ***Neonates:*** Neonatal *Chlamydia* infection can occur during the birthing process if the mother is infected. Infection may affect mucous membranes of the eye, oropharynx, urogenital tract, and rectum while the patient remains asymptomatic. Symptoms most often present as conjunctivitis appearing 5 to 12 days after birth or afebrile pneumonia appearing between ages 1 and 3 months. These complications further highlight the importance of prenatal screening and treatment as the most favorable for preventing neonatal infection.[18]

— ***Rectal* Chlamydia *treatment:*** Rectal *Chlamydia*, like urogenital and oropharyngeal *Chlamydia*, can be treated with azithromycin or doxycycline. However, providers should consider doxycycline as the treatment of choice for patients engaging in receptive anal sexual contact because of an increase in treatment failure and persistent/recurrent infection when treated with azithromycin, particularly when treating patients from known high-risk populations (eg, men having sex with men, transgender persons, sex workers) or if there is genital coinfection.[27-30]

— ***Coinfection:*** Studies have shown that women between the ages of 15 to 25 years who are sexually active and infected with gonorrhea have a high probability of being coinfected with *Chlamydia*.[31]

Case Studies

Adult Case Study 6-1

JD is a 21-year-old transgender man who presents to the primary care clinic for STD testing. He is sexually active with men and women and reports multiple partners in the last 12 months. He reports oral sex (fellatio and cunnilingus), receptive anal sex, and penile-vaginal sex. The last sexual contact was 3 days ago, and no protective barriers were used. A partner from 1 month ago contacted him to tell him he should get tested for STDs. He denies any symptoms at this time. JD uses self-prescribed hormone therapy and has no significant medical history and no known drug allergies.

Examination

Physical and anogenital examination are normal.

Laboratory Testing

Urine NAAT for *Chlamydia trachomatis* and *Neisseria gonorrhoeae* (CT/NG) is negative. Pharyngeal NAAT for CT/NG is positive for *C. trachomatis*. Rectal NAAT for CT/NG is negative. Dipstick urinalysis is normal. HIV antibody–negative *Treponema pallidum* total antibody screen is negative. Acute hepatitis panel is negative.

Treatment

JD returns to the clinic and is administered azithromycin 1 g orally in a single dose. Abstention from sexual contact for 7 days after treatment to avoid reinfection and transmission of infection is discussed, and JD's questions about transmission of infection are addressed. The local public health district is notified per mandatory reporting requirements, and the patient is informed regarding disease investigation follow-up procedures. Patient education discussions include consistent condom use, safe sex practices, and sexual health. Condoms are provided. JD expresses interest in meeting with a local provider who specializes in community-based transgender care. Appointment assistance is provided.

Child Case Study 6-2

AJ is a 10-year-old prepubertal girl who presents to the child advocacy center for a scheduled clinical forensic examination. Her history includes disclosing penile-oral contact and digital-vaginal contact by a 16-year-old boy who lives in the same apartment complex. The disclosure is made to the mother and the forensic interviewer. The last known contact was approximately 2 months ago.

Examination

Complete head-to-toe physical examination, including anogenital structures, is normal.

Laboratory Testing

Urine human chorionic gonadotropin is negative (performed on all female children demonstrating premenarchal development, as early as 8 years or older).[32] Urine NAAT for CT/NG is negative. Pharyngeal NAAT for CT/NG is positive. Dipstick urinalysis is normal.

Treatment

AJ is given azithromycin 1 g orally in a single dose. Child protective services and law enforcement are notified of the laboratory results and treatment status. The local public health district is notified per mandatory reporting requirements; patient and patient's guardian are informed regarding disease investigation follow-up procedures. AJ is given an opportunity to speak with the provider alone and with her mother, and the patient does not have any questions. KC (patient's biological mother) meets separately with the provider, and follow-up recommendations are provided, an advocate's name and contact information are provided, and school and work excuse forms are printed and provided to KC.

References

1. Sexually transmitted disease surveillance 2017. Centers for Disease Control and Prevention Web site. https://www.cdc.gov/std/stats17/2017-STD-Surveillance-Report_CDC-clearance-9.10.18.pdf. Published September 2018. Accessed October 2, 2019.
2. Chlamydia: detailed fact sheet. Centers for Disease Control and Prevention Web site. https://www.cdc.gov/std/chlamydia/stdfact-chlamydia-detailed.htm. Updated October 4, 2016. Accessed July 20, 2019.
3. Bell TA, Stamm WE, Wang SP, Kuo CC, Holmes KK, Grayston JT. Chronic Chlamydia trachomatis infections in infants. *JAMA*. 1992;267(3):400-402.
4. Barry PM, Kent CK, Philip SS, Klausner JD. Results of a program to test women for rectal chlamydia and gonorrhea. *Obstet Gynecol.* 2010;115(4):753-759.
5. Thompson CI, MacAulay AJ, Smith IW. Chlamydia trachomatis infections in the female rectums. *Genitourin Med.* 1989;65(4):269-273.
6. Kalayoglu MV. Ocular chlamydial infections: pathogenesis and emerging treatment strategies. *Curr Drug Targets Infect Disord.* 2002;2(1):85-91.
7. Jones RB, Rabinovitch RA, Katz BP, et al. Chlamydia trachomatis in the pharynx and rectum of heterosexual patients at risk for genital infection. *Ann Intern Med.* 1985;102(6):757-762.
8. Fleming DT, Wasserheit JN. From epidemiological synergy to public health policy and practice: the contribution of other sexually transmitted diseases to sexual transmission of HIV infection. *Sex Transm Infect*. 1999;75(1):3-17.

9. Farley TA, Cohen DA, Elkins W. Asymptomatic sexually transmitted diseases: the case for screening. *Prev Med.* 2003;36(4):502-509.

10. Korenromp EL, Sudaryo MK, de Vlas SJ, et al. What proportion of episodes of gonorrhoea and chlamydia becomes symptomatic? *Int J STD AIDS.* 2002;13(2):91-101.

11. Wiesenfeld HC, Sweet RL, Ness RB, Krohn MA, Amortegui AJ, Hillier SL. Comparison of acute and subclinical pelvic inflammatory disease. *Sex Transm Dis.* 2005;32(7):400-405.

12. Haggerty CL, Gottlieb SL, Taylor BD, Low N, Xu F, Ness RB. Risk of sequelae after Chlamydia trachomatis genital infection in women. *J Infect Dis.* 2010;201(suppl 2):S134-S155.

13. Oakeshott P, Kerry S, Aghaizu A, et al. Randomized controlled trial of screening for Chlamydia trachomatis to prevent pelvic inflammatory disease: the POPI (prevention of pelvic infection) trial. *BMJ.* 2010;340:c1642.

14. Cates W Jr., Wasserheit JN. Genital chlamydial infections: epidemiology and reproductive sequelae. *Am J Obstet Gynecol.* 1991;164(6 pt 2):1771-1781.

15. Weström L, Joesoef R, Reynolds G, Hagdu A, Thompson SE. Pelvic inflammatory disease and fertility. A cohort study of 1,844 women with laparoscopically verified disease and 657 control women with normal laparoscopic results. *Sex Transm Dis.* 1992;19(4):185-192.

16. Carter JD, Inman RD. Chlamydia-induced reactive arthritis: hidden in plain sight? *Best Pract Res Clin Rheumatol.* 2011;25(3):359-374.

17. Berger RE, Alexander ER, Monda GD, Ansell J, McCormick G, Holmes KK. Chlamydia trachomatis as a cause of acute "idiopathic" epididymitis. *N Engl J Med.* 1978;298(6):301-304.

18. 2015 sexually transmitted diseases treatment guidelines: chlamydial infections. Centers for Disease Control and Prevention Web site. https://www.cdc.gov/std/tg2015/chlamydia.htm. Updated June 4, 2015. Accessed July 24, 2019.

19. Papp JR, Schachter J, Gaydos C, Van Der Pol B. Recommendations for the laboratory-based detection of Chlamydia trachomatis and Neisseria gonorrhoeae—2014. *MMWR Recomm Rep.* 2014;63(RR-02):1-19.

20. Masek BJ, Arora N, Quinn N, et al. Performance of three nucleic acid amplification tests for detection of Chlamydia trachomatis and Neisseria gonorrhoeae by use of self-collected vaginal swabs obtained via an Internet-based screening program. *J Clin Microbiol.* 2009;47(6):1663-1667.

21. Knox J, Tabrizi SN, Miller P, et al. Evaluation of self-collected samples in contrast to practitioner-collected samples for detection of Chlamydia trachomatis, Neisseria gonorrhoeae, and Trichomonas vaginalis by polymerase chain reaction among women living in remote areas. *Sex Transm Dis.* 2002;29(11):647-654.

22. Bachmann LH, Johnson RE, Cheng H, et al. Nucleic acid amplification tests for diagnosis of Neisseria gonorrhoeae and Chlamydia trachomatis rectal infections. *J Clin Microbiol.* 2010;48(5):1827-1832.

23. Mimiaga MJ, Mayer KH, Reisner SL, et al. Asymptomatic gonorrhea and chlamydial infections detected by nucleic acid amplification tests among Boston area men who have sex with men. *Sex Transm Dis.* 2008;35(5):495-498.

24. Schachter J, Moncada J, Liska S, Shayevich C, Klausner JD. Nucleic acid amplification tests in the diagnosis of chlamydial and gonococcal infections of the oropharynx and rectum in men who have sex with men. *Sex Transm Dis.* 2008;35(7):637-642.

25. FDA clears first diagnostic tests for extragenital testing for chlamydia and gonorrhea. Food and Drug Administration Web site. https://www.fda.gov/news-events/press-announcements/fda-clears-first-diagnostic-tests-extragenital-testing-chlamydia-and-gonorrhea. Published May 23, 2019. Accessed May 11, 2020.

26. LeFevre ML; U.S. Preventive Services Task Force. Screening for Chlamydia and gonorrhea: U.S. Preventive Services Task Force recommendation statement. *Ann Intern Med.* 2014;161(12):902–910.

27. WHO guidelines for the treatment of *Chlamydia trachomatis*. World Health Organization Web site. https://apps.who.int/iris/bitstream/handle/10665/246165/9789241549714-eng.pdf;jsessionid=C08F294384D418BF693C0BB412207848?sequence=1. Accessed October 2, 2019.

28. Khsropour CM, Dombrowski JC, Barbee LA, Manhart LE, Golden MR. Comparing azithromycin and doxycycline for the treatment of rectal chlamydia infection: a retrospective cohort study. *Sex Transm Dis.* 2015;41(2):79-85.

29. Hocking JS, Kong FY, Timms P, Huston WM, Tabrizi SN. Treatment of rectal chlamydia infection may be more complicated than we originally thought. *J Antimicrob Chemother.* 2015;70(4):961-964.

30. Kong FY, Tabrizi SN, Fairley CK, et al. The efficacy of azithromycin and doxycycline for the treatment of rectal chlamydia infection: a systematic review and meta-analysis. *J Antimicrob Chemother.* 2015;70(5):1290-1297.

31. Dicker LW, Mosure DJ, Berman SM, Levine WC. Gonorrhea prevalence and coinfection with chlamydia in women in the United States, 2000. *Sex Transm Dis.* 2003;30(5):472-475.

32. Sexual assault and abuse and STDs. Centers for Disease Control and Prevention Web site. https://www.cdc.gov/std/tg2015/sexual assault.htm. Updated June 4, 2015. Accessed April 13, 2020.

Chapter 7

Gonorrhea

Lauren Traveller, DNP, APRN, FNP-C
Kelsey Kincaid, BA
Rachell A. Ekroos, PhD, APRN-BC, AFN-BC, FAAN

Disease and Mimics

— Gonorrhea is the second most common reportable disease in the United States.[1]

— The highest rates of gonorrhea are among adolescents and young adults ages 15 to 24 years.[1,2]

— Gonorrhea is caused by *Neisseria gonorrhoeae*, a gram-negative *diplococcus* (**Figure 7-1**) bacterium that infects the mucous membranes of the reproductive tract, urethra, pharynx, eyes, and rectum. It can be spread through direct contact (eg, sexual contact) or perinatally during childbirth.[2]

— In high-risk populations, gonococcal and chlamydial coinfection may be present.[3-5]

— Most gonococcal infections are asymptomatic. When present, the clinical manifestations may include dysuria; vaginal, urethral, or rectal discharge; anal itching, soreness, and bleeding; painful bowel movements; and swollen lymph nodes. Although typically asymptomatic, a pharyngeal infection may present as a sore throat with swollen cervical lymph nodes.[2]

— Untreated gonococcal infections can develop into pelvic inflammatory disease (PID) among women or epididymitis among men and lead to infertility in both. In women with PID, there is a risk of ectopic pregnancy, tubo-ovarian abscess, and chronic pelvic pain.[1]

— Gonococcal infections increase susceptibility to infection with human immunodeficiency virus (HIV), particularly in men who have sex with men (MSM).[6,7]

Figure 7-1. *Intracellular gram-negative diplococci of* Neisseria gonorrhoeae.

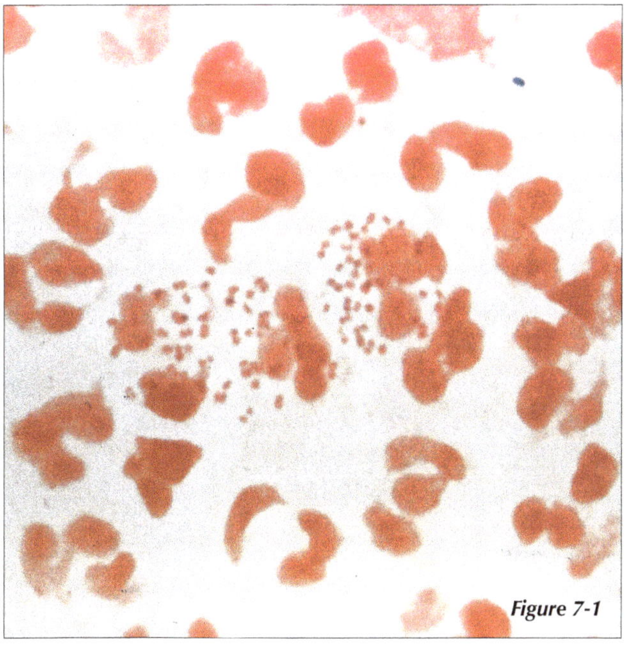

Epidemiology

The national rate of gonococcal infections is currently on the rise; however, this may be because of changes in screening practices, diagnostic tests, and reporting practices. The prevalence of infection is highest among males, with a rate increase of 86.3% from 2013 to 2017, although this may be because of increased extragenital screening (eg, throat, rectum). The rate of gonococcal infections among non-Hispanic blacks is 8.3 times higher than among whites, demonstrating racial disparity.[1]

Risk factors related to the acquisition of gonococcal infection include community prevalence, new or multiple sexual partners, young age, a history of prior gonococcal infection, drug use, sex work, and social determinants of health, such as minority ethnicity, lower education attainment, and socioeconomic levels.[1,8] Transmission may occur through contact with the penis, vagina, anus, or mouth. Individuals are at risk for serial gonococcal infections if they continue to have sexual contact with untreated infected persons.[1] Proper condom use is protective against the transmission of gonorrhea.[8,9]

Gonococcal infections are often asymptomatic.[2,10] Common infection sites include the genitals, but infection may occur at extragenital locations including the rectum, oropharynx, conjunctiva, and joints.[2] Urogenital symptoms in men can include dysuria, a pus-like penile discharge, unilateral testicular pain, and inguinal lymph node swelling. Urogenital symptoms in women can include an increase in vaginal discharge (**Figure 7-2**), dysuria, bleeding between menstrual cycles or after vaginal coitus, dyspareunia, and abdominal or pelvic pain. On pelvic examination, the cervix may be friable and show frank, mucopurulent discharge; however, these findings demonstrate cervicitis (**Figure 7-3**) and are nonspecific to gonococcal infection. Adnexal and cervical motion tenderness may also be present. Anorectal symptoms may include pruritus ani (anal itching), pus-like rectal discharge, and reports of blood on toilet paper after bowel movements. In the case of eye infection, the patient may report eye pain, light sensitivity, and unilateral or bilateral pus-like discharge (**Figure 7-4**). Oropharyngeal infection symptoms may present as a sore throat with swollen lymph nodes. Additional serious complications include disseminated gonococcal infection (DGI), presenting with polyarthritis, tenosynovitis, dermatitis, and septic arthritis (infection in the joints). Infected joints may appear swollen, red, and warm and be very painful on movement.[10]

***Figure 7-2**. Vaginal discharge in a 6-year-old girl who disclosed attempted penile penetration with ejaculation. Culture positive for* Neisseria gonorrhoeae.

***Figure 7-3**. Gonococcal cervicitis. (Courtesy of CDC, Atlanta, GA.)*

***Figure 7-4**. Gonococcal ophthalmia. (Courtesy of CDC, Atlanta, GA.)*

Gonococcal infections may be diagnosed by nucleic acid amplification testing (NAAT) or by a culture of urethral, endocervical, vaginal, rectal, pharyngeal, or conjunctival specimens. Extragenital NAATs (eg, throat, rectum, vagina) have demonstrated increased sensitivity and specificity in detecting gonorrhea compared with cultures. In March 2019, the Food and Drug Administration approved the first diagnostic tests for extragenital testing for gonorrhea.[10-12]

Gonorrhea screening is recommended for all sexually active persons younger than 25 years of age or considered to be at high risk for infection. Risk factors include a history of sexually transmitted infections (STIs), engaging in sexual activity with

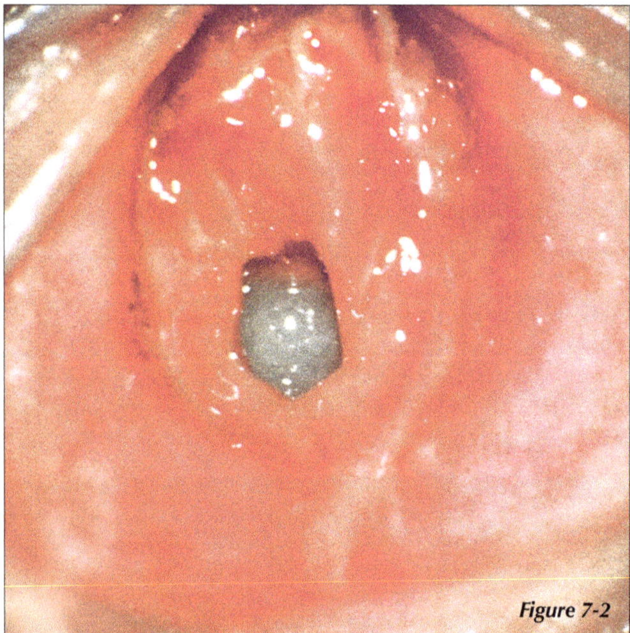

Figure 7-2

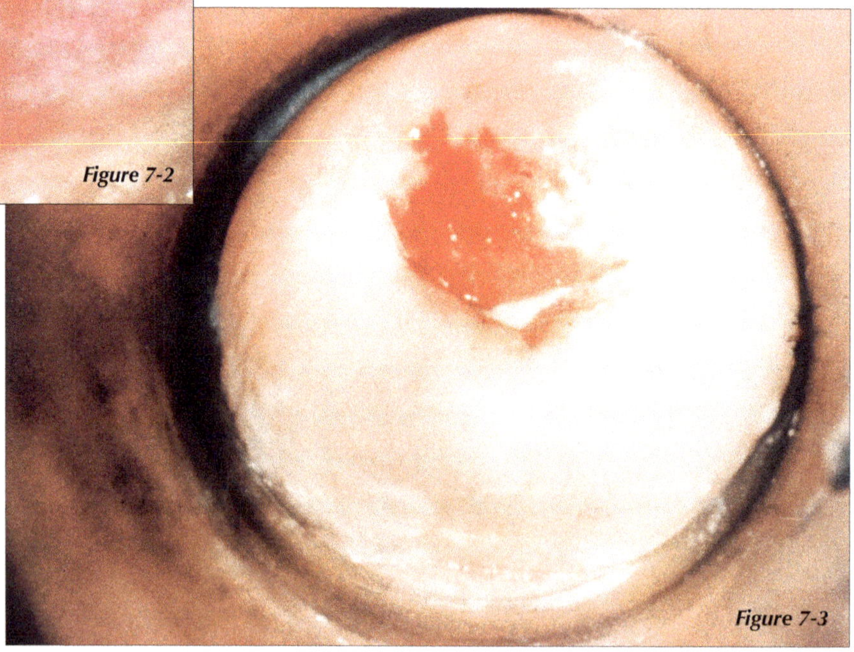

Figure 7-3

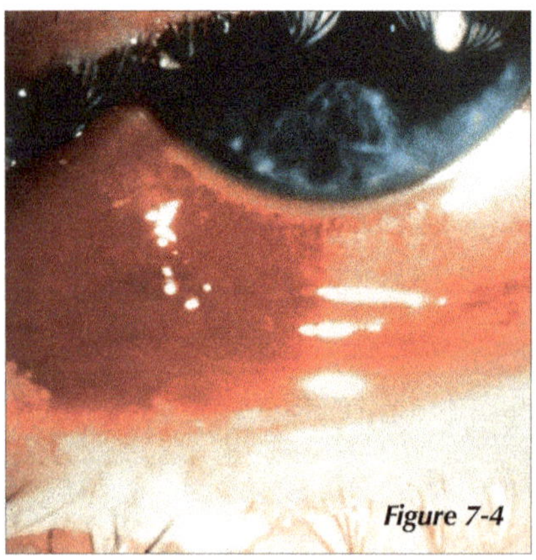

Figure 7-4

new or multiple partners or a sex partner who is known to have an STI, inconsistent condom use, sex work, drug use, MSM, and high community prevalence.[2,8] All individuals diagnosed with gonorrhea should also be screened for other STIs.[10]

A positive gonococcal infection in an infant or prepubertal child is diagnostic evidence for sexual abuse if congenital infection has been ruled out and is reportable per mandated reporting regulations. It is important to use high-specificity tests for diagnosis given the legal, psychological, and social ramifications of a false-positive test. Any child with a gonococcal infection should receive testing for other STIs, including *Chlamydia*, syphilis, and HIV. In prepubescent females, the most common presentation is vaginitis; anorectal and pharyngeal gonococcal infections in sexually abused children are most often asymptomatic.[10]

Treatment Guidelines

Dual therapy with a single dose of ceftriaxone 250 mg intramuscularly (IM) and azithromycin 1 g orally is the recommended treatment for uncomplicated gonococcal infection as a result of increasing antibiotic resistance and to provide coverage for potential *Chlamydia* coinfection. Patients should refrain from sexual activity for at least 1 week after treatment. Treatment of partners is necessary to prevent complications for asymptomatic partners and reinfection of the patient. In patients who develop a complicated gonococcal infection, such as DGI, hospitalization is recommended to ensure treatment adherence. In any complicated gonococcal infection, an infectious disease consult is recommended.[10] **Table 7-1** provides a summary of treatment guidelines.

Table 7-1. Summary of Treatment Guidelines for Gonorrhea[10]

Infection	Population	Recommended Treatment	Alternative Treatment*
Uncomplicated gonococcal infections of the vagina, cervix, urethra, rectum, or pharynx	Adults	Ceftriaxone 250 mg IM in a single dose ***PLUS*** Azithromycin 1 g PO in a single dose	If ceftriaxone is not available: Cefixime 400 mg PO in a single dose ***PLUS*** Azithromycin 1 g PO in a single dose
	Infants and children ≥ 45 kg	Ceftriaxone 250 mg IM in a single dose ***PLUS*** Azithromycin 1 g PO in a single dose	If ceftriaxone is not available: Cefixime 400 mg PO in a single dose ***PLUS*** Azithromycin 1 g PO in a single dose
	Infants and children ≤ 45 kg	Ceftriaxone 25-50 mg/kg IV or IM in a single dose, not to exceed 125 mg IM	
	Pregnant	Same regimen as nonpregnant persons	Same regimen as nonpregnant persons
	HIV infection	Same regimen as those without HIV infection	Same regimen as those without HIV infection
	Suspected treatment failure	Re-treat with the recommended regimen	
Maternal gonococcal exposure	Neonates (1-30 days)	Ceftriaxone 25-50 mg/kg IV or IM in a single dose, not to exceed 125 mg (given regardless of signs of infection)	

(continued)

Table 7-1. Summary of Treatment Guidelines for Gonorrhea[10] *(continued)*

Infection	Population	Recommended Treatment	Alternative Treatment*
Gonococcal conjunctivitis	Adults	Ceftriaxone 1 g IM in a single dose ***PLUS*** Azithromycin 1 g PO in a single dose	
Ophthalmia neonatorum prophylaxis	Neonates (1-30 days)	Erythromycin (0.5%) ophthalmic ointment in each eye in a single application at birth	
Ophthalmia neonatorum	Neonates (1-30 days)	Ceftriaxone 25-50 mg/kg IV or IM in a single dose, not to exceed 125 mg	
DGI: Arthritis and arthritis-dermatitis syndrome	Adults	Ceftriaxone 1 g IM or IV every 24 hours ***PLUS*** Azithromycin 1 g PO in a single dose	Cefotaxime 1 g IV every 8 hours ***OR*** Ceftizoxime 1 g IV every 8 hours ***PLUS*** Azithromycin 1 g PO in a single dose
DGI: Meningitis and endocarditis	Adults	Ceftriaxone 1-2 g IV every 12-24 hours ***PLUS*** Azithromycin 1 g PO in a single dose	
DGI: Pediatric bacteremia or arthritis	Child > 45 kg	Ceftriaxone 1 g IM or IV in a single dose daily every 24 hours for 7 days	
	Child < 45 kg	Ceftriaxone 50 mg/kg (maximum dose: 1 g) IM or IV in a single dose daily for 7 days	
DGI and scalp abscesses in neonates	Neonates (1-30 days)	Ceftriaxone 25-50 mg/kg/day IV or IM in a single daily dose for 7 days, with a duration of 10-14 days if meningitis is documented ***OR*** Cefotaxime 25 mg/kg IV or IM every 12 hours for 7 days, with a duration of 10-14 days if meningitis is documented	

IM, intramuscularly; IV, intravenously; PO, per os (orally).
For more information on treatment, see the Centers for Disease Control and Prevention's (CDC's) sexually transmitted disease guidelines at https://www.cdc.gov/std/tg2015/gonorrhea.htm.
**Per the 2015 CDC guidelines, patients with pharyngeal gonorrhea who receive an alternative treatment regimen should return 14 days after treatment for a test of cure using either culture or NAAT. A positive NAAT should be followed by a confirmatory culture before retreatment and a positive culture should include antimicrobial susceptibility testing.*[10]

Special Considerations

— ***Pregnancy:*** Treatment of uncomplicated gonococcal infection in pregnant women is with the dual therapy of ceftriaxone and azithromycin. Prenatal screening ensures adequate treatment of infection before delivery.[10]

— ***HIV infection:*** HIV-positive individuals should receive the same standard dual therapy for gonococcal infections as those without HIV infection. There are no special treatment considerations among this population.[10]

— ***Neonates:*** It is a legal mandate in most states for all neonates to receive prophylactic erythromycin ointment in each eye regardless of delivery method or gonococcal infection status of the mother. If a neonate is born vaginally to a mother with untreated gonococcal infection, provide prophylactic treatment. Screening for infection should be performed at exposed sites. Additionally, provide screening for *Chlamydia* infection.[10]

— ***Allergy:*** Cephalosporin use is contraindicated in patients with a history of immunoglobulin E (IgE)–mediated penicillin allergy.[13,14] Alternative therapy includes dual treatment with azithromycin 2 g orally plus either gemifloxacin 320 mg orally or gentamicin 240 mg IM; another option is spectinomycin if available.[10]

— ***Treatment failure:*** In cases of treatment failure as a result of reinfection, re-treat with the same medication combination and have patient return for a test of cure in 7 to 14 days.[10] If infection is suspected not to be a result of reexposure to an infected partner or if treatment again fails, consultation by an infectious disease specialist should be requested.

Case Studies

Adult Case Study 7-1

AT is an 18-year-old woman in the process of moving out of state for college. She presents to the primary care clinic requesting a birth control prescription plus a physical and meningitis immunizations, which are required for college admission. The human papillomavirus (HPV) vaccination is offered, and patient education is provided about STI screening. AT states she has never had any STI screening or the HPV vaccinations. She reports a sexual history of 6 different partners, with 1 male partner in the past 3 months. Exposure risks include fellatio, cunnilingus, penile-vaginal intercourse, and inconsistent condom use. AT is currently using unspecified oral birth control. No significant medical history and no drug allergies are reported.

Examination

The physical examination and anogenital examination are both normal.

Laboratory Testing

Urine NAAT for *Chlamydia trachomatis* and *N. gonorrhoeae* (CT/NG) is negative. Pharyngeal NAAT for CT/NG is positive for *N. gonorrhoeae*. HIV antibody screen is negative. Syphilis antibody screen (IgM and IgG) is nonreactive.

Treatment

The patient returns to the clinic for treatment and is administered ceftriaxone 250 mg IM and azithromycin 1 g orally taken with food offered in the clinic to avoid upset stomach, and she is advised of possible nausea and vomiting. Patient education discussions include consistent condom use, safe sex practices, and sexual health. Condoms are provided. The local public health district is notified per mandatory reporting requirements and AT is notified regarding disease investigation follow-up procedures. The patient is advised to avoid all sexual contact with persons or objects for at least 7 days. The patient is advised to notify any recent sexual partners about the need to also be tested.

Child Case Study 7-2

OL is a 9-year-old boy presenting to the local child advocacy center for concerns regarding sexual abuse by an unknown adult male. The patient discloses penile contact to "my mouth" and "my butt." The last contact was 1 month ago.

Examination

A complete head-to-toe examination, including anogenital structures, was normal.

Laboratory Testing

Urine NAAT for CT/NG is negative. Pharyngeal NAAT for CT/NG is negative. Anorectal NAAT is positive for *N. gonorrhoeae*. HIV antibody screen is negative. Syphilis antibody screen (IgM and IgG) is nonreactive.

Treatment

Patient returns to the clinic for treatment and is administered ceftriaxone 250 mg IM to the left buttock and azithromycin 1 g orally taken with food offered in the clinic to avoid upset stomach. The parents are advised of possible nausea and vomiting. Local public health district is notified per mandatory reporting requirements and patient's guardian is informed regarding disease investigation follow-up procedures.

References

1. Sexually transmitted disease surveillance 2017. Centers for Disease Control and Prevention Web site. https://www.cdc.gov/std/stats17/default.htm. Updated October 15, 2018. Accessed October 1, 2019.

2. Gonorrhea: detailed fact sheet. Centers for Disease Control and Prevention Web site. https://www.cdc.gov/std/gonorrhea/stdfact-gonorrhea-detailed.htm. Updated October 25, 2016. Accessed July 24, 2019.

3. Kent CK, Chaw JK, Wong W, et al. Prevalence of rectal, urethral, and pharyngeal chlamydia and gonorrhea detected in 2 clinical settings among men who have sex with men: San Francisco, California, 2003. *Clin Infect Dis.* 2005;41(1):67-74.

4. Dicker LW, Mosure DJ, Berman SM, Levine WC. Gonorrhea prevalence and coinfection with chlamydia in women in the United States, 2000. *Sex Transm Dis.* 2003;30(5):472-476.

5. Nsuami M, Cammarata CL, Brooks BN, Taylor SN, Martin DH. Chlamydia and gonorrhea co-occurrence in a high school population. *Sex Transm Dis.* 2004;31(7):424-427.

6. Jin F, Prestage G, Imrie J, et al. Anal sexually transmitted infections and risk of HIV infection in homosexual men. *J Acquir Immune Defic Syndr.* 2010;53(1):144-149.

7. Fleming DT, Wasserheit JN. From epidemiological synergy to public health policy and practice: the contribution of other sexually transmitted diseases to sexual transmission of HIV infection. *Sex Transm Infect.* 1999;75(1):3-17.

8. U.S. Preventive Services Task Force. Screening for gonorrhea: recommendation statement. *Ann Fam Med.* 2005;3(3):263-267.

9. Holmes KK, Levine R, Weaver M. Effectiveness of condoms in preventing sexually transmitted infections. *Bull World Health Organ.* 2004;82(6):454-461.

10. Workowski KA, Bolan GA; Centers for Disease Control and Prevention. Sexually transmitted diseases treatment guidelines, 2015. *MMWR Recomm Rep.* 2015;64(RR-03):1-137.

11. Van Der Pol B, Ferraro DV, Buck-Barrington L, et al. Multicenter evaluation of the BDProbeTec ET system for detection of *Chlamydia trachomatis* and *Neisseria gonorrhoeae* in urine specimens, female endocervical swabs, and male urethral swabs. *J Clin Microbiol.* 2001;39(3):1008-1016.

12. FDA clears first diagnostic tests for extragenital testing for chlamydia and gonorrhea. Food and Drug Administration Web site. https://www.fda.gov/news-events/press-announcements/fda-clears-first-diagnostic-tests-extragenital-testing-chlamydia-and-gonorrhea. Published May 23, 2019. Accessed May 11, 2020.

13. Ahmed KA, Fox SJ, Frigas E, Park MA. Clinical outcome in the use of cephalosporins in pediatric patients with a history of a penicillin allergy. *Int Arch Allergy Immunol.* 2012;158(4):405-410.

14. Park MA, Koch CA, Klemawesch P, Joshi A, Li JT. Increased adverse drug reactions to cephalosporins in penicillin allergy patients with positive penicillin skin test. *Int Arch Allergy Immunol.* 2010;153(3):268-273.

Section III

Viral Infections

Chapter 8

Human Papillomavirus

Nancy R. Downing, PhD, RN, SANE-A, SANE-P, FAAN

Disease and Mimics

- Human papillomavirus (HPV) is the most common sexually transmitted infection (STI) in the United States[1] and is associated with anogenital warts (**Figure 8-1**) and several types of cancer.
- HPV is a double-stranded viral DNA particle that resides in squamous epithelium cells that make up outer skin layers.[2]
- There are more than 150 identified HPV types.[3] HPV types are categorized by risk for cancer development: high (16, 18), intermediate (31, 33, 35, 39, 45, 51, 52, 56, 58, 59), and low (6, 11).[4]
- Most people with HPV are asymptomatic but can still spread the infection through skin-to-skin contact, most commonly through sexual activity.[5]
- Many cases resolve spontaneously[6] or are dormant at undetectable levels.[7, 8]
- HPV is associated with 91% of cervical cancers, 75% of vaginal cancers, 69% of vulvar cancers, 63% of penile cancers, 91% of anal cancers, and 70% of oropharyngeal cancers.[6]
- HPV 9-valent vaccine (Gardasil 9) targets HPV types 6, 11, 16, 18, 31, 33, 45, 52, and 58.[9]
- HPV infection rates are declining because of availability of safe and effective HPV vaccines; however, in the United States, fewer than half of adolescents aged 13 to 17 years complete the vaccine series.[11]
- Mimics include anal skin tags[12] and vulvar vestibular papillomatosis,[13] which are normal variants.

Epidemiology

HPV is primarily spread through sexual contact.[4] Although HPV rates are decreasing in response to the HPV vaccine, HPV remains a prevelant STI.[14] HPV infections can resolve spontaneously,[6] although it is unknown whether the virus clears completely or remains latent in cells at undetectable levels.[8] Latent HPV may resurge, especially in immunocompromised individuals.[7] Although most visible HPV infections, such as anogenital and oral warts, are associated with low-risk HPV types, more than 42 000 HPV-related cancers are diagnosed in the United States annually,[15] including an average of 11 866 cases of cervical cancer and 18 226 cases of oropharyngeal cancer.[16] HPV diagnosis is based on clinical inspection of the anogenital area or oral cavity and by cervical Papanicolaou (Pap) test and colposcopic examination in women.[17] HPV is not a reportable STI in most states.[4]

Figure 8-1. Condyloma acuminata, adult female anogenital and perineal area. (Courtesy of CDC, Atlanta, GA; and Joe Millar.)

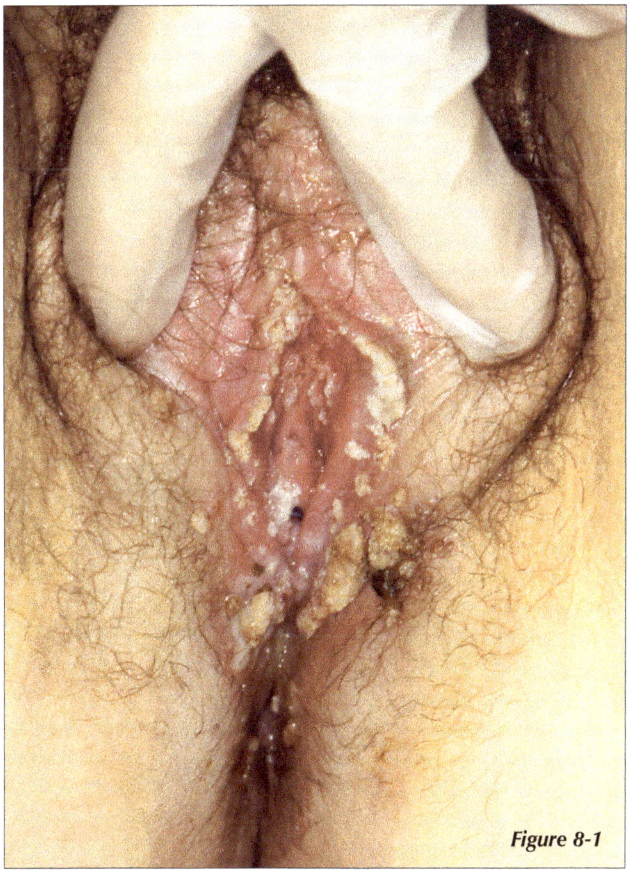

Figure 8-1

Anogenital warts associated with HPV infection have been declining since the advent of HPV vaccines; they affect approximately 5.9% of males who have sex with females, 4.6% of males who have sex with males (MSM), and 1.6% of females.[18] Prevalence of penile HPV continues to increase with age.[19] Visible symptoms do not need to be present to spread the infection.[5] HPV types 6 and 11 are associated with 90% of cases of anogenital warts.[20,21] High-risk anogenital HPV types have been found in the highest rates in females and MSM.[22] Although most anogenital warts are associated with low-risk HPV types, they can cause pain and discomfort, disfigurement, and emotional distress.[23] HPV testing of anogenital warts is not recommended by the Centers for Disease Control and Prevention (CDC) unless the warts do not respond to treatment or the person is immunocompromised.[24]

Figure 8-2. *Condyloma acuminata, adult male anal area. (Courtesy of CDC, Atlanta, GA; and Dr. Wiesner.)*

Figure 8-3. *Condyloma acuminata, 2-year-old female genital and perineal area.*

Figure 8-4. *Condyloma acuminata, oral cavity, HIV-positive adult (Courtesy of CDC, Atlanta, GA; and Sol Silverman, Jr., DDS.)*

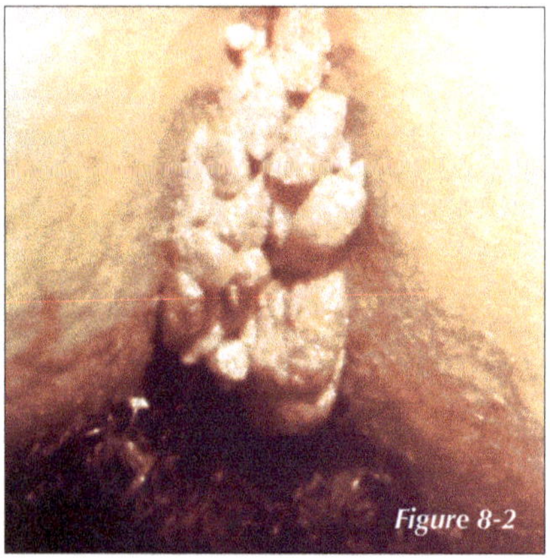

Figure 8-2

The incubation period for anogenital warts postexposure ranges from 3 weeks to 8 months, but the warts can remain dormant for much longer periods.[7] Persons with anogenital warts might also have intravaginal and/or intra-anal warts (**Figure 8-2**).[25] Anogenital warts are often called Condylomata acuminata regardless of appearance, although there are 4 major morphologic types[20]:

— ***Condylomata acuminata:*** Caulîflower-like appearance; may be skin-colored, pink, or hyperpigmented (**Figure 8-3**)

— ***Smooth papules:*** Usually dome-shaped and skin-colored

— ***Flat papules:*** Macular to slightly raised, skin-colored, and have a smooth surface

— ***Keratotic warts:*** With a thick keratinized layer that can resemble common warts or seborrheic keratosis

HPV is most likely transmitted to oral and oropharyngeal cavities through genital-oral contact.[26] In the United States, the prevalence of oral HPV infection, with or without visible lesions, is approximately 7% to 11 %.[26,27] Although most types of visible oral lesions are associated with low-risk HPV types 6 and 11,[22] high-risk HPV 16 was the most prevalent type found in oral rinse samples.[27] Oral prevalence in women is bimodal, with peaks around ages 25 and 55 years, whereas in men there does not appear to be an age-related prevalence.[19] Rates of HPV-related oral and oropharyngeal cancer have been increasing steadily in the United States.[28] The most common morphological types of oral warts include the following[29]:

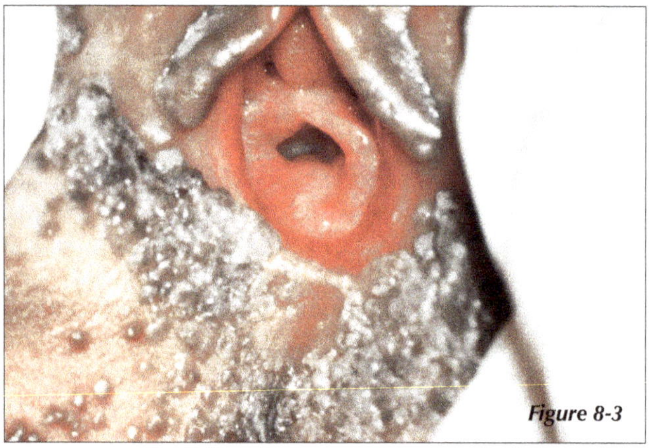

Figure 8-3

— ***Squamous papilloma:*** Benign tumor on soft palate, tongue, frenulum, lower lip, or uvula; mostly associated with HPV 6 and 11

— ***Condylomata acuminata:*** Pink or white nodules on the tongue, lips, palate, or floor of the mouth; mostly associated with HPV 6 and 11 (**Figure 8-4**)

— ***Verruca vulgaris:*** Mostly seen in children; associated with HPV 1, 2, 4, 6, 7, 11, and 16

— ***Oral leukoplakia:*** Premalignant white patch or plaque most commonly caused by HPV 6, 11, and 16

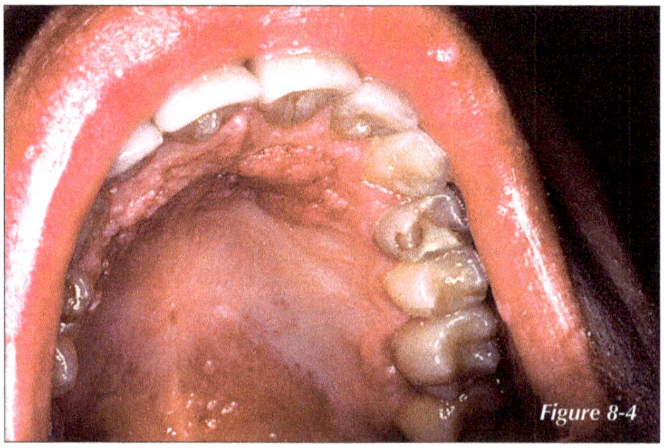

Figure 8-4

Prevalence of cervical HPV is estimated to be more than 11% worldwide, with the highest prevalence in women younger than age 25 years.[17] Prevalence peaks around age 20.[19] Persistent cervical HPV infection is associated with cervical cancer, with onset typically occurring several years to decades after initial infection.[3]

Treatment Guidelines

Most cases of HPV are asymptomatic and resolve spontaneously.[6] If left untreated, warts can either spontaneously resolve, stay the same, or increase in size and number.[24] Recommended treatment is based on patient preference, size and number of warts, cost, convenience, adverse effects, and health care provider experience.[24]

Various treatments for anogenital warts include topical treatments, which can be applied at home by patients, and topical or mechanical removal by a health care provider. There is no preferred treatment method; if one method is not effective, another method can be tried.[24] Treatment for internal warts (including urethral meatus, vaginal, cervical, and intra-anal) should be conducted by an experienced health care provider. No topical treatment has been validated for use in children, but sinecatechins (Veregen) ointment has shown promise as a safe and effective treatment that needs randomized clinical trial validation.[30]

The recommended treatment for oral warts is to either monitor for spontaneous resolution or surgical removal.[31] There are no validated topical treatment methods, in part because of low prevalence of oral warts. See **Table 8-1** for treatment guidelines.

Table 8-1. 2015 CDC Wart Treatment Guidelines

Anogenital[24]

Patient-Applied

Treatment	*Regimen*	*Notes*
Imiquimod 3.75% or 5% cream	— Apply 3.75% cream at bedtime every night *OR* Apply 5% cream at bedtime 3 times per week — Wash with soap and water 6 to 10 hours after application	— Might weaken condoms and vaginal diaphragms — May cause local irritation or hypopigmentation — May worsen other preexisting skin conditions (eg, psoriasis, vitiligo, lichenoid dermatoses) — Poses low risk in pregnancy, though CDC recommends avoiding use until more data are available
Podofilox 0.5% solution or gel	— Apply 2 times a day for 3 days, followed by 4 days with no treatment — Repeat cycle, if needed, for up to 4 cycles	— Total wart area should not be >10 cm^2 — Total volume used should be ≤ 0.5 mL/day — Should not be used in pregnancy
Sinecatechins 15% ointment (green tea extract)	— Apply 3 times a day in a thin layer until warts are gone — Do not use longer than 16 weeks — Wash after use	— Might weaken condoms and vaginal diaphragms — Avoid sexual contact while ointment is on the skin — May cause local irritation — Not recommended if patient is HIV positive, is immunocompromised, or has genital herpes — Safety unknown in pregnancy

(continued)

Table 8-1. 2015 CDC Wart Treatment Guidelines *(continued)*

ANOGENITAL[24]

Provider-Applied

Treatment	*Regimen*	*Notes*
Cryotherapy	— Liquid nitrogen or cryoprobe application by health care provider — More than one application may be necessary; warts may reoccur	— Ensure health care provider is trained in proper use — May cause pain, necrosis, and blistering — Local anesthesia may be helpful
Surgical removal	— Tangential scissor or shave excision, curettage, CO^2 laser, or electrosurgery — 1 visit; warts may reoccur	— Can be most efficient method of eliminating warts at 1 time — May be preferable if warts cover large surface area — Typically does not require suturing — Recurrence possible
Trichloroacetic acid (TCA) or bichloroacetic acid (BCA) 80%-90% solution	— Chemically destroys warts — Repeat weekly if necessary	— May cause chemical burns, damage to adjacent tissue — Cover with sodium bicarbonate if pain occurs

URETHRAL MEATUS[24]

— Cryotherapy (liquid nitrogen)
— Surgical removal

VAGINAL/CERVICAL/INTRA-ANAL[24]

— Cryotherapy (liquid nitrogen)
— Surgical removal
— TCA and BCA 80%-90% solution

ORAL[31]

— No validated, accepted topical treatment
— Surgical removal

HIV, Human immunodeficiency virus.
For more information on treatment, see the CDC's sexually transmitted disease guidelines at https://www.cdc.gov/std/tg2015/hpv.htm.

SPECIAL CONSIDERATIONS

— ***Pregnancy:*** Positive cervical HPV tests during pregnancy have been associated with a small increase in preterm prelabor rupture of membranes.[32,33] The CDC does not recommend HPV vaccine during pregnancy.[9]

— ***Immunocompromised patients/HIV infection:*** There is evidence that persons who are immunocompromised might experience HPV-related symptoms either because they are more susceptible to all types of infection or because latent viruses become reactivated.[34] Persons with HPV who also test positive for human immunodeficiency virus (HIV) are at higher risk for HPV-related cancers.[35,36] There is evidence that HPV infection increases susceptibility to HIV infection because of changes in skin cell integrity.[35]

— ***Neonates:*** Vertical transmission of HPV from mothers to neonates has been documented.[37-39] Most infants were no longer positive when retested 2 to 6 months later. It is unclear whether this indicates resolution or latency of HPV infection.[37]

— *Children:* HPV can be transmitted to children by nonsexual contact and can be self-inoculated from warts on other areas of the body, especially fingers (**Figure 8-5**).[40] Information about maternal HPV history can identify risk of vertical transmission; presence of warts on a caretaker's fingers may increase risk of nonsexual transmission.[40] Warts in the anogenital area in children older than 5 years of age are more suggestive of sexual contact[12,41] and warrant assessment for sexual abuse.

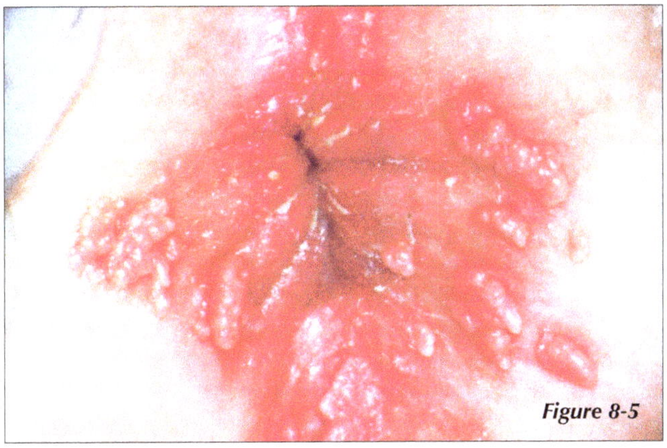

Figure 8-5. *Condyloma acuminata, 4-year-old female perianal area, no sexual abuse outcry.*

Prevention and Screening

Gardasil 9-valent HPV vaccine provides protection against HPV types that cause the majority of HPV-associated warts and cancers (HPV 6, 11, 16, 18, 31, 33, 45, 52, and 58).[9] Gardasil 9 is the only HPV vaccine currently available in the United States. CDC guidelines[24] recommend that HPV vaccination starts at age 11 or 12; the HPV vaccine series can be started at age 9, which is recommended in cases of suspected or known sexual abuse or assault.[42] HPV vaccine is recommended for males and females 13 to 26 years, if not previously vaccinated, and up to age 45 based on shared clinical decision making with a health care provider.[43] See **Table 8-2** for age, number of doses, and dose timing recommendations.

Table 8-2. HPV Vaccine Age, Follow-Up, Dose, and Timing Recommendations[24,43]

Age for Dose #1	Dose #2	Dose #3
9 to 14 years	6 to 12 months	Not indicated
15 to 26 years (9 to 14 years and immunocompromised)	1 to 2 months	6 months
27 to 45 years (based on shared clinical decision making)	1 to 2 months	6 months

Universal asymptomatic screening for HPV is not recommended because of high rates of spontaneous resolution and the possibility of viral latency.[24] If anogenital warts are present, the CDC recommends screening for other STIs.[24] Patients should be instructed to use condoms, because they can reduce risk of anogenital[44] and oral transmission.[24]

Pap tests are cytologic tests that examine cervical cell samples for abnormal cells.[45] The cervix can also be tested for HPV. Neither the Pap nor HPV tests have perfect sensitivity and specificity.[46] The US Preventive Services Task Force currently recommends cervical cancer screening for women ages 21 to 65 years, with cervical cytologic testing alone every 3 years and high-risk HPV testing every 5 years with or without cytology for women ages 30 to 65.[45]

Case Studies

Adult Case Study 8-1

ML is a 22-year-old man who presents to the public health department with perianal warts. He states he first noticed them about a month ago when showering and became concerned when he had bleeding after a bowel movement. He has had 4 male sex partners, with first sexual activity starting at age 17.

Examination

Bilateral 1-cm x 1.5-cm vertical clusters of condyloma acuminata on the inferior half of the anus. Anoscopy reveals no internal anal lesions.

Laboratory Testing

Nucleic acid amplification tests (NAATs) for *Chlamydia trachomatis* and *Neisseria gonorrhoeae* are negative; rapid plasma reagin for syphilis is nonreactive; HIV-1/HIV-2 antibody test is negative; tests are also negative for HSV-1 and HSV-2. HPV testing is not indicated.

Treatment

ML elects to try sinecatechins 15% ointment first and is instructed to apply it 3 times a day and wash after use. ML is instructed to avoid sexual contact while ointment is on the skin and is told that sinecatechins can weaken condoms. ML is counseled that he can spread HPV to sex partners even if the warts disappear, that he should inform sex partners about his anogenital warts, and to use condoms during intercourse. He is instructed to use the ointment no longer than 16 weeks and to return after that if the anogenital warts do not respond to treatment. HPV vaccine series is started. Patient is to return for dose 2 in 1 to 2 months and dose 3 in 6 months.

Child Case Study 8-2

JB is a 10-year-old girl whose mother brings her to the pediatric clinic after the patient complains of itching and bumps in her "underwear area." The child has no outcry of sexual assault or abuse to the mother or health care provider, and the mother expresses no immediate concern for sexual abuse. The mother is asked about her own history of HPV and denies knowledge of HPV history. The patient is questioned without the mother present and denies anyone is harming her. Other household members include her father and 6-year-old brother.

Examination

A 1 cm x 0.5 cm area of smooth papules on her perineum just below the posterior fourchette and a 0.5 cm x 0.3 cm area on the inferior end of the left labia majora.

Laboratory Testing

HPV testing is not indicated. STI testing for signs of sexual abuse include urine NAAT for *Chlamydia trachomatis*, urine NAAT for *Neisseria gonorrhoeae,* and urine NAAT for *Trichomonas vaginalis*, which are all negative.

Treatment

JB is referred to a child advocacy center for a forensic interview and medical forensic examination. Law enforcement and child protective services are notified. A referral is made to pediatric dermatology for appropriate treatment of anogenital warts. JB is advised to take warm baths without soap or bubble bath for relief from itching and is instructed not to scratch herself. HPV vaccine series is started. Patient to return for final dose in 6 to 12 months.

References

1. Satterwhite CL, Torrone E, Meites E, et al. Sexually transmitted infections among US women and men: prevalence and incidence estimates, 2008. *Sex Transm Dis.* 2013;40(3):187-193.
2. Carter JR, Ding Z, Rose BR. HPV infection and cervical disease: a review. *Aust N Z J Obstet Gynaecol.* 2011;51(2):103-108.
3. Serrano B, Brotons M, Bosch FX, Bruni L. Epidemiology and burden of HPV-related disease. *Best Pract Res Clin Obstet Gynaecol.* 2018;47:14-26.
4. Gargano J, Elissa M, Watson M, Unger E, Markowitz L. Chapter 5: human papillomavirus. In: Roush SW, Baldy LM, Hall MAK, eds. *Manual for the Surveillance of Vaccine-Preventable Diseases*. Atlanta, GA: Centers for Disease Control and Prevention; 2017:43-54.
5. Kerkar SC, Latta S, Salvi V, Mania-Pramanik J. Human papillomavirus infection in asymptomatic population. *Sex Reprod Healthc.* 2011;2(1):7-11.
6. Viens LJ, Henley SJ, Watson M. Human papillomavirus-associated cancers: United States, 2008-2012. *MMWR Morb Mortal Wkly Rep.* 2016;65(26):661-666.

7. Gravitt PE, Winer RL. Natural history of HPV infection across the lifespan: role of viral latency. *Viruses*. 2017;9(10):e267.
8. Rositch AF, Burke AE, Viscidi RP, Silver MI, Chang K, Gravitt PE. Contributions of recent and past sexual partnerships on incident human papillomavirus detection: acquisition and reactivation in older women. *Cancer Res*. 2012;72(23):6183-6190.
9. Petrosky E, Bocchini JA Jr, Hariri S, et al; Centers for Disease Control and Prevention. Use of 9-valent human papillomavirus (HPV) vaccine: updated HPV vaccination recommendations of the advisory committee on immunization practices. *MMWR Morb Mortal Wkly Rep*. 2015;64(11):300-304.
10. Joura EA, Giuliano AR, Iversen OE, et al. A 9-valent HPV vaccine against infection and intraepithelial neoplasia in women. *N Engl J Med*. 2015;372(8):711-723.
11. Walker TY, Elam-Evans LD, Yankey D, et al. National, regional, state, and selected local area vaccination coverage among adolescents aged 13-17 years: United States, 2017. *MMWR Morb Mortal Wkly Rep*. 2018;67(33):909-917.
12. Adams JA, Farst KJ, Kellogg ND. Interpretation of medical findings in suspected child sexual abuse: an update for 2018. *J Pediatr Adolesc Gynecol*. 2018;31(3):225-231.
13. Muhammed RT, Afra TP, De D. Vestibular papillomatosis: a normal variation commonly misdiagnosed as genital condylomata. *Am J Obstet Gynecol*. 2019;220(4):403.
14. Shi R, Devarakonda S, Liu L, Taylor H, Mills G. Factors associated with genital human papillomavirus infection among adult females in the United States, NHANES 2007-2010. *BMC Res Notes*. 2014;7:544.
15. United States cancer statistics (USCS): cancers associated with human papillomavirus, United States—2011-2015. Centers for Disease Control and Prevention Web site. https://www.cdc.gov/cancer/uscs/about/data-briefs/no4-hpv-assoc-cancers-United-States-2011-2015.htm. Updated October 31, 2018. Accessed August 1, 2019.
16. HPV and cancer: how many cancers are linked with HPV each year? Centers for Disease Control and Prevention Web site. https://www.cdc.gov/cancer/hpv/statistics/cases.htm. Updated August 15, 2018. Accessed August 1, 2019.
17. Bruni L, Diaz M, Castellsagué M, Ferrer E, Bosch FX, de Sanjosé S. Cervical human papillomavirus prevalence in 5 continents: meta-analysis of 1 million women with normal cytological findings. *J Infect Dis*. 2010;202(12):1789-1799.
18. Mann LM, Llata E, Flagg EW, et al. Trends in the prevalence of anogenital warts among patients at sexually transmitted disease clinics: Sexually Transmitted Disease Surveillance Network, United States, 2010-2016. *J Infect Dis*. 2018;219(9):1389-1397.
19. Brouwer AF, Eisenberg MC, Carey TE, Meza R. Multisite HPV infections in the United States (NHANES 2003-2014): an overview and synthesis. *Prev Med*. 2019;123:288-298.
20. Patel H, Wagner M, Singhal P, Kothari S. Systematic review of the incidence and prevalence of genital warts. *BMC Infect Dis*. 2013;13(1):39.
21. Yanofsky VR, Patel RV, Goldenberg G. Genital warts: a comprehensive review. *J Clin Aesthet Dermatol*. 2012;5(6):25-36.
22. Lisboa C, Santo I, Azevedo J, et al. High prevalence of human papillomavirus on anal and oral samples from men and women with external anogenital warts: the HERCOLES Study. *Acta Derm Venereol*. 2019;99(6):557-563.
23. Drolet M, Brisson M, Maunsell E, et al. The impact of anogenital warts on health-related quality of life: a 6-month prospective study. *Sex Transm Dis*. 2011;38(10):949-956.
24. Workowski KA, Bolan GA; Centers for Disease Control and Prevention. Sexually transmitted diseases treatment guidelines, 2015. *MMWR Recomm Rep*. 2015;64(RR-03):1-137.
25. 2015 sexually transmitted diseases treatment guidelines: anogenital warts. Centers for Disease Control and Prevention Web site. https://www.cdc.gov/std/tg2015/warts.htm. Updated June 4, 2015. Accessed August 2, 2019.
26. Gillison ML, Broutian T, Pickard RK, et al. Prevalence of oral HPV infection in the United States, 2009-2010. *JAMA*. 2012;307(7):693-703.

27. Deshmukh KS, Suk R, Chiao EY, et al. Differences in prevalence between sexes and concordance with genital human papillomavirus infection, NHANES 2011 to 2014. *Ann Intern Med.* 2017;167(10):714-724.
28. Van Dyne EA, Henley SJ, Saraiya M, Thomas CC, Markowitz LE, Benard VB. Trends in human papillomavirus–associated cancers—United States, 1999-2015. *MMWR Morb Mortal Wkly Rep.* 2018;67(33):918-924.
29. Bharti AH, Chotaliya K, Marfatia YS. An update on oral human papillomavirus infection. *Indian J Sex Transm Dis AIDS.* 2013;34(2):77-82.
30. Deeb M, Levy R, Pope E, Lara-Corrales I. Sinecatechins ointment for the treatment of warts in children. *Pediatr Dermatol.* 2019;36(1):121-124.
31. Jaiswal R, Pandey M, Shukla M, Kumar M. Condyloma acuminatum of the buccal mucosa. *Ear Nose Throat J.* 2014;93(6):219-223.
32. Cotton-Caballero A, Dudley D, Ferguson J, Pettit K, Boyle A. Maternal human papillomavirus infection increases the risk of premature rupture of membranes. *Obstet Gynecol.* 2017;129(5):S137.
33. Pandey D, Solleti V, Jain G, et al. Human papillomavirus (HPV) infection in early pregnancy: prevalence and implications. *Infect Dis Obstet Gynecol.* 2019;2019:437602.
34. Maglennon GA, McIntosh PB, Doorbar J. Immunosuppression facilitates the reactivation of latent papillomavirus infections. *J Virol.* 2014;88(1):710-716.
35. Houlihan CF, Larke NL, Watson-Jones D, et al. Human papillomavirus infection and increased risk of HIV acquisition. A systematic review and meta-analysis. *AIDS.* 2012;26(17):2211-2222.
36. Videla S, Darwich L, Cañadas MP, et al; HIV-HPV Study Group. Natural history of human papillomavirus infections involving anal, penile, and oral sites among HIV-positive men. *Sex Transm Dis.* 2013;40(1):3-10.
37. Freitas AC, Mariz FC, Silva MA, Jesus AL. Human papillomavirus vertical transmission: review of current data. *Clin Infect Dis.* 2013;56(10):1451-1456.
38. Hahn HS, Kee MK, Kim HJ, et al. Distribution of maternal and infant human papillomavirus: risk factors associated with vertical transmission. *Eur J Obstet Gynecol Reprod Biol.* 2013;169(2):202-206.
39. Park H, Lee SW, Lee IH, et al. Rate of vertical transmission of human papillomavirus from mothers to infants: relationship between infection rate and mode of delivery. *Virol J.* 2012;9:80.
40. Bacopoulou F, Karakitsos P, Kottaridi C, et al. Genital HPV in children and adolescents: does sexual activity make a difference? *J Pediatr Adolesc Gynecol.* 2016;29(3):228-233.
41. Unger ER, Fajman NN, Maloney EM, et al. Anogenital human papillomavirus in sexually abused and nonabused children: a multicenter study. *Pediatrics.* 2011;128(3):e658-665.
42. Markowitz LE, Dunne EF, Saraiya M, et al; Centers for Disease Control and Prevention. Human papillomavirus vaccination: recommendations of the Advisory Committee on Immunization Practices (ACIP). *MMWR Recomm Rep.* 2014;63(RR-05):1-30.
43. Advisory Committee on Immunization Practices. 2019 childhood and adult immunization schedules. Centers for Disease Control and Prevention Web site. https://www.cdc.gov/vaccines/acip/index.html. Updated March 21, 2019. Accessed August 2, 2019.
44. Lam JU, Rebolj M, Dugué PA, Bonde J, von Euler-Chelpin M, Lynge E. Condom use in prevention of Human Papillomavirus infections and cervical neoplasia: systematic review of longitudinal studies. *J Med Screen.* 2014;21(1):38-50.
45. Cervical cancer: screening. U.S. Preventive Services Task Force Web site. https://www.uspreventiveservicestaskforce.org/uspstf/recommendation/cervical-cancer-screening. Published August 21, 2018. Accessed August 2, 2019.
46. Koliopoulos G, Nyaga VN, Santesso N, et al. Cytology versus HPV testing for cervical cancer screening in the general population. *Cochrane Database Syst Rev.* 2017;8:CD008587.

Chapter 9

Herpes Simplex Virus

Cindy Weston, DNP, APRN, CCRN, CNS-CC, FNP-BC

Disease and Mimics

- Herpes simplex virus (HSV) infections are a common, lifelong sexually transmitted infection (STI) and are the leading cause of recurrent genital ulcers (**Figure 9-1**).[1,2]
- HSV is caused by 2 DNA virus subtypes. HSV-1 is typically orolabial and is acquired in childhood, and HSV-2 is typically genital or perianal and is acquired through sexual contact as a young adult. However, transmission of both types may occur through sexual contact (ie, genital to genital, genital to anal, genital to oral, oral to genital, direct transfer through fingers).
- The clinical manifestations of HSV are characterized by recurrent, painful oral, genital, and/or anal vesicular, ulcerative lesions.
- Genital HSV infection facilitates both the acquisition and transmission of human immunodeficiency virus (HIV).[2]
- The majority of persons infected with genital herpes are unaware of their infection, and asymptomatic shedding of HSV in these persons accounts for the majority of transmitted genital HSV infections.[3,4]
- Neonatal HSV infection is rare but often fatal or neurologically debilitating. The risk is highest among infants of women who develop primary HSV infection at or near the time of delivery.[5]
- Any HSV infection in prepubertal children warrants assessment for sexual abuse.[6]

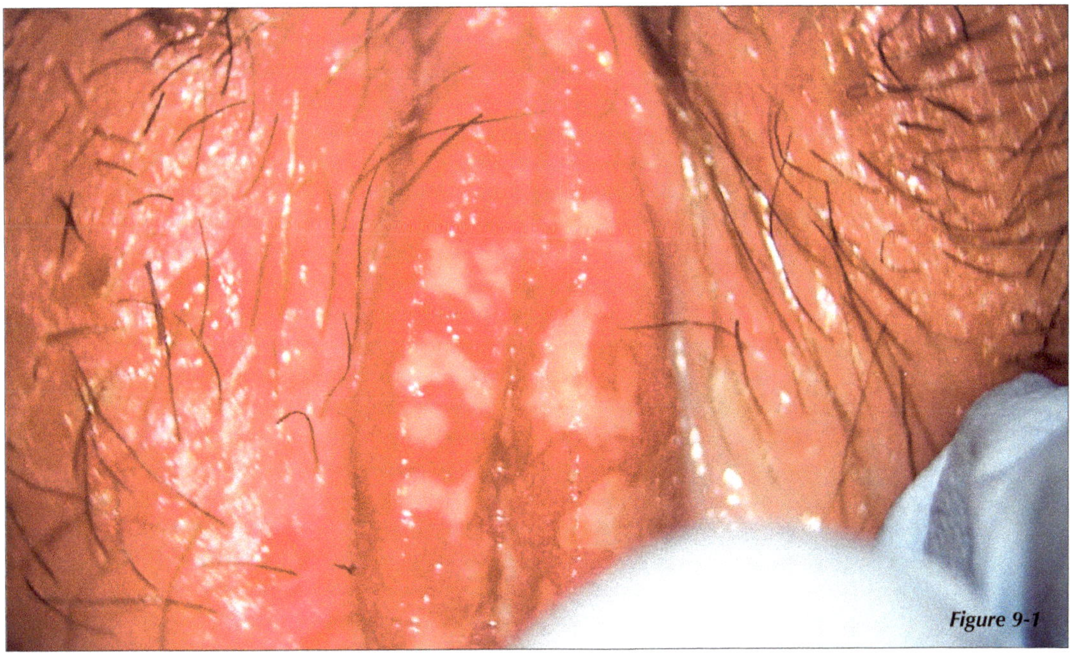

Figure 9-1. *14-year-old sexual assault victim 10 days after primary HSV infection. (Courtesy of Diana Faugno, MSN, RN, CPN, SANE-A, SANE-P, FAAFS, DF-IAFN, DF-AFN.)*

Epidemiology

The age-adjusted prevalence for the total United States population with HSV-1 is 48.1%, and the prevalence of HSV-2 is 12.1%. Both HSV-1 and HSV-2 affect more females than males.[4] Racial disparity also exists, with the highest prevalence of HSV-1 in Mexican Americans and the highest prevalence of HSV-2 in non-Hispanic black persons.[4] Transmission of HSV usually occurs through close contact with a person who is shedding HSV at a mucosal or epithelial surface, or in genital or oral secretions. The shedding of HSV is often independent of visible HSV lesions. Most individuals who are shedding HSV are asymptomatic, and up to 85% are unaware they have HSV infection.[3,7] Other areas of autoinnoculation include broken skin on hands and fingers (ie, herpetic whitlow) and mucus membrane (ie, occular). When symptoms of occular transmission are present, a visit to the ophthalmologist is imperative in order to prevent blindness.

Although HSV-2 is the primary cause of genital herpes, an increase in HSV-1 genital infections has been associated with oral sexual contact, particularly in young women and in men who have sex with men.[8] Lesion recurrences and asymptomatic viral shedding are more frequent with genital HSV-2 infection than for genital HSV-1 infection.[3] Condom use is protective against heterosexual HSV transmission, particularly from men to women (96%) but less so from women to men (65%).[9] The best method for reducing the risk of transmitting infection is antiviral suppression therapy in addition to routine condom use and avoiding contact when herpetic lesions are present.[10]

A symptomatic primary infection presents with a painful vesicular (cluster of small blisters) or ulcerative lesion that occurs 2 to 14 days after exposure and persists for, on average, 3 weeks (**Figures 9-2** and **9-3**).[10] Systemic symptoms including fever, headache, body aches, and lymphadenopathy may accompany the first outbreak.[11,12] Female patients often report dysuria and sometimes vaginal discharge. Some individuals have mild symptomatic presentation with itching or a singular "sore" that often gets mistaken for a pimple or ingrown hair.[12] The lesion progresses from vesicle to ulcer to crusted during the recovery process. A viral swab of the lesion with confirmatory diagnostic type-specific virologic testing through cell culture or polymerase chain reaction (PCR) amplification is recommended to identify HSV-1 and HSV-2.[8] Serologic blood tests are available to detect prior infection of HSV-1 and HSV-2 but may have a false negative up to 3 months after the primary infection and are not recommended for asymptomatic population screening.[10] Recurrent HSV infections are typically milder than the primary infection, but viral shedding may still persist up to 2 weeks after each occurrence, along with intermittent asymptomatic shedding episodes.[3,10] Recurrence can be triggered by emotional stress, fever, exposure to sunlight, and menstruation. Complications of HSV infections include keratoconjunctivitis, encephalitis, and disseminated disease.

Genital herpes in prepubertal children is rare and should always involve assessment for sexual abuse.[6] Nonabuse mechanisms of genital HSV transmission are possible, including autoinoculation with HSV-1 or inoculation by an infected caregiver during routine care. Findings of HSV-2 in a prepubertal child who presents with oral or genital herpetic lesions strengthens the evidence for sexual abuse.[6]

Figure 9-2-a and b. *Primary herpes infection in a male patient. (Courtesy of CDC, Atlanta, GA.)*

Figure 9-3-a. *Primary herpes infection in a female patient. (Courtesy of CDC, Atlanta, GA.)*

Figure 9-3-b. *Same patient, 4 days later. (Courtesy of CDC, Atlanta, GA.)*

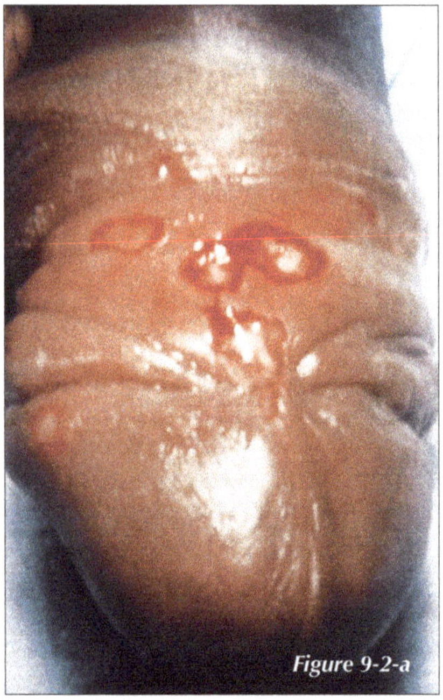
Figure 9-2-a

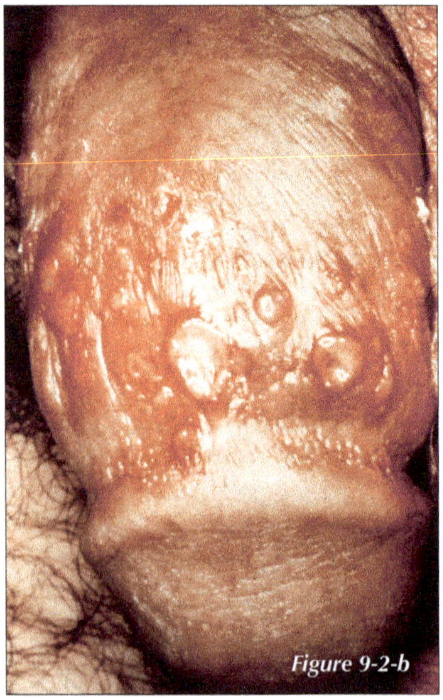
Figure 9-2-b

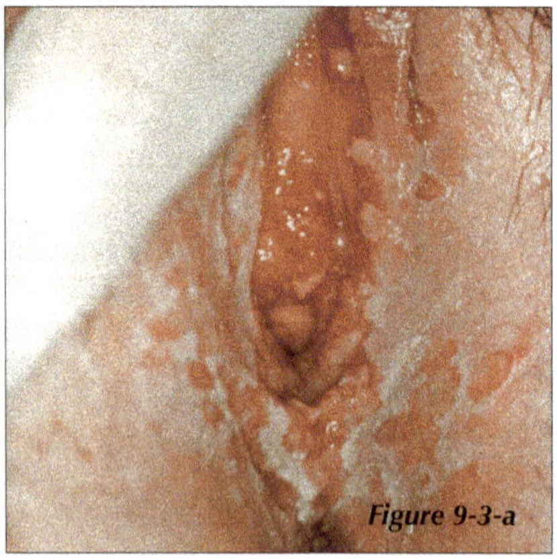
Figure 9-3-a

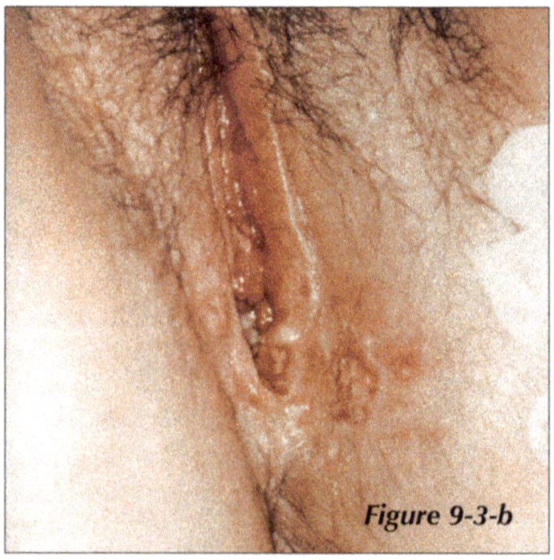
Figure 9-3-b

Treatment Guidelines

HSV is treated with antiviral medication. Pediatric HSV treatment with acyclovir is weight-based and dependent on immunocompetence. Valacyclovir has approved indication to treat HSV in the mouth or lips (orolabial) for children older than age 12 years. For adults, the Centers for Disease Control and Prevention recommends antiviral therapy with acyclovir, valacyclovir, or famciclovir to treat symptoms (primary infection or episodic therapy) and to prevent recurrences and reduce viral shedding and transmission (suppressive therapy) (**Table 9-1**).[8,10]

In rare cases, HSV infection presents with severe disseminated disease necessitating hospitalization. The recommendation for adults with severe HSV infection or complication is acyclovir at 5 to 10 mg/kg intravenously (IV) every 8 hours for 2 to 7 days until clinical improvement is observed, followed by oral antiviral therapy for at least 10 days.[8] Counseling plays an integral role in the management of a patient diagnosed with HSV infection because of the significant psychological burden of HSV related to the need for behavioral changes and disclosure to sexual partners.

Table 9-1. Summary of Treatment Guidelines for Herpes Simplex Virus

	Age	Acyclovir	Valacyclovir	Famciclovir
Primary Infection	<12 years[13]	75 mg/kg/day PO divided 5 times a day for 7 days *OR* 5 mg/kg/dose IV every 8 hours for 5-7 days (orolabial) *OR* 40-80 mg/kg/day PO divided every 6-8 hours for 5-10 days (anogenital) **Maximum dose 1000 mg/day**		
	≥12 years[13]	1000 mg/day PO divided 5 times a day for 7-10 days *OR* 1200 mg/day PO divided every 8 hours for 7-10 days *OR* 5 mg/kg/dose IV every 8 hours for 5-7 days	1 g PO twice daily for 7-10 days	
	Adult[8*]	400 mg PO 3 times a day for 7-10 days *OR* 200 mg PO 5 times a day for 7-10 days	1 g PO twice daily for 7-10 days	250 mg PO 3 times a day for 7-10 days *OR* 500 mg PO twice daily for 7 days
Recurrent Infection	≥12 years[13]	1000 mg/day PO divided 5 times a day for 5 days *OR* 400 mg PO 3 times a day for 5 days	2 g PO twice daily for 1 day (orolabial)	
	Adult[8]	400 mg PO 3 times a day for 5 days *OR* 800 mg PO twice daily for 5 days *OR* 800 mg PO 3 times a day for 2 days	500 mg PO twice daily for 3 days *OR* 1 g PO once daily for 5 days	125 mg PO twice daily for 5 days *OR* 1 g PO twice daily for 1 day *OR* 500 mg PO once, followed by 250 mg PO twice daily for 2 days

(continued)

Table 9-1. Summary of Treatment Guidelines for Herpes Simplex Virus *(continued)*

	Age	Acyclovir	Valacyclovir	Famciclovir
Suppressive Therapy	<12 years[13]	40-80 mg/kg/day PO divided 3 times a day **Maximum dose 1000 mg/day**		
	≥12 years[13]	400 mg PO twice daily, may continue for 12 months then reevaluate need	1 g PO twice daily for 7-10 days	
	Adult[8,*]	400 mg PO twice daily	500 mg PO once daily† *OR* 1 g PO once daily	250 mg PO twice daily
Immuno-suppressed	<12 years[13]	30 mg/kg/day IV divided 3 times a day for 7-14 days		
	≥12 years[13]	15 mg/kg/day IV divided 3 times a day for 7-14 days		
Severe HSV Complication	Adult[8]	5-10 mg/kg IV every 8 hours for 2-7 days followed by oral antiviral therapy for at least 10 days		

IV, intravenously. PO, per os (orally).
For more information on treatment, see the CDC's sexually transmitted disease guidelines at https://www.cdc.gov/std/tg2015/herpes.htm.
**Treatment can be extended if healing is incomplete after 10 days of therapy.*
†Valacyclovir 500 mg once daily might be less effective than other valacyclovir or acyclovir dosing regimens in persons who have very frequent recurrences (ie, ≥10 episodes per year).[8]

Special Considerations

— ***Pregnancy:*** Prophylactic therapy with acyclovir or valacyclovir beginning at 36 weeks gestation should be offered to all women with a personal history of genital herpes.[14] This prophylactic approach has been shown to reduce the risk of HSV shedding at delivery, reduce the risk of HSV recurrence at delivery by 75%, and reduce the need for cesarean delivery because of recurrent genital herpes by 40%.[14]

— ***HIV infection:*** Higher doses of antiviral medication for treatment and suppression of HSV are required for efficacy in persons with HIV. Recurrent outbreaks and viral shedding might be more frequent and prolonged. Suppressive therapy in persons with HIV infection may reduce clinical manifestations of HSV but does not reduce the risk for either HIV or HSV-2 transmission to susceptible partners.[15]

— ***Neonates:*** Asymptomatic infants born through vaginal delivery in the presence of maternal HSV genital lesions should undergo close monitoring, testing, and treatment according to the Pediatric Committee on Infectious Diseases.[16] The incidence of neonatal HSV infection has increased 56% from 2009 to 2015 with a stable mortality rate when guideline treatment and recommendations are followed.[17] When applicable, maternal prophylaxis is the optimal approach.

— ***Allergy or resistance to antiviral therapy:*** Although rare, reports of allergic or adverse reactions to acyclovir, valacyclovir, and famciclovir exist. In the case of allergy, desensitization to acyclovir has been described.[8,18] Antiviral resistance is suspected when lesions persist in individuals who received extended antiviral therapy. All suspected cases of antiviral resistance should be referred to an infectious disease specialist.[8]

Case Studies

Adult Case Study 9-1

AB is a 21-year-old male college student who presents to the urgent care clinic requesting STI testing. He reports a new-onset painful penile lesion 5 days after a sexual encounter with a new partner. He states he feels like he has "the flu" and reports generalized body aches.

Examination

A 1-cm circular cluster of intact vesicular lesions is identified on the lateral shaft of the circumcised penis, with mild erythema.

Laboratory Testing

HSV PCR type-specific swab of lesion is performed; HSV-1 is negative and HSV-2 is positive. Nucleic acid amplification test (NAAT) for *Chlamydia trachomatis* is negative; NAAT for *Neisseria gonorrhoeae* is negative; rapid plasma reagin is nonreactive; HIV antibody test is negative. No HSV serological test is performed because of presentation with primary infection.

Treatment

AB is started on valacyclovir 1000 mg orally twice daily for 7 days. He is counseled on consistent condom use and avoiding sexual activity when lesions are present. The possibility of recurrence is discussed along with suppression therapy options as indicated.

Child Case Study 9-2

CD is a 4-year-old girl who is brought to the emergency department by her mother and maternal grandmother for concerns of oral lesions present for 2 days, along with decreased oral intake. No reports of fever, nausea, or vomiting. The child attended preschool and was picked up by a male relative each day who provided childcare until the mother and maternal grandmother returned home from work. The child is up to date on immunizations and has no chronic health conditions.

Examination

Small clusters of blisters, ulcers, and crusted lesions are identified circumferentially around the mouth on both the upper and lower lip extending past the vermillion border, with small ulcerative lesions in the inferior and superior oral labium.

Laboratory Testing

Complete blood cell count and complete metabolic panel are within normal limits without findings of severe dehydration. Viral HSV type-specific PCR swab of the lesion is collected.

Treatment

The child receives a 20 mg/kg IV bolus of 0.9% sodium chloride solution and acyclovir 100 mg IV once, and is then started on acyclovir 200 mg/5 mL orally 5 times a day for 7 days. The health care provider files a formal child safety report for suspected abuse with the state child protective agency. The following day, results confirm HSV-2 infection.

References

1. Looker KJ, Garnett GP, Schmid GP. An estimate of the global prevalence and incidence of herpes simplex virus type 2 infection. *Bull World Health Organ.* 2008;86(10):805-812.
2. Barnabas RV, Wasserheit JN, Huang Y, et al. Impact of herpes simplex virus type 2 on HIV-1 acquisition and progression in an HIV vaccine trial (the Step study). *J Acquir Immune Defic Syndr.* 2011;57(3):238-244.
3. Tronstein E, Johnston C, Huang ML, et al. Genital shedding of herpes simplex virus among symptomatic and asymptomatic persons with HSV-2 infection. *JAMA.* 2011;305(14):1441-1449.

4. McQuillan G, Kruszon-Moran D, Flagg EW, Paulose-Ram R; National Center of Health Statistics. Prevalence of herpes simplex virus type 1 and type 2 in persons aged 14–49: United States, 2015–2016. https://www.cdc.gov/nchs/data/databriefs/db304.pdf. Published February 2018. Accessed July 9. 2019.

5. Knezevic A, Martic J, Stanojevic M, et al. Disseminated neonatal herpes caused by herpes simplex virus types 1 and 2. *Emerg Infect Dis*. 2007;13(2):302-304.

6. Reading R, Hughes G, Hill J, Debelle G. Genital herpes in children under 11 years and investigations for sexual abuse. *Arch Dis Child*. 2011;96(8):752-757.

7. Fanfair R, Zaidi A, Taylor LD, Xu F, Gottlieb S, Markowitz L. Trends in seroprevalence of herpes simplex virus type 2 among non-Hispanic blacks and non-Hispanic whites aged 14 to 49 years—United States, 1988 to 2010. *Sex Transm Dis*. 2013;40(11):860-864.

8. 2015 sexually transmitted diseases treatment guidelines: genital HSV infections. Centers for Disease Control and Prevention Web site. https://www.cdc.gov/std/tg2015/herpes.htm. Published June 4, 2015. Accessed July 9, 2019.

9. Margaret AS, Mujugira A, Hughes JP, et al. Effect of condom use on per-act HSV-2 transmission risk in HIV-1, HSV-2-discordant couples. *Clin Infect Dis*. 2016;62(4):456-461.

10. Glass N, Nelson HD, Huffman L. Screening for genital herpes simplex: brief update for the U.S. preventive services task force. US Preventive Services Task Force Web Site. https://www.uspreventiveservicestaskforce.org/Home/GetFile/1/733/herpesup/pdf. Accessed July 9, 2019.

11. Corey L, Wald A. Genital herpes. In: Holmes KK, Sparling PF, Stamm WE, et al, eds. Sexually Transmitted Diseases. 4th ed. New York, NY: McGraw-Hill; 2008:399-437.

12. Genital herpes: basic fact sheet. Center for Disease Control and Prevention Web site. https://www.cdc.gov/std/herpes/stdfact-herpes.htm. Updated August 28, 2017. Accessed July 9, 2019.

13. James SH, Whitley RJ. Treatment of herpes simplex virus infections in pediatric patients: current status and future needs. *Clin Pharmacol Ther*. 2010;88(5):720-724.

14. The American College of Obstetricians and Gynecologists. Practice bulletin no. 82: management of herpes in pregnancy. *Obstet Gynecol*. 2007;109(6):1489-1498.

15. Mujugira A, Magaret AS, Celum C, et al. Daily acyclovir to decrease herpes simplex virus type 2 (HSV-2) transmission from HSV-2/HIV-1 coinfected persons: a randomized controlled trial. *J Infect Dis*. 2013;208(9):1366-1374.

16. Kimberlin DW, Baley J; Committee on Infectious Diseases, Committee on Fetus and Newborn. Guidance on management of asymptomatic neonates born to women with active genital herpes lesions. *Pediatrics*. 2013;131(2):383-386.

17. Mahant, S, Hall M, Schondelmeyer AC, Berry JG, Kimberlin DW, Shah SS; Pediatric Research in Inpatient Settings Network and the Collaborative Antiviral Study Group. Neonatal herpes simplex virus infection among Medicaid-enrolled children: 2009-2015. *Pediatrics*. 2019;143(4):e20183233.

18. Henry RE, Wegmann JA, Hartle JE, Christopher GW. Successful oral acyclovir desensitization. *Ann Allergy*. 1993;70(5):386-388.

Chapter 10

HIV AND AIDS

Melanie Gibbons Hallman, DNP, CRNP, CEN, FNP-BC, ACNP-BC, ENP-C, TCRN, FAEN
Sallie Johnson Shipman, EdD, MSN, RN, CNL, NHDP-BC
Kelsey Tucker Geer, MSN, FNP-C
Patricia M. Speck, DNSc, CRNP, FNP-BC, DF-IAFN, FAAFS, DF-AFN, FAAN

DISEASE AND MIMICS

- Human immunodeficiency virus (HIV) is an RNA retrovirus that causes acquired immunodeficiency syndrome (AIDS).[1]
- The 2 types of HIV are type 1 and type 2, the latter being extremely uncommon in the United States.[1]
- Opportunistic infections are common in HIV infection and can include tuberculosis, *Pneumocystis jiroveci* pneumonia, *Mycobacterium* infection, cytomegalovirus infection, *Cryptosporidium* infection, or candidiasis.[2-4]
- Coexisting, curable frequent sexually transmitted infections (STIs) include syphilis, *Neisseria gonorrhoeae*, *Chlamydia trachomatis*, and others.
- Common HIV mimics include the following[2,5,6]:
  - ***Constitutional symptoms:*** Catarrhal, flu, malaise
  - ***Malignancies and autoimmune diseases***
  - ***Head, eye, ear, nose, and throat/immune system:*** Pharyngitis from streptococcal infection, Epstein-Barr (mononucleosis), cytomegalovirus, toxoplasmosis, or influenza; oral or genital ulcers (such as herpes simplex virus [HSV]); coxsackievirus; aphthous stomatitis; or Behçet's disease
  - ***Gastrointestinal and urinary systems:*** Persistent diarrhea from viral or bacterial gastroenteritis; or laboratory elevation of transaminase from viral hepatitis (B & C), cytomegalovirus, Epstein-Barr, or drug reaction
  - ***Integumentary system:*** Rash from primary HSV infection, secondary syphilis infection, enterovirus, rubella, rickettsial diseases, roseola, parvovirus B19, allergic reaction, or rheumatological disease
  - ***Neurological system***: Meningitis/encephalitis from enterovirus infection, HSV, West Nile, or other viral encephalitis
- HIV infection is percutaneously and sexually transmitted through contact with large quantities of the virus, which is present in early and late infection.[7]
- Individuals are at increased risk for developing acute infection through transmission if they have been sexually exposed, are a nursing mother or have household contact with someone who is HIV positive, or have an occupational hazard (eg, police, health care professionals).[8]

EPIDEMIOLOGY

As of 2017, approximately 25% of the estimated 36.9 million persons with HIV infection globally are unaware of their infection.[9] Approximately 50% to 90% of persons with acute HIV infection are symptomatic and many seek medical care.[10,11]

The estimated prevalence of HIV includes both the number living with diagnosed HIV infection and the estimated number of persons living with undiagnosed HIV.[12,13] By 2016, the Centers for Disease Control and Prevention (CDC) estimated that 1 140 400 persons 13 years of age and older were living with diagnosed or undiagnosed HIV infection in the United States.[13] The number of persons living with diagnosed or undiagnosed HIV (estimated HIV prevalence) increased each year from 2010 to 2016 and corresponds with the number of new HIV infections.[12,13] The lifetime risk for developing HIV in the United States is 1:68 in males and 1:253 in females.[12,13] New infections outpace HIV deaths.

By the end of 2016, of the persons living with diagnosed or undiagnosed HIV in the United Sates, the CDC estimated that 77% were male and 23% were female.[13] An estimated 57% acquired HIV through male-to-male sexual contact, 26% through heterosexual contact, 12% by injection drug use, and 5% had combined risk factors for male-to-male sexual contact[14] and injection drug use.[15] HIV prevalence among transgender persons is 13.7%.[16] Transgender women who have addictions, which are a barrier to adherence, have elevated rates of HIV infection.[17]

As of 2016, among those living with HIV in the United States, approximately 42% are black/African American; 30% are white; 22% are Hispanic/Latino; and 6% are of other races, including American Indian/Alaska Native, Asian, Native Hawaiian/Pacific Islander, and persons who identify as multiple races.[13] African Americans comprise 12% of the United States population but are 42% of persons living with HIV. Of the persons living with HIV in the United States who were 13 years old or older in 2016, 61% were 45 years of age or older.[13]

In 2016, the highest HIV prevalence rate in the United States per 100 000 people was in the South, with the second highest in the Northeast.[13] Forty-five percent of persons with HIV resided in the South, 23% in the Northeast, 20% in the West, and 12% in the Midwest.[13]

HIV Disease Definitions

— ***Acute infection*** refers to the body's seroconversion process, often with an acute retroviral syndrome.

— ***Early infection*** refers to those with documented infection in the recent past, usually within the preceding 6 months, pinpointing the date of exposure.

— ***Conversion*** typically occurs within the first 6 to 12 months of the disease, creating a false negative on less sensitive HIV tests. Conventional sensitive testing eliminates false negatives.

Pathogenesis

During the first days and weeks of HIV infection, there is a modest decline in peripheral blood $CD4^+$ T-cells with a dramatic decline in gastrointestinal $CD4^+$ T-cells.[18] Recent studies suggest that the pathogenicity of HIV is not restricted to immune suppression. HIV causes chronic inflammation, which in turn may contribute to a variety of diseases in the neurological, cardiovascular, renal, and hepatic systems.[18] After contact with large quantities of virus, if a person is infected, symptoms include a brief acute retroviral syndrome of unexplained fever and lymph node tenderness and swelling.[18]

Without treatment, HIV transitions to a multiyear chronic illness that progressively depletes CD4 T lymphocytes. CD4 T lymphocytes maintain effective immune function.[18] When immune cells are depleted, the patient is symptomatic, with a life-threatening immunodeficiency known as AIDS.[18] The late stage of infection develops over months to years (median time of approximately 11 years) and is diagnosed as AIDS.[18] In the absence of treatment, persons with AIDS will die from AIDS-related causes, including organ failure and opportunistic infections.[19-21]

Early Treatment Outcomes

Early antiretroviral treatment substantially reduces infection transmission, improves laboratory disease markers, decreases severity of acute symptoms, lowers viral load, decreases the rate of mutation through viral replication suppression, and preserves immune system function.[19] Persons provided early antiretroviral therapy can expect to live a near-normal life approximating other chronic diseases.[20-22]

Preparation for Those Wishing to Work With HIV-Positive Patients

Any provider choosing to work with patients who are at risk for HIV should complete the CDC's training on HIV prevention, detection, and treatment (https://www.cdc.gov/hiv/training/programs.html).

Notifying Partners of Patients with HIV

Partner notification is an important component of disease management. Disease management provides:

- — Early diagnosis, early treatment, and reduced risk for HIV transmission
- — A decrease in individual morbidity and mortality risk
- — Opportunity to modify risk behaviors

Determine if a partner exists, then determine if the partner should be notified concerning exposure. The term ***partner*** includes sex partners and persons with whom syringes or other injection equipment is shared. Partner notification for HIV infection should be confidential. Specific guidance regarding spousal notification varies by jurisdiction. Detailed recommendations concerning identification, notification, screening,[23] diagnosis, and treatment of exposed partners are available via the CDC's Recommendations for Partner Services Programs for HIV Infection, Syphilis, Gonorrhea, and Chlamydial Infections.[24-26]

Partner-notification procedures include explaining the processes, benefits, and risks of treatment and referral to counseling and testing. If persons with HIV infection are unwilling to notify their partners or cannot ensure their partners will seek counseling, HIV care staff or health department personnel should use confidential partner notification procedures.

Health department staff are trained to employ public health investigation strategies to confidentially locate persons who are hard to reach or unwilling to seek treatment. When found, partners should be offered postexposure prophylaxis (PEP) with combination antiretrovirals if they were exposed to genital secretions or blood of a partner with HIV infection through sex or injection drug use. Offer PEP if the contact was in the preceding 72 hours.[27] Research demonstrates that if started after 72 hours, there is no HIV prevention impact.[2]

Patient Presentation

Early symptoms of HIV infection include the following[8]:

- — Fever and flu-like symptoms, including night sweats, chills, fatigue, lethargy/malaise, and myalgia, present in 50% to 70% of patients within 2 to 4 weeks after exposure
- — Skin rash that is variable in severity and presentation, often mimicking drug eruptions, secondary syphilis, and other viral exanthems, present in 50% of patients
- — Neurological symptoms that include mild to moderate headache and, infrequently, severe meningitis, encephalitis, and/or Guillain-Barré syndrome, present in nearly 50% of patients
- — Sore throat, diagnosed as pharyngitis with cervical adenopathy but usually without tonsillar exudates in 50% of patients, mimicking Epstein-Barr viral infection (mononucleosis) and esophageal candidiasis or *Pneumocystis jiroveci* pneumonia
- — Oral ulcers, present in 10% to 20% of patients

— Cervical adenopathy, which can exist along with adenopathy in other locations, present in about 30% to 40% of patients

— Diarrhea , present in about 20% of patients

Laboratory findings in early symptoms include the following[8]:

— Leukopenia, anemia, thrombocytopenia, and transaminase elevation

— Transient reduction in $CD4^+$ T-cell counts, but not less than 200 cells/mm

— Elevation in creatinine, laboratory evidence of rhabdomyolysis, and cerebrospinal fluid pleocytosis, although these findings are less common

Antibody testing for HIV-1 and HIV-2 and virological testing to detect HIV antigens and RNA should be performed. Viral counts are inaccurate up to 6 weeks but are useful in percutaneous transmission to establish a baseline for job-related injury.

Initial workup includes a basic metabolic panel (BMP) with a liver function panel, complete blood cell count (CBC) with differential, erythrocyte sedimentation rate, C-reactive protein, pregnancy test in fertile female patients, and chest x-ray examination. Also rule out other STIs and tuberculosis (TB). If in a primary care setting, follow up laboratory tests with abnormal findings for differential diagnosis. Other testing may be necessary in the management of the patient beyond the scope of the acute discovery and referral of disease.

Late symptoms include weight loss, weakness, chills, fever, lymphadenopathy, diaphoresis, and fatigue. Laboratory findings in late symptoms include CD4 count less than 200 cells/mm.[8] In addition, although opportunistic infections are uncommon today, some patients present with oral pharyngeal or esophageal candidiasis or *Pneumocystis* pneumonia.

Workup for patients with late symptoms should include:

— Antibody testing for HIV-1 and HIV-2

— Virological testing to detect HIV antigens and RNA

Treatment Guidelines

Treatment of HIV infection falls into 3 categories:

1. PEP for HIV infection has recently been recommended in adults.
2. Treatment of HIV infection with antiretroviral therapy (ART) reduces the morbidity and mortality and helps prevent HIV transmission for all HIV-infected individuals, regardless of CD4 T lymphocytes count. When addressing strategies to optimize adherence to ART, it is important to educate patients regarding the benefits and side effects of ART. Clinical and/or psychosocial factors may delay starting ART or PEP, but therapy should be initiated as soon as possible, depending on exposure or active disease.[28]
3. Early diagnosis and aggressive treatment of opportunistic infections are also important.[29]

Treatment Regimens

There are many different classes of drugs used to treat HIV. Therapy is individualized based on viral load, strain, resistance, and chronicity of disease. All people with HIV need more than 1 drug to control viral replication and reduce viral load. Medication prevents resistance by slowing the RNA replication. As of 2017, research supports treatment of acute and chronic HIV infection with the same antiretroviral therapy. However, consider the following issues:

— In the naive patient who has no evidence of genotypic drug-resistant virus, consider any treatment option (eg, dual nucleoside reverse transcriptase inhibitors [NRTIs] with a non-nucleoside reverse transcriptase inhibitor [NNRTI], a ritonavir-boosted protease inhibitor [PI/r], or an integrase strand transfer inhibitor [INSTI]).

— Present resistance is a consideration in treatment decisions. If patient has drug resistance, select 3 fully active agents at a minimum.

— If patient started therapy before the availability of drug resistance testing, consideration of initiating a dual NRTI plus PI/r-based regimen is prudent, because resistance to PIs is relatively infrequent. Additionally, resistance to these drugs is less likely to occur if NRTI resistance is unknowingly present.[30]

Table 10-1 outlines the recommended schedule of laboratory evaluations of source and exposed persons for providing nonoccupational PEP (nPEP) with preferred regimens.

Side Effects

Patients experience side effects for protracted times, which makes adherence difficult. These effects can include diarrhea, dizziness, headaches, fatigue, fever, muscle aches, nausea, and vomiting. Persistence of side effects should lead to a consideration of antiretroviral medication change.

Counseling and Referral

For many patients, the first reaction after being informed of a positive HIV test result is distress. There are adaptive challenges, including coping with other people's reactions, learning strategies for maintaining physical and emotional health, initiating changes in behavior, and reducing the risk for acquiring additional STIs. Persons testing positive for HIV infection have unique needs, including behavioral interventions (eg, a substance abuse program), mental health disorders (eg, depression) and emotional distress, and requiring assistance with securing and maintaining employment and housing. Behavioral, psychological, and social services are integral to adaptive health responses.

Provider-Specific Recommendations for HIV Counseling and Linkage to Services

Counsel the patient, either on site or through referral, concerning the behavioral, psychosocial, and medical implications of HIV infection. Assess the need for immediate medical care and psychosocial support. Link newly diagnosed persons with services provided by health care personnel experienced in the management of HIV infection. Consider substance abuse counseling and treatment, treatment for mental health disorders or emotional distress, reproductive counseling, risk-reduction counseling, and case management.

Providers should follow up to ensure that patients have received services for any identified needs. Providers should implement trauma-informed care principles to create safety, trustworthiness and transparency, openness, collaboration and mutuality, voice, choice, and empowerment in the context of culture, history, and gender in micro, mezzo, and macro systems.[31]

In summary, several successful, innovative interventions to assist persons with HIV infection and reduce the possibility of transmission to others have been developed for diverse at-risk populations, and these can be locally replicated or adapted.[32-37] Involvement of nongovernmental and community-based organizations might complement such efforts in the clinical setting, where coordinated community responses and peer groups exist to support the patient.[38]

Table 10-1. Recommended Schedule of Laboratory Evaluations of Source and Exposed Persons for Providing nPEP With Preferred Regimens

Test	Source	Exposed Persons			
	Baseline	Baseline	4–6 Weeks After Exposure	3 Months After Exposure	6 Months After Exposure
For all persons considered for or prescribed nPEP for any exposure					
HIV Ag/Ab testing[a] (or antibody testing if Ag/Ab test unavailable)	X	X	X	X	X[b]
Hepatitis B serology, including: – Hepatitis B surface antigen – Hepatitis B surface antibody – Hepatitis B core antibody	X	X			X[c]
Hepatitis C antibody test	X	X			X[d]
For all persons considered for or prescribed nPEP for sexual exposure					
Syphilis serology[e]	X	X	X		X
Gonorrhea[f]	X	X	X[g]		
Chlamydia[f]	X	X	X[g]		
Pregnancy[h]		X	X		
For persons prescribed tenofovir DF+ emtricitabine + raltegravir OR tenofovir DF + emtricitabine + dolutegravir					
Serum creatinine (for calculating estimated creatinine clearance[i])		X	X		
Alanine transaminase, aspartate aminotranferase		X	X		
For all persons with HIV infection confirmed at any visit					
HIV viral load	X	X[j]			
HIV genotypic resistance	X	X[j]			

Abbreviations: Ag/Ab, antigen/antibody combination test; HIV, human immunodeficiency virus; nPEP, nonoccupational postexposure prophylaxis; tenofovir DF, tenofovir disoproxil fumarate.

[a] *Any positive or indeterminate HIV antibody test should undergo confirmatory testing of HIV infection status.*

[b] *Only if hepatitis C infection was acquired during the original exposure; delayed HIV seroconversion has been seen in persons who simultaneously acquire HIV and hepatitis C infection.*

[c] *If exposed person susceptible to hepatitis B at baseline.*

[d] *If exposed person susceptible to hepatitis C at baseline.*

[e] *If determined to be infected with syphilis and treated, should undergo serologic syphilis testing 6 months after treatment.*

[f] *Testing for chlamydia and gonorrhea should be performed using nucleic acid amplification tests. For patients diagnosed with a chlamydia or gonorrhea infection, retesting 3 months after treatment is recommended.*

- *For men reporting insertive vaginal, anal, or oral sex, a urine specimen should be tested for chlamydia and gonorrhea.*
- *For women reporting receptive vaginal sex, a vaginal (preferred) or endocervical swab or urine specimen should be tested for chlamydia and gonorrhea.*
- *For men and women reporting receptive anal sex, a rectal swab specimen should be tested for chlamydia and gonorrhea.*
- *For men and women reporting receptive oral sex, an oropharyngeal swab should be tested for gonorrhea. (http://www.cdc.gov/std/tg2015/tg-2015-print.pdf)*

[g] *If not provided presumptive treatment at baseline, or if symptomatic at follow-up visit.*

[h] *If woman of reproductive age, not using effective contraception, and with vaginal exposure to semen.*

[i] *eCrCl = estimated creatinine clearance calculated by the Cockcroft-Gault formula; eCrClCG= [(140 – age) x ideal body weight] ÷ (serum creatinine x 72) (x 0.85 for females).*

[j] *At first visit where determined to have HIV infection.*

Updated Guidelines for Antiretroviral Postexposure Prophylaxis After Sexual, Injection Drug Use, or Other Nonoccupational Exposure to HIV— United States, 2016 from the Centers for Disease Control and Prevention, U.S. Department of Health and Human Services (CDC, 2016). https://www.cdc.gov/hiv/pdf/programresources/cdc-hiv-npep-guidelines.pdf.

Special Considerations

Pregnancy and Neonates

— After a pregnant woman has been identified as having HIV infection, she should be educated about the benefits of antiretroviral treatment for her health and for reducing the risk for transmission to her infant. In the absence of antiretroviral treatment, a mother's risk of transmitting HIV to her neonate is approximately 30% but can be reduced to less than 2% through antiretroviral treatment, obstetrical interventions (ie, elective cesarean section at 38 weeks of pregnancy), and breastfeeding avoidance.[39]

— Pregnant women who have HIV infection should be linked to an HIV care provider and given appropriate antenatal and postpartum treatment and advice.

— Detailed and regularly updated recommendations for the initial management of persons who are pregnant and HIV positive are available at https://aidsinfo.nih.gov/guidelines/html/3/perinatal/488/overview.

— Transmission of HIV to infants and children can occur by 1 of 4 means:

  — Vertical transmission

  — Breastfeeding[39]

  — Percutaneous exposure

  — Mucous membrane exposure to infected blood or body fluids, through sexual contact

— All pregnant women should be tested for HIV infection during the first prenatal visit and during the third trimester, preferably before 36 weeks gestation.[40,41]

— Pregnant women should be informed about being tested for HIV as part of the panel of prenatal tests and provided with the opportunity to decline. If the patient declines, encourage testing at subsequent prenatal visits.[40-42]

— Retesting during each pregnancy is recommended, even if the woman's previous HIV test results are negative.

— Testing pregnant women improves knowledge and facilitates receipt of interventions (ART and obstetrical), substantially reducing the risk of perinatal transmission of HIV.

— All women with no prenatal care should be tested for HIV at the time of delivery.

Children

— Antiretroviral therapy is indicated for most HIV-infected children.

— Consultation with a pediatric HIV specialist is suggested to choose a treatment regimen.

— Children with HIV or AIDS may manifest growth failure for various reasons, including esophagitis; diarrhea from parasitic, viral, or bacterial infections; and malabsorption.

— Other manifestations include central nervous system disease, cardiomyopathy, hepatitis, and recurrent invasive infections.

— If PEP is being considered for a child sexual abuse victim, consultation with a pediatric HIV specialist is recommended to choose the appropriate treatment regimen.

— Before testing is done, pretest counseling must be performed, and posttest counseling must also be arranged. If the abuse was recent, seroconversion may not have occurred, which may produce a false-negative result. Because of this, all patients should have repeat testing ideally at 6 weeks and at 3 and 6 months after the initial test.

— Testing for HIV is done first with an enzyme immunoassay, which serves as a screening test. If this is positive, Western blot or immunofluorescent antibody tests should be used for confirmation.

— The incidence of HIV infection acquired by pediatric victims of sexual abuse from HIV-infected perpetrators is unknown.

Under- and Uninsured

The Ryan White HIV/AIDS Program provides a comprehensive system of care that includes primary medical care and essential support services for people living with HIV who are uninsured or underinsured. Data about the treatment of those individuals can be found at https://hab.hrsa.gov/data/data-reports.

Legal Considerations

The HIV Law and Policy organization provides a state-by-state list of regulations related to confidentiality and disclosure at http://www.hivlawandpolicy.org/state-hiv-laws.

Nonoccupational Postexposure Prophylaxis

The algorithm for nPEP should be used when making decisions related to prophylaxis (**Figure 10-1**).

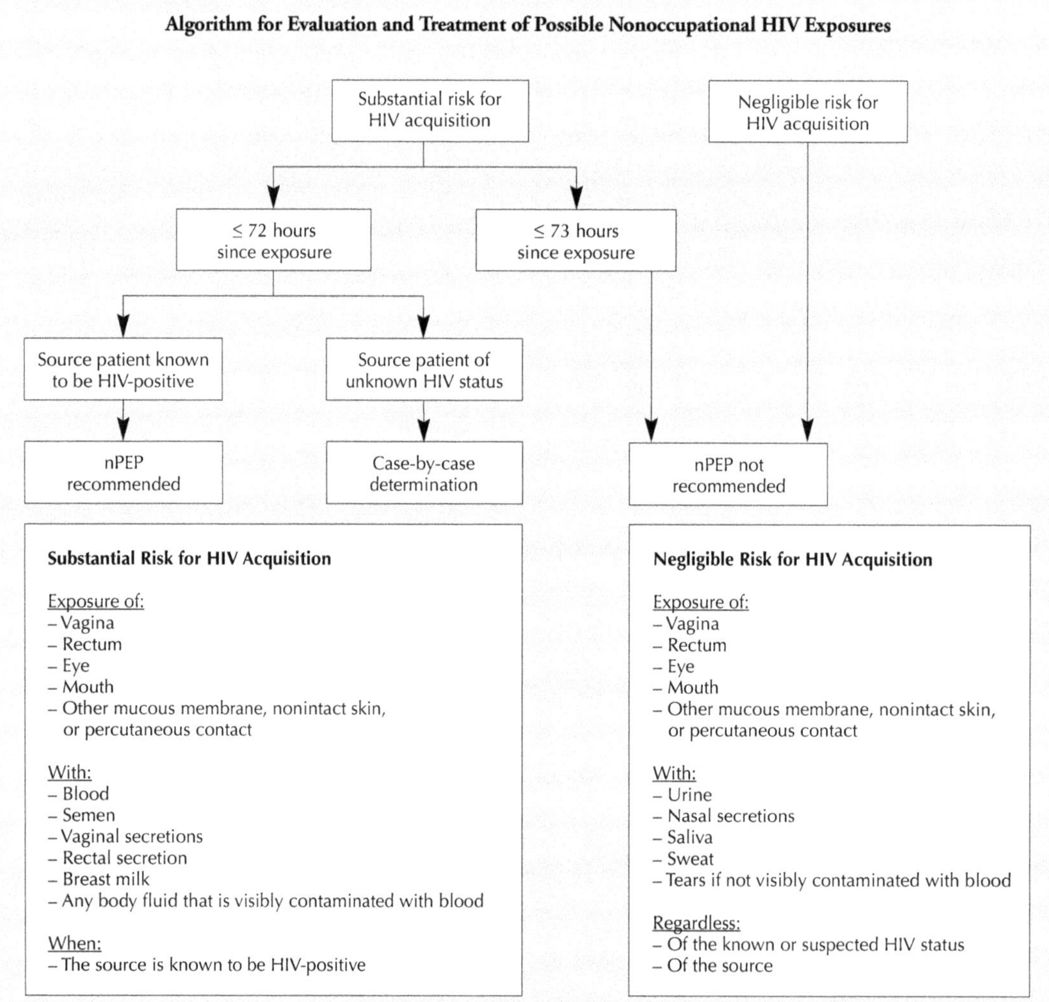

Source: www.cdc.gov/hiv/pdf/programresources/cdc-hiv-nPEP-guidelines.pdf **Figure 10-1**

Figure 10-1. *Algorithm for evaluation and treatment of possible nonoccupational HIV exposures.*

Case Studies

Adult Case Study 10-1

A sanitation worker in the hospital is cleaning the emergency department (ED) waiting room and is stuck by a needle from an unknown source. He reports the injury to the ED charge nurse, who alerts the hospital needlestick team. The patient has baseline laboratory drawn by ED personnel.

Examination

The examination of the injury consists of documenting puncture wound, amount of bleeding, risk history for prior exposure, and underlying medical history.

Laboratory Testing

A BMP, baseline renal and hepatic function panels, CBC with differential, and hepatitis panel with baseline HIV are done.

Treatment

The patient is given nPEP with instructions to begin until laboratory results return.

Child Case Study 10-2

A 10-year-old girl with frequent upper respiratory infections and mouth sores presents to the ED during paternal visitation. The paternal grandmother is concerned because the child is lethargic and appears sick. The grandmother believes the child is being abused by her mother's boyfriend.

The triage nurse calls child protective services and law enforcement to begin an investigation. The advanced practice provider begins the medical history interview and delays a medical workup for symptoms until after the medical forensic evaluation.

Examination

The evaluation indicates that the anogenital area is without acute or previous injury, but the patient has significant white patches over vestibular tissue, and in the mouth a thick white coating on the posterior tongue and soft palate (painful to swallow) is identified.

Laboratory Testing

All laboratory tests are completed after the medical forensic evaluation. Tests include urinalysis; CBC; cultures for all orifices; drug screen; STI screening with nucleic acid amplification testing (NAAT) for *Chlamydia*, gonorrhea, and HIV; and bloodwork plus chest x-ray examination.

The NAATs for *Chlamydia* and gonorrhea are negative, and the NAAT for HIV is positive. Further testing for CD4 count, HIV type, TB skin test, and other opportunistic infections is ordered.

Treatment

The patient is given antifungal medication to treat thrush and genital lesions. She is referred to a pediatric HIV clinic for management.

References

1. Cloyd MW. Human retroviruses. In: Baron S, ed. *Medical Microbiology,* 4th ed. Galveston, TX; University of Texas Medical Branch at Galveston: 1996:Chapter 62.

2. HIV: AIDS and opportunistic infections. Centers for Disease Control and Prevention Web site. https://www.cdc.gov/hiv/basics/livingwithhiv/opportunisticinfections.html. Updated August 6, 2019. Accessed November 1, 2019.

3. Dufaur L, Matin N. Important opportunistic infections in HIV. *Medicine.* 2018;46(6):352-355.

4. Sørensen A, Jespersen S, Katzenstein TL, et al. Clinical presentation and opportunistic infections in HIV-1, HIV-2 and HIV-1/2 dual seropositive patients in Guinea-Bissau. *Infect Dis (Lond).* 2016;48(8):604-611.

5. Javadi S, Menias CO, Karbasian N, et al. HIV-related malignancies and mimics: imaging findings and management. *Radiographics.* 2018;38(7):2051-2068.

6. Roszkiewicz J, Smolewska E. Kaleidoscope of autoimmune diseases in HIV infection. *Rheumatol Int.* 2016;36(11):1481-1491.

7. Krause KH, Lewis-O'Connor A, Berger A, et al. Current practices of HIV postexposure prophylaxis treatment for sexual assault patients in an emergency department. *Womens Health Issues.* 2014;24(4):e407-e412.

8. Hirschel B. Infectious diseases: evaluation and management of acute HIV. Infectious Disease Advisor Web site. https://www.infectiousdiseaseadvisor.com/home/decision-support-in-medicine/infectious-diseases/evaluation-and-management-of-acute-hiv/. Accessed September 18, 2019.

9. Monitoring selected national HIV prevention and care objectives by using HIV surveillance data. Centers for Disease Control and Prevention Web site. https://www.cdc.gov/hiv/pdf/library/reports/surveillance/cdc-hiv-surveillance-supplemental-report-vol-23-4.pdf. Accessed September 18, 2019.

10. Weintrob AC, Giner J, Menezes P, et al. Infrequent diagnosis of primary human immunodeficiency virus infection: missed opportunities in acute care settings. *Arch Intern Med.* 2003;163(17):2097-2100.

11. Schacker T, Collier AC, Hughes J, Shea T, Corey L. Clinical and epidemiologic features of primary HIV infection. *Ann Intern Med.* 1996;125(4):257-264.

12. Hall HI, An Q, Tang T, et al; Centers for Disease Control and Prevention. Prevalence of diagnosed and undiagnosed HIV infection—United States, 2008-2012. *MMWR Morb Mortal Wkly Rep.* 2015;64(24):657-662.

13. Diagnoses of HIV infection in the United States and dependent areas, 2017. Centers for Disease Control and Prevention. Web site. https://www.cdc.gov/hiv/pdf/library/reports/surveillance/cdc-hiv-surveillance-report-2017-vol-29.pdf. Accessed September 19, 2019.

14. de Oliveira T, Kharsany ABM, Gräf T, et al. Transmission networks and risk of HIV infection in KwaZulu-Natal, South Africa: a community-wide phylogenetic study. *Lancet.* 2017;4(1):e41-e50.

15. Shiau S, Arpadi SM, Yin MT, Martins SS. Patterns of drug use and HIV infection among adults in a nationally representative sample. *Addict Behav.* 2017;68:39-44.

16. Becasen JS, Denard CL, Mullins MM, Higa DH, Sipe TA. Estimating the prevalence of HIV and sexual behaviors among the US transgender population: a systematic review and meta-analysis, 2006-2017. *Am J Public Health.* 2018;29:e1-e8.

17. Santos GM, Rapues J, Wilson EC, et al. Alcohol and substance use among transgender women in San Francisco: prevalence and association with human immunodeficiency virus infection. *Drug Alcohol Rev.* 2014;33(3):287-295.

18. Smit C, Geskus R, Walker S; CASCADE Collaboration. Effective therapy has altered the spectrum of cause-specific mortality following HIV seroconversion. *AIDS.* 2006;20(5):741-749.

19. Panel on Antiretroviral Guidelines for Adults and Adolescents. Guidelines for the use of antiretroviral agents in adults and adolescents with HIV. Department of Health and Human Services Web site. https://aidsinfo.nih.gov/contentfiles/lvguidelines/adultandadolescentgl.pdf. Accessed November 4, 2019.

20. Wada N, Jacobson LP, Cohen M, French A, Phair J, Muñoz A. Cause-specific life expectancies after 35 years of age for human immunodeficiency syndrome-infected and human immunodeficiency syndrome-negative individuals followed simultaneously in long-term cohort studies, 1984-2008. *Am J Epidemiol.* 2013;177(2):116-125.

21. Engsig FN, Zangerle R, Katsarou O, et al; Antiretroviral Therapy Cohort Collaboration (ART-CC) and the Collaboration of Observational HIV Epidemiological Research Europe (COHERE) in EuroCoord. Long-term mortality in HIV-positive individuals virally suppressed for >3 years with incomplete CD4 recovery. *Clin Infect Dis.* 2014;58(9):1312-1321.

22. Samji H, Cescon A, Hogg RS, et al; North American AIDS Cohort Collaboration on Research and Design (NA-ACCORD) of IeDEA. Closing the gap: increases in life expectancy among treated HIV-positive individuals in the United States and Canada. *PLoS One.* 2013;8(12):e81355.

23. Carter JW Jr, Hart-Cooper GD, Butler MO, Workowski KA, Hoover KW. Provider barriers prevent recommended sexually transmitted disease screening of HIV-infected men who have sex with men. *Sex Transm Dis.* 2014;41(2):137-142.

24. HIV: partner notification services. Centers for Disease Control and Prevention Web site. https://www.cdc.gov/hiv/clinicians/screening/partner-notification-services.html. Updated September 3, 2019. Accessed September 19, 2019.

25. US Preventive Services Task Force. Screening for bacterial vaginosis in pregnancy to prevent preterm delivery: US Preventive Task Force recommendation statement. *Ann Intern Med.* 2008;148(3):214-219.

26. Centers for Disease Control and Prevention. Recommendations for partner services programs for HIV infection, syphilis, gonorrhea, and chlamydial infection. *MMWR Recomm Rep.* 2008;57(RR-9):1-83.

27. Smith DK, Grohskopf LA, Black RJ, et al; US Department of Health and Human Services. Antiretroviral postexposure prophylaxis after sexual, injection drug use, or other nonoccupational exposure to HIV in the United States: recommendations from the U.S. Department of Health and Human Services. *MMWR Recomm Rep.* 2005;54(RR-2):1-20.

28. Kelley CF, Kahle E, Siegler A, et al. Applying a PrEP continuum of care for men who have sex with men in Atlanta, Georgia. *Clin Infect Dis.* 2015;61(10):1590-1597.

29. Kaplan JE, Benson C, Holmes KK, et al; Centers for Disease Control and Prevention, National Institutes of Health, HIV Medicine Association of the Infectious Diseases Society of America. Guidelines for prevention and treatment of opportunistic infections in HIV-infected adults and adolescents: recommendations from CDC, the National Institutes of Health, and the HIV Medicine Association of the Infectious Diseases Society of America. *MMWR Recomm Rep.* 2009;58(RR-4):1-207.

30. Bangsberg DR, Hecht FM, Charlebois ED, et al. Adherence to protease inhibitors, HIV-1 viral load, and development of drug resistance in an indigent population. *AIDS.* 2000;14(4):357-366.

31. Bloom SL. *Creating Sanctuary: Toward the Evolution of Sane Societies.* New York, NY; Routledge: 1997.

32. Centers for Disease Control and Prevention, Health Resources and Services Administration, National Institutes of Health, American Academy of HIV Medicine, Association of Nurses in AIDS Care, International Association of Providers of AIDS Care, the National Minority AIDS Council, Urban Coalition for HIV/AIDS Prevention Services. Recommendations for HIV prevention with adults and adolescents with HIV in the United States, 2014. Centers for Disease Control and Prevention Web site. https://stacks.cdc.gov/view/cdc/44064. Amended December 30, 2016. Accessed September 19, 2019.

33. Fisher JD, Cornman DH, Osborn CY, Amico KR, Fisher WA, Friedland GA. Clinician-initiated HIV risk reduction intervention for HIV-positive persons: formative research, acceptability, and fidelity of the Options Project. *J Acquir Immune Defic Syndr.* 200437(suppl 2):S78-S87.

34. Wingood GM, DiClemente RJ, Mikhail L, et al. A randomized controlled trial to reduce HIV transmission risk behaviors and sexually transmitted diseases among women living with HIV: the WiLLOW Program. *J Acquir Immune Defic Syndr.* 2004;37(suppl 2):S58-S67.

35. Richardson JL, Milam J, Stoyanoff S, et al. Using patient risk indicators to plan prevention strategies in the clinical care setting. *J Acquir Immune Defic Syndr.* 2004;37(suppl 2):S88-S94.

36. Myers JJ, Shade SB, Rose CD, et al. Interventions delivered in clinical settings are effective in reducing risk of HIV transmission among people living with HIV: results from the Health Resources and Services Administration (HRSA)'s Special Projects of National Significance initiative. *AIDS Behav.* 2010;14(3):483-492.

37. Marks G, Crepaz N, Senterfitt JW, Janssen RS. Meta-analysis of high-risk sexual behavior in persons aware and unaware they are infected with HIV in the United States: implications for HIV prevention programs. *J Acquir Immune Defic Syndr.* 2005;39(4):446-453.

38. National standards for peer support in HIV. HIV Peer Support Web site. http://hivpeersupport.com/wp-content/uploads/2017/08/national_standards_final_web.pdf. Accessed November 4, 2019.

39. Panel on Treatment of Pregnant Women with HIV Infection and Prevention of Perinatal Transmission. Recommendations for use of antiretroviral drugs in pregnant women with HIV infection and interventions to reduce perinatal HIV transmission in the United States. AIDSinfo Web site. https://aidsinfo.nih.gov/contentfiles/lvguidelines/perinatalgl.pdf. Accessed September 19, 2019.

40. US Preventive Services Task Force. Screening for chlamydial infection: U.S. Preventive Services Task Force recommendation statement. *Ann Intern Med.* 2007;147(2):128-134.

41. Branson BM, Handsfield HH, Lampe MA, et al; Centers for Disease Control and Prevention. Revised recommendations for HIV testing of adults, adolescents, and pregnancy women in health-care settings. *MMWR Recomm Rep.* 2006;55(RR-14):1-17.

42. Chou R, Cantor A, Bougatsos C, Zakher B. Screening for HIV in pregnant women: systematic review to update the U.S. Preventive Services Task Force recommendation. *Ann Intern Med.* 2012;157:719-728.

Chapter 11

Hepatitis A

David T. House, DNP, CRNP, ENP-C, FNP-BC, CNS
Rebecca Suttle, DNP, CRNP, AGACNP-BC
Kathy Gill-Hopple, PhD, RN, SANE-A, SANE-P, DF-AFN

Disease and Mimics

— Hepatitis A is one of the most prevalent forms of viral hepatitis and the most common cause of foodborne infection in the world.[1]

— Hepatitis A is an extremely contagious disease caused by the hepatitis A virus (HAV) and can lead to liver infection and inflammation.

— Diagnosis is made through detection of anti-HAV–specific immunoglobulin (IgG and IgM) antibodies.

— Since the availability of the hepatitis A vaccine in 1995, the rate of HAV in the United States has decreased more than 95%.[2] However, several HAV outbreaks have been recorded in the United States within the past 3 to 4 years as a result of person-to-person transmission and contaminated foods.[1,3,4]

— HAV is endemic in areas of Asia (except Japan), Africa, South and Central America, the Middle East, and the Western Pacific.

— HAV is transmitted through the fecal-oral route or exposure to contaminated food or water.

— The incubation period for HAV ranges between 15 to 50 days, with an average of 28 days.[2,5] HAV is replicated in the liver and passes into feces through the biliary system, typically 10 to 12 days after exposure.[5]

— The clinical presentation of HAV in adults is symptomatic, whereas the majority of children may be, and often are, asymptomatic.[2] Symptoms may present 2 to 6 weeks after exposure and include fever, nausea, vomiting, diarrhea, anorexia, abdominal pain, dark urine, jaundice, fatigue, and joint pain.[2] Symptoms typically last less than 2 months.[2,4,5]

Epidemiology

In 2016 there were an estimated 4000 new hepatitis A infections in the United States, with 70 cases identifying HAV as the cause of death.[2] The group with the highest prevalence of HAV was non-Hispanic white men between the ages 55 and 64 years.[2] Worldwide there were 7134 deaths from HAV, which accounted for 0.5% of the total mortality as a result of viral hepatitis.[1] As of May 2019, 34 countries either used or are planning on introducing the HAV vaccine as a routine immunization for at-risk children.[1]

The transmission of HAV may occur through several different mechanisms. Fecal-oral person-to-person transmission is common between infected children and adults, in homeless populations, as a result of high-risk behaviors such as injection drug use and men having sex with men (MSM), and because of travel to countries where HAV is common.[2,3,5] Improper food handling and preparation (eg, food not cooked to 185°F for 1 minute) is a common source.[2,5] In the United States, waterborne outbreaks are unlikely because of the chlorination of water.[2]

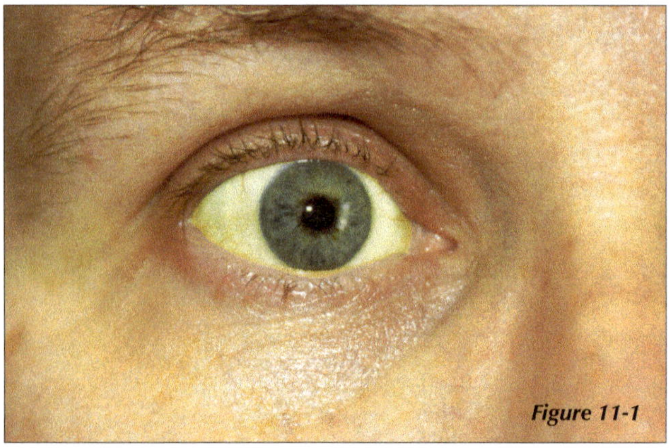

Those infected with HAV have a wide range of signs and symptoms. Signs and symptoms are more often seen in adults than children. Approximately 70% of children younger than age 6 years will be asymptomatic.[2] Acute symptoms may be mild to severe and consist of fever, nausea, vomiting, diarrhea, abdominal discomfort, hepatomegaly, loss of appetite, dark urine, jaundice, scleral icterus, fatigue, joint pain, and clay-colored bowel movements (**Figures 11-1** and **11-2**).[2,5] Acutely symptomatic children and adolescents may complain of fatigue, anorexia, nausea, fever, right upper quadrant pain, myalgia, and arthralgias.[2] Jaundice occurs in more than 70% of adolescents and adults.[1,5] HAV can lead to extrahepatic complications such as glomerulonephritis, arthritis, myocarditis, aplastic anemia, optic neuritis, and thrombocytopenia.[5] Hepatitis A is rarely fatal and does not cause chronic liver disease; however, it may cause fulminant hepatitis or debilitating symptoms.[1] In rare cases, patients will suffer severe acute liver damage; however, liver transplantation is an option.[5] Symptoms typically last less than 2 months, but 10% to 15% of symptomatic patients may relapse or experience prolonged symptoms for up to 6 months.[2]

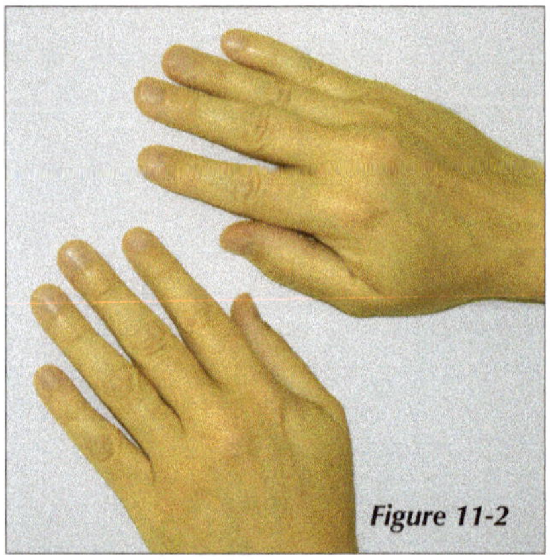

Figure 11-1. Conjunctival icterus.

Figure 11-2. Jaundice.

Identifying hepatitis A based on clinical presentation is difficult to differentiate from other types of acute viral hepatitis. Diagnosis is made through detection of anti-HAV–specific immunoglobulin antibodies (IgG and IgM).[1,2] Before the onset of symptoms (5 to 10 days) IgM becomes positive, and it may be detectable for up to 1 year.[5] A positive IgG is typically identified in the initial recovery phase or may indicate previous exposure or HAV immunization.[5] Additional tests to detect HAV RNA, such as reverse transcriptase polymerase chain reaction, may be used for diagnosis.[1,5]

Treatment Guidelines

There is no specific treatment for HAV. HAV is a self-limiting disease, and therapy is aimed at supportive measures, such as replacement of fluids lost from vomiting and diarrhea.[1,2] Avoid medications with hepatic metabolism, such as acetaminophen, and alcohol to prevent further liver damage. Hospitalization may be necessary as a result of dehydration or symptoms of acute liver failure.[2]

HAV treatment is aimed at prevention through good hand hygiene, sanitation practices, food and water precautions, and vaccination.[2,5,6] Active vaccination consists of either a 2-dose series of hepatitis A vaccine or a 3-dose series of hepatitis A and hepatitis B vaccine, which provides lifelong immunity (**Table 11-1**).[2,5] Almost 100% of patients vaccinated with the hepatitis A vaccine develop protective levels of antibodies within 1 month after only 1 dose.[1,2]

Vaccination Recommendations

— Children older than 12 months and children adopted from HAV-endemic countries[1,2,3]

— Individuals at risk for infection (eg, homeless populations, inmates in jails and drug treatment facilities)[1,2,3,5,7]

— MSM[1,2,3,5,7]

— Illicit injection and noninjection drug users[3,5,7]

— Individuals traveling to HAV-endemic areas, such as Asia, Africa, South and Central America, the Middle East, and the Western Pacific[1,2,3,5]

— Immunocompromised individuals and those with chronic liver disease and clotting disorders[2,3,5]

— Individuals who work with HAV-infected animals[2,3,5]

— Individuals diagnosed with hepatitis B or C[8]

Immune globulin IM (IGIM; GamaSTAN S/D) is approved by the US Food and Drug Administration for hepatitis A prophylaxis and provides immediate, passive short-term protection both before and after exposure (**Table 11-2**).[2,5]

Table 11-1. Hepatitis A Vaccination Recommendations

Vaccine	Age	Schedule (months)*	No. of Doses	Volume (mL)	Dose (U)	Description
HAVRIX†	12 months to 18 years	0, 6-12	2	0.5	720	Hepatitis A inactivated vaccine; approved for ages ≥ 1 year
	≥19 years	0, 6-12	2	1	1440	
VAQTA‡	12 months to 18 years	0, 6-18	2	0.5	25	Hepatitis A inactivated vaccine; approved for ages ≥ 1 year
	≥19 years	0, 6-18	2	1	50	
TWINRIX§	≥18 years	0, 1, 6	3	1	720	Hepatitis A (inactivated) & B (recombinant); ages ≥18 years

For more information on treatment, see the CDC's sexually transmitted disease guidelines at https://www.cdc.gov/hepatitis/hav/havfaq.htm.
**0 months represents timing of the initial dose; subsequent numbers represent months after the initial dose.*
†Hepatitis A vaccine, inactivated, GlaxoSmithKline.
‡Hepatitis A vaccine, inactivated, Merck & Co., Inc.
§Combined hepatitis A and hepatitis B vaccine, inactivated, GlaxoSmithKline.
mL, Milliliters; U, Enzyme-linked immunosorbent assay (ELISA) units
Data from CDC.[9]

Table 11-2. Immune Globulin IM (GamaSTAN S/D) (Grifols Therapeutics, Inc.)

Indication	Dose
Preexposure Prophylaxis	
Up to 1 month of travel	0.1 mL/kg
Up to 2 months of travel	0.2 mL/kg
2 months of travel or longer	0.2 mL/kg (repeat every 2 months)
Postexposure Prophylaxis	0.1 mL/kg

Data from CDC.[9]

Special Considerations

— Patients with a history of severe allergic reaction or hypersensitivity to alum or the preservative 2-phenoxyethanol in HAVRIX should not receive the hepatitis A vaccine.[2]

— ***Children and adolescents:*** Children and adolescents are generally asymptomatic and may serve as a source of infection.[2] Children younger than 6 years of age can shed HAV for up to 10 weeks longer than adults.[5] Therefore, the HAV vaccine is part of the immunization schedule for children in the United States. However, vaccination is not recommended for children younger than 12 months.[2,5]

— ***Household members caring for a child from an endemic area:*** It is recommended that caregivers be vaccinated at least 2 weeks before exposure to the child.[6]

— ***Pregnancy:*** No identified transmission from mother to fetus has been discovered.[2,5] However, HAV infection during pregnancy has been associated with premature rupture of membranes, preterm labor, and placental abruption.[2] Therefore, it is recommended that pregnant women who are at risk receive the hepatitis A vaccine.[2]

— ***Individuals with blood disorders:*** Although rare, patients with blood clotting disorders such as hemophilia could potentially acquire HAV through the administration of blood products such as solvent/detergent–treated factor VIII and IX concentrates.[2]

— ***Animal handlers:*** Outbreaks have been reported in individuals who work with nonhuman primates infected with HAV as a result of contact with animal saliva.[2,5]

— ***International travel:*** Those traveling internationally to highly or intermediately endemic areas such as Asia (except Japan), Africa, South and Central America, the Middle East, and the Western Pacific are encouraged to get the hepatitis A vaccination or immune globulin.[1,2] Travelers should receive education on hygiene (hand washing), sanitation, food, and water precautions.[2]

— ***Postexposure prophylaxis:*** Within 2 weeks of exposure to HAV, patients who have not previously received the hepatitis A vaccine should be administered immune globulin (0.02 mL/kg) or a single dose of monovalent hepatitis A vaccine (HAVRIX or VAQTA).[2] It is recommended that immune globulin be used for children younger than 12 months of age, patients with chronic liver disease, older persons, or those with severe cases of hepatitis A. Additionally, a dose of the vaccine should be given at the same time as the immune globulin, followed by a scheduled second vaccine dose.[2]

— ***Immunocompromised, HIV, and chronic liver disease:*** Antibody response is directly related to $CD4^+$ levels in patients with human immunodeficiency virus (HIV).[2] Patients with advanced HIV and chronic liver disease have lower antibody concentrations and lower efficacy after vaccination for hepatitis.[2] It is recommended that patients who are immunocompromised, have acquired immunodeficiency syndrome, are on hemodialysis, or have chronic liver disease receive the hepatitis A vaccine.

Case Studies

Adult Case Study 11-1

PM is a 20-year-old man who recently arrived home from his first year of college. He had previously been in good health, was taking no medications, and had not traveled outside of the United States. Ten days after arriving home, he began to complain of unusual fatigue, generalized malaise, minimal appetite, nausea, and was unable to eat without vomiting. He goes to his primary care provider after 2 days of feeling ill. He denies sexual activity, drug use, or getting tattoos. He does report partying heavily with friends the night after he returned home.

Examination

PM's temperature is 100.6°F (38.6°C), pulse 100 beats per minute, and blood pressure 110/58 mm Hg. He is well developed and well nourished, with skin that is pink, warm, and dry. The abdomen is soft without tenderness or hepatomegaly.

Laboratory Testing

Complete blood cell count and metabolic panel are within normal limits. Anti-HAV IgM is positive. Anti-HAV IgG and hepatitis B panel are negative.

Treatment

Instructions for supportive care are given, with no restrictions on activity or diet. PM is instructed to return if the nausea and vomiting continue. The patient receives a combined hepatitis A and B vaccine.

Child Case Study 11-2

BK is a 5-year-old child from Central America, brought to the United States by her mother. Two weeks after arriving in the country, she became fatigued while playing and had a significant decrease in appetite. After 2 days, her mother became concerned when the child began vomiting and complaining of generalized pain in her extremities, so she took the child to the emergency department of the nearest hospital.

Examination

The child appears to be of normal growth and development for her age. Her abdomen is soft, yet she complains of right upper quadrant tenderness and mild pruritus, and she exhibits mild scleral icterus and intermittent vomiting. The liver edge is palpated well below the right costal margin, and there is no splenomegaly present. BK has a low-grade fever of 99.9°F (37.7°C) axillary, pulse 110 beats per minute, and blood pressure 90/64 mm Hg.

Laboratory Testing

Anti-hepatitis A surface antigen, anti-HBc, anti-HCV, and IgM anti-HEV tests are completed. Results are positive for anti-HAV IgM. A complete blood cell count, metabolic panel, and coagulation profile are within normal limits. Stool is guaiac negative, and urinalysis is negative for bilirubin.

Treatment

BK is hospitalized for 3 days and receives intravenous hydration and an antiemetic. She is released after a successful course of treatment. The child's mother receives a hepatitis A vaccine, as do the other family members she will be staying with.

References

1. Hepatitis A. World Health Organization Web site. https://www.who.int/news-room/fact-sheets/detail/hepatitis-a. Published July 9, 2019. Accessed July 21, 2019.

2. Viral hepatitis: hepatitis A information. Centers for Disease Control and Prevention Web site. https://www.cdc.gov/hepatitis/hav/index.htm. Updated June 13, 2019. Accessed July 21, 2019.

3. Campos-Outcalt D. CDC provides advice on recent hepatitis A outbreaks. *J Fam Prac.* 2018;67(1):30-32.

4. Linder KA, Malani PN. Hepatitis A. *JAMA.* 2017;318(23):2393.

5. O'Neil J. Issues leading to the recent outbreaks of hepatitis A. *J Nurse Pract.* 2018;14(9):639-644.

6. Nelson NP. Travelers' health: travel-related infectious diseases. Centers for Disease Control and Prevention Web site. https://wwwnc.cdc.gov/travel/yellowbook/2020/travel-related-infectious-diseases/hepatitis-a. Updated June 1, 2019. Accessed July 22, 2019.

7. Kuehn B. Shifting hepatitis A epidemiology. *JAMA.* 2018;320(24):2522.

8. Workowski K, Bolan GA; Centers for Disease Control and Prevention. Sexually transmitted diseases treatment guidelines, 2015. *MMWR Recomm Rep.* 2015;64(RR-03):1-137.

9. Viral hepatitis: hepatitis A questions and answers for health professionals. Centers for Disease Control and Prevention Web site. https://www.cdc.gov/hepatitis/hav/havfaq.htm#general. Updated July 27, 2019. Accessed August 6, 2019.

Appendix 11-1. Hepatitis A, B, and C: Learn the Differences

Appendix 11-1. Hepatitis A, B, and C: Learn the Differences

	Hepatitis A - Caused by the Hepatitis A Virus (HAV)	Hepatitis B - Caused by the Hepatitis B Virus (HBV)	Hepatitis C - Caused by the Hepatitis C Virus (HCV)
How is it spread?	HAV is found in the feces of people with hepatitis A and is usually spread by close personal contact (including sex or living in the same household). It can also be spread by eating food or drinking water contaminated with HAV.	HBV is found in blood and certain body fluids. The virus is spread when blood or body fluid from an infected person enters the body of a person who is not immune. HBV is spread through having unprotected sex with an infected person, sharing needles or "works" when shooting drugs, exposure to needlesticks or sharps on the job, or from an infected mother to her baby during birth. Exposure to infected blood in ANY situation can be a risk for transmission.	HCV is found in blood and certain body fluids. The virus is spread when blood or body fluid from an HCV-infected person enters another person's body. HCV is spread through sharing needles or "works" when shooting drugs, through exposure to needlesticks or sharps on the job, or sometimes from an infected mother to her baby during birth. It is possible to transmit HCV during sex, but it is not common.
Who should be vaccinated?	— People who wish to be protected from HAV infection — All children at age 1 year (12–23 months) — Men who have sex with men — Users of street drugs (injecting and non-injecting) — People who travel or work in any area of the world except the United States, Canada, Western Europe, Japan, New Zealand, and Australia — People who will have close personal contact with an international adoptee from a country where HAV infection is common during the first 60 days following the adoptee's arrival in the United States — People with chronic liver disease, including HCV — People working with HAV in a laboratory — People with clotting factor disorders (eg, hemophilia)	— All infants, children, and teens ages 0 through 18 years — Any adult who wants to be protected from HBV infection — Sexually active people who are not in long-term, mutually monogamous relationships — Men who have sex with men — People seeking evaluation or treatment for a sexually transmitted disease — Health care or public safety workers who might be exposed to blood or body fluids — Residents and staff of facilities for developmentally disabled people — Adults younger than 60 years of age with diabetes — Dialysis and pre-dialysis patients — People infected with HIV — People in close personal contact (ie, household or sexual) with someone who has chronic HBV infection — Current or recent injection-drug users — Travelers to regions of the world where hepatitis B is common (Asia, Africa, the Amazon Basin in South America, the Pacific Islands, Eastern Europe, or the Middle East) — People with chronic liver disease	**Who should be tested?** There is no vaccine to prevent HCV. Testing for HCV is recommended for the following groups of people. — People born during 1945–1965 — Injecting drug users — Recipients of clotting factors made before 1987 — Hemodialysis patients — Recipients of blood or solid organ transplants before 1992 — Infants born to HCV-infected mothers — People with undiagnosed abnormal liver test results — People with HIV infection Although HCV is not commonly spread through sex, individuals having sex with multiple partners or with an infected steady partner may be at increased risk of HCV infection.

(continued)

Appendix 11-1. Hepatitis A, B, and C: Learn the Differences *(continued)*

	Hepatitis A - Caused by the Hepatitis A Virus (HAV)	Hepatitis B - Caused by the Hepatitis B Virus (HBV)	Hepatitis C - Caused by the Hepatitis C Virus (HCV)
Symptoms	Viral hepatitis symptoms are similar no matter which type of hepatitis you have. If symptoms occur, you might experience any or all of the following: jaundice (yellowing of the skin and whites of the eyes), fever, loss of appetite, fatigue, dark urine, joint pain, abdominal pain, diarrhea, nausea, and vomiting. Very rarely, a recently acquired case of viral hepatitis can cause liver failure and death. Sometimes in these instances, a liver transplant (if a liver is available) can save a life. Note: For all types of viral hepatitis, symptoms are less common in children than in adults, and for people of any age with HCV infection, they are less likely to experience symptoms.		
	Incubation period: 15 to 50 days, average 28 days	**Incubation period:** 60 to 150 days, average 90 days	**Incubation period:** 14 to 180 days, average 45 days
Chronic infection	There is no chronic infection. Once you have had HAV infection, you cannot get it again. About 15 out of 100 people infected with HAV will have prolonged illness or relapsing symptoms over a 6–9 month period.	Chronic infection occurs in up to 90% of infants infected at birth; in about 30% of children infected at ages 1–5 years; and less than 5% of people infected after age 5 years. In the United States, about 2 000 people die each year from hepatitis B. Death from chronic liver disease occurs in 15%–25% of chronically infected people. People who have chronic HBV infection have a much higher risk of liver failure and liver cancer.	Chronic infection occurs in 75%–85% of newly infected people and 70% of chronically infected people go on to develop chronic liver disease. In the United States, about 20 000 people die each year from HCV. People who have chronic HCV infection have a much higher risk of liver failure and liver cancer. Chronic HCV-related liver disease is the leading cause for liver transplant.
What treatment helps?	— There is no treatment for HAV other than supportive care. — Avoid alcohol. It can worsen liver disease.	— People with chronic HBV infection should have a medical evaluation for liver disease every 6–12 months. Several antiviral medications are currently licensed for the treatment of individuals with chronic HBV. These drugs are effective in preventing serious liver problems in up to 40% of patients, but the drugs do not get rid of the virus. Liver transplant is the last resort, but livers are not always available. — Avoid alcohol. It can worsen liver disease. — There is no medication to treat recently acquired HBV infection.	— People with chronic HCV infection should have a medical evaluation for liver disease every 6–12 months. There are drugs licensed for the treatment of individuals with chronic HCV infection. Combination therapy is currently the treatment of choice and can eliminate the virus in approximately 40–50% of patients with genotype 1 (the most common genotype in the United States). — Get vaccinated against hepatitis A and B. — Avoid alcohol. It can worsen liver disease. — There is no medication for the treatment of recently acquired HCV infection.

(continued)

Appendix 11-1. Hepatitis A, B, and C: Learn the Differences ***(continued)***

	Hepatitis A - Caused by the Hepatitis A Virus (HAV)	Hepatitis B - Caused by the Hepatitis B Virus (HBV)	Hepatitis C - Caused by the Hepatitis C Virus (HCV)
How is it prevented?	— Get vaccinated! Safe and effective vaccines to prevent HAV infection have been available in the United States since 1995. — Always wash your hands with soap and water after using the toilet, changing a diaper, and before preparing or eating food. — For a recent exposure to someone with HAV or if traveling soon (leaving in less than 2 weeks) to an area of the world where hepatitis A is common, see your health care provider about your need for hepatitis A vaccine or a dose of immune globulin (IG).	— Get vaccinated! Hepatitis B vaccination is the best protection. Two or 3 shots are given over a period of 1 to 6 months, depending on brand. — Whenever a woman is pregnant, she should be tested for hepatitis B (HBsAg blood test); infants born to HBV-infected mothers should be given HBIG (hepatitis B immune globulin) and vaccine within 12 hours of birth. — Tell your sex partner(s) to get vaccinated too, and always follow "safer sex" practices (eg, using condoms).	— There is no vaccine to prevent HCV infection. — HCV can be spread by sex, but this is not common. If you are not in a mutually monogamous relationship, use latex condoms correctly and every time to prevent the spread of sexually transmitted diseases. (The efficacy of latex condoms in preventing HCV infection is unknown, but their proper use may reduce transmission.) In addition to getting hepatitis A vaccine, you should also get hepatitis B vaccine.

Adapted from Immunization Action Coalition, Saint Paul, MN. www.immunize.org/catg.d/p4075.pdf. Updated October 2018. Accessed November 26, 2019.

Chapter 12

Hepatitis B

Rebecca Suttle, DNP, CRNP, AGACNP-BC
David T. House, DNP, CRNP, ENP-C, FNP-BC, CNS

Disease and Mimics

— Hepatitis B virus (HBV) can cause serious acute viral illness that can lead to chronic liver disease, including cirrhosis and hepatocellular cancer and, in some cases, death.

— HBV is a partly double-stranded DNA virus with many serological markers: HBsAg and anti-HBs, HBeAg and anti-HBe, and anti-HBc immunoglobulin M (IgM) and G (IgG).

— HBV is transmitted via the blood, semen, or other body fluid of an infected person by sexual contact, through sharing of drug injection equipment, or via perinatal transmission at birth.[1] It can survive outside the body for at least 7 days and can cause infection during that time.[2]

— Individual patient outcomes vary, including severity of symptoms and progression to chronic infection. Outcomes depend on the interaction between the virus and the host's immune response.[3]

— Infants and children have a much higher risk for progression to chronic infection compared with adults.[1]

— Screening is recommended for at-risk groups, and vaccination can prevent infection.

— There is no treatment for acute infection other than supportive care; however, long-term antiviral therapy for chronic infection decreases hepatic inflammation and can reverse cirrhosis, as well as reduce risk for hepatocellular carcinoma.[3]

— Chronic HBV infection has 3 distinct phases, including immune tolerance, immune clearance, and inactive phases with risk for reactivation.[4]

Epidemiology

HBV infection is the most common chronic viral infection in the world, with an estimated 2 billion people infected and more than 350 million chronic carriers.[3] Hepatitis B vaccine became available in 1981.[3] The rate of new HBV infections in the United States declined from 1990 to 2014, mostly because of the initiation of routine hepatitis B vaccinations in children in 1991.[2,3,5] A slight increase in 2014 occured because of increasing illicit injected drug use.[5] An estimated 20 900 acute hepatitis B diagnoses occurred in 2016, although only 3218 were actually reported cases.[5] It is estimated that there are approximately 850 000 to 2.2 million chronic cases of hepatitis B in the United States.[5] From 2001 through 2016, the incidence of HBV cases reported in the United States was consistently highest among those aged 30 to 39 years and lowest among those aged 0 to 19 years.[6] The reported incidence of acute hepatitis B was higher for males than for females during this period, with the rate for males being approximately 1.5 times higher than that of females in 2016.[6]

Until 2013, historical data showed that non-Hispanic blacks had the highest incidence rate of acute hepatitis B in the United States.[6] In 2016 the rate of acute hepatitis B was highest for non-Hispanic whites.[6] Non-Hispanic whites were the only ethnic group to have increasing rates of infection beginning in 2009, whereas all other ethnic groups had declining rates from 2001 to 2016.[6] About 90% of acutely infected infants will develop chronic HBV compared with 25% to 50% of children (aged 1 to 5 years) and 2% to 6% of adults.[1] Approximately 40% of men and 15% of women with HBV will die as a result of liver cirrhosis or hepatocellular carcinoma.[3]

Transmission and Prevention

HBV is transmitted via contact with infected blood or semen. The major modes of transmission include sexual interaction, use of infected drug injection equipment, and perinatal transmission.[6] Risk for infection is higher in infants born to infected mothers, sex partners of infected persons, men who have sex with men (MSM), injection drug users, household contacts or sexual partners of those with chronic HBV infection, health care and public safety workers at risk for occupational exposure to blood or body fluids, and hemodialysis patients.[2] Screening for HBV should test for 3 HBV seromarkers (hepatitis B surface antigen [HBsAg], antibody to HBsAg [anti-HBs], and antibody to hepatitis B core antigen [anti-HBc]). Screening should include those born in countries with a high HBV prevalence (2% or higher), MSM, injection drug users, people positive for human immunodeficiency virus (HIV), household and sexual contacts of HBV-infected persons, those on immunosuppressive therapy, those with end-stage renal disease, blood and tissue donors, or those with elevated aminotransferase levels.[2] Pregnant women and infants born to HBV-infected mothers should also be screened for infection.[2]

Prevention of HBV infection depends on 2 key actions: avoiding transmission and inducing immunity in people who have not been exposed.[3] Universal precautions and the screening of donated blood have significantly reduced transmission of HBV in health care settings.[3] Transmission can also be reduced by counseling individuals who are infected, identifying at-risk individuals and providing screening and vaccination, and employing universal vaccination of neonates.[3] Prevention of HBV infection in neonates and children is vital given the increased risk of progression to chronic infection in these groups. Routine vaccination of neonates is recommended by the Centers for Disease Control and Prevention (CDC); however, vaccination can also be performed in childhood or later.[2] There are currently 3 single-agent vaccines and 2 combination vaccines available in the United States. Vaccine schedule and dosing should be followed per the CDC recommendations.

Diagnosis and Treatment

Symptoms during acute infection and individual outcomes depend on the age at infection and the host's immune response.[3] Infants and children younger than 5 years of age, as well as immunosuppressed adults, are often asymptomatic.[6] Approximately 70% of adults with acute HBV infection will not have symptoms.[3] When present, signs and symptoms can include fever, fatigue, anorexia, nausea, vomiting, abdominal pain, dark urine (**Figure 12-1**), clay-colored bowel movements, joint pain, or jaundice (**Figure 12-2**).[1]

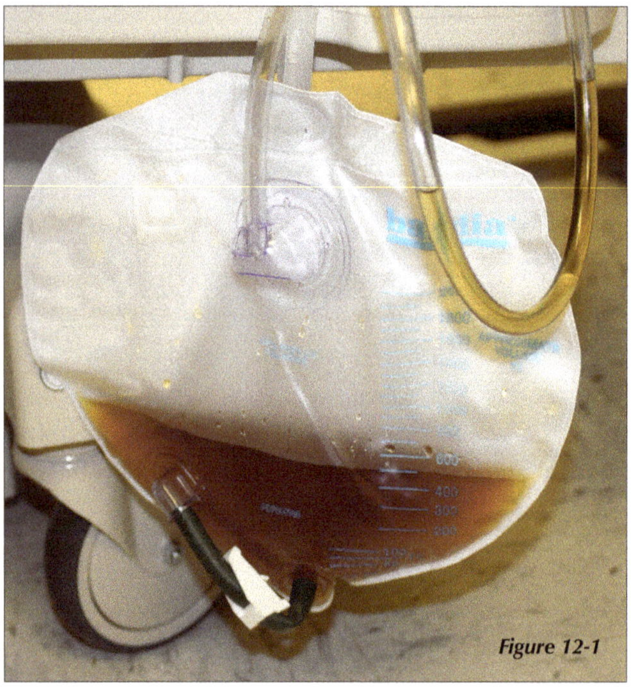

Figure 12-1

Figure 12-1. *Dark urine is symptomatic of hepatitis B infection.*

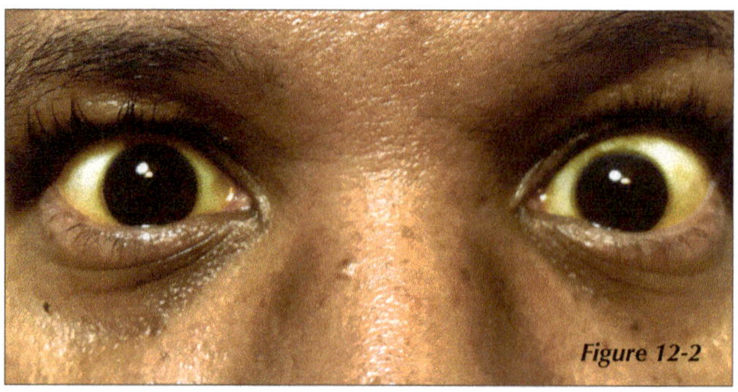

Figure 12-2

Figure 12-2. *Jaundiced eyes.*

Most individuals with chronic infection are asymptomatic. Chronic hepatitis B infection may progress to cirrhosis or hepatocellular carcinoma. The incidence of hepatocellular carcinoma is slightly higher in individuals with cirrhosis.[3] Progression to these conditions is often first noticeable on liver function tests such as alanine aminotransferase (ALT) and aspartate aminotransferase (AST). Factors associated with an increased risk of hepatocellular carcinoma include age greater than 50 years, male gender, family history of hepatocellular carcinoma, African or Asian race, obesity, diabetes mellitus, use of alcohol, and concurrent infection with hepatitis C (HCV) or D (HDV) virus.[3]

HBV has several serological markers that are known to be present or absent in varying combinations depending on the chronicity and timing of infection (**Table 12-1**). These markers include HBsAg, anti-HBs, HBeAg (hepatitis B e antigen), anti-HBe (hepatitis B e antibody), and anti-HBc, anti-HBc IgM (IgM antibody to hepatitis B core antigen), and anti-HBc IgG (IgG antibody to hepatitis B core antigen).[2,3] HBV DNA can be used to directly measure the viral load and can help the provider assess the activity of the virus as well as monitor response to treatment when taken into consideration with other laboratory values. The patterns that the serological markers follow are predictable throughout the progression of both acute and chronic infections (**Figure 12-3**). Accurate clinical interpretation of the markers is essential for proper diagnosis and treatment. For more information on treatment, see the CDC's sexually transmitted disease guidelines at https://www.cdc.gov/vaccines/vpd/hepb/hcp/index.html.

Table 12-1. Interpretations for Screening Tests for HBV Infection

Interpretation	Screening Test Results			Management
	HBsAG	**Anti-HBc**	**Anti-HBs**	
Chronic hepatitis B	+	+	–	Additional testing and management needed
Past HBV infection, resolved	–	+	+	No further management unless immunocompromised or undergoing chemotherapy or immunosuppressive therapy
Past HBV infection, resolved *OR* false positive	–	+	–	HBV DNA testing if immunocompromised patient
Immune	–	–	+	No further testing
Uninfected and not immune	–	–	–	No further testing
Acute infection	+	+ (IgM anti-HBc)		Monitor
Isolated core antibody*	–	–	–	Dependent on situation

**Can be a result of the following:*
- *— False positive: Repeat testing required.*
- *— Past infection: No action needed.*
- *— Occult HBV infection: Needs to be known if the patient ever became immunosuppressed or was given chemotherapy or treated with antiviral therapy for HCV infection. Consider monitoring HBV DNA.*
- *— Passive transfer to infant born to HBsAg-positive mother. No specific action needed.*

Data from Terrault NA, et al[4]; and CDC.[2]

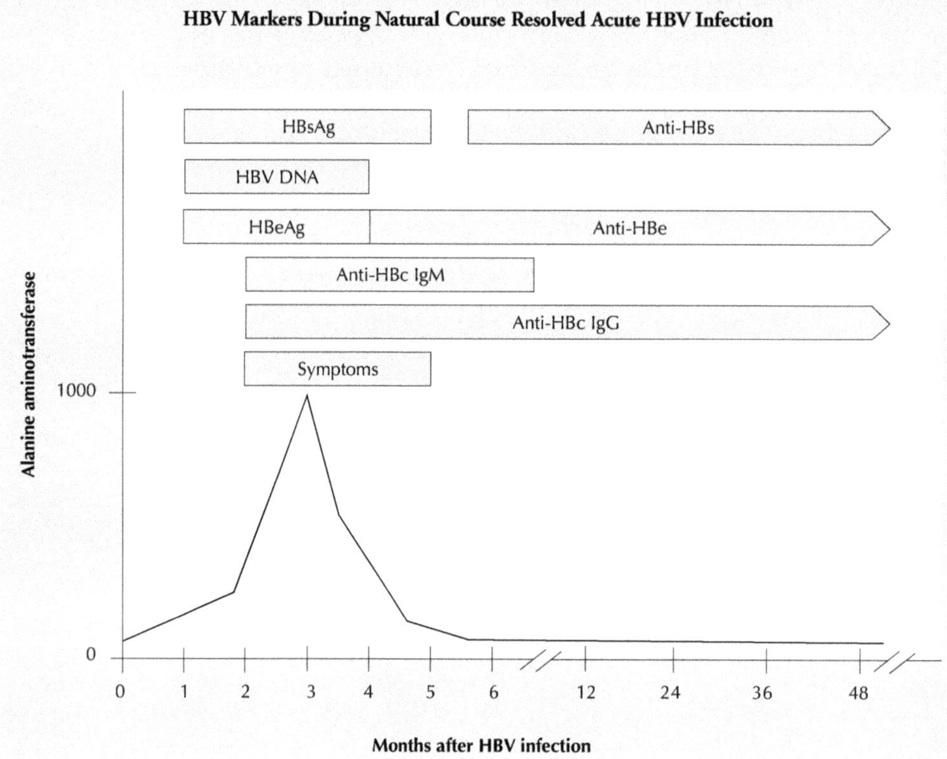

Figure 12-3-a

Figure 12-3-a. *HBV markers during natural course resolved acute HBV infection.*

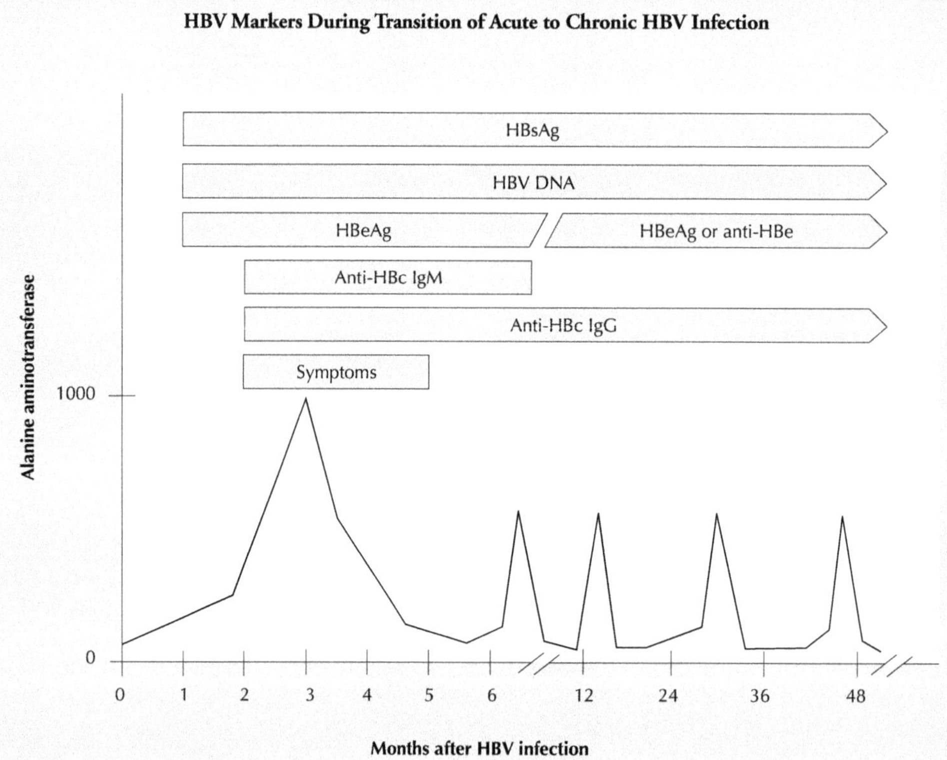

Figure 12-3-b

Figure 12-3-b. *HBV markers during transition of acute to chronic HBV infection.*

Acute hepatitis B infection is typically a self-limiting illness in individuals who are otherwise immunocompetent. Treatment during acute infection consists of supportive care. Rarely, patients will have severe courses of acute HBV or will have resulting liver failure. In these cases, management with antiviral therapy is indicated.[4]

Management of chronic infection should include screening for other diseases, such as HIV, HCV, and HDV. The severity of the liver disease should be established using blood counts and liver enzymes as well as invasive or noninvasive methods as indicated to assess the liver more directly (ie, biopsy) and alfa-fetoprotein and ultrasound to screen for hepatocellular carcinoma.[4]

The decision to treat chronically infected patients is typically based on ALT levels, along with patient age, HBV DNA levels, and severity of liver disease and symptoms.[4] The goal of treatment is to prevent cirrhosis, hepatic failure, and hepatocellular carcinoma; suppress HBV replication; and induce remission of liver disease that is present.[4] HBeAg status is also used as a guide for treatment-based decisions because prolonged HBeAg positivity is a risk factor for progression to cirrhosis and hepatocellular carcinoma.[1,4] HBeAg seroconversion (conversion from HBeAg to anti-HBe) is often used as a therapeutic endpoint because this conversion indicates a change from the active phase of the disease to the inactive carrier state.[4]

Antiviral therapies available for the treatment of chronic HBV infection include conventional and pegylated interferon alfa and nucleos(t)ide analogues (NAs), which include lamivudine, adefovir, and telbivudine (less preferred options) and entecavir and tenofovir, which have 3 preparations.[4] As a result of increasing issues with resistance to NAs, individuals who have minimal disease or those who are unlikely to achieve a sustained response, should not be treated with NA, especially when younger than age 30.[4]

Patient education is critical to ensure that infected individuals understand the need for lifelong monitoring, transmission prevention, and the appropriate lifestyle changes.[4] Lifestyle changes should include limiting or abstaining from alcohol intake. Caution should be exercised when taking drugs that are metabolized by the liver, such as acetaminophen. Those with HBsAg positivity should be counseled on transmission prevention.

Special Considerations

— ***Coinfection with HCV:*** All individuals with HBV infection should be screened for HCV coinfection by testing for the presence of anti-HCV. HBsAg-positive patients are at risk of HBV DNA and ALT flares while on HCV direct-acting antiviral (DAA) therapy. Because of this, those who do not meet treatment standards for HBV but are being treated for HCV should have regular monitoring of their HBV DNA levels. HBsAg-negative patients with HCV are at very low risk of reactivation with HCV-DAA therapy and only infrequent monitoring of ALT levels is recommended, with HBV DNA and HBsAg testing being limited to those whose ALT levels increase or fail to normalize during or after treatment.[4]

— ***Patients who receive immunosuppressive or cytotoxic therapy:*** Individuals who have had a previous and resolved acute HBV infection are at risk of HBV reactivation if they begin immunosuppressive or cytotoxic therapy for treatment of a different medical condition. Reactivation will cause an increase in HBV DNA compared with baseline and reverse seroconversion from HBsAg negativity to HBsAg positivity for HBsAg-negative and anti-HBc–positive individuals. If HBV reactivates, a hepatitis flare can occur and would be manifested by an ALT elevation. Routine screening for HBV in individuals before the start of immunosuppressive therapy has become standard in many areas. Prophylactic treatment for HBV reactivation is recommended in certain at-risk groups. Close HBV monitoring is recommended in other groups, with on-demand treatment started if necessary.[4]

— ***Pregnancy:*** The American Association for the Study of Liver Disease (AASLD) suggests antiviral therapy to reduce the risk of perinatal transmission of HBV in HBsAg-positive pregnant women with an HBV DNA level greater than 200 000 IU/mL. Infants born to HBsAg-positive mothers should receive immunoprophylaxis using the HBV vaccination with or without hepatitis B immunoglobulin. Tenofovir disoproxil fumarate (TDF) is the preferred antiviral therapy in this group, with lamivudine and telbivudine being the other pregnancy-approved options. Treatment is typically started at 28 to 32 weeks and stopped at birth or shortly after with monitoring for ALT flares (every 3 months for 6 months) after the end of treatment. Breastfeeding is not contraindicated.[4]

— ***Children:*** The AASLD suggests antiviral therapy in HBeAg-positive children (aged 2 to <18 years) with both elevated ALT and measurable HBV DNA levels, with the goal of achieving sustained HBeAg seroconversion. Providers should keep in mind that the upper limit of normal values for ALT in healthy children are not firmly established and appear to vary based on multiple factors. Interferon alfa-2b is approved for children 1 year and older, whereas lamivudine and entecavir are approved for children 2 years and older. TDF is approved for children 12 years and older. Resistance patterns to NAs should be considered when choosing treatment. Children who stop antiviral therapy should be monitored every 3 months for at least 1 year. The AASLD recommends against the use of antiviral therapy in HBeAg-positive children (aged 2 to <18 years) with persistently normal ALT, regardless of HBV-DNA level.[4]

Case Studies

Adult Case Study 12-1

CD is a 36-year-old Caucasian man who presents to the emergency department (ED) with extreme fatigue and nausea and vomiting over the past 4 weeks, as well as dark urine over the past few days. He reports a year-long history of injection drug abuse after a failed marriage, although he has been clean for 2 months. He reports smoking cigarettes at a rate of half a pack per day and denies current use of alcohol or any illegal drugs. He identifies as heterosexual and reports having multiple female sexual partners. He lives with his brother at this time. He denies any recent sick contacts and has no family history of any chronic illnesses or infectious diseases. He denies having any other medical problems, including a history of HIV and hepatitis, as well as a history of any surgical procedures. On review of symptoms, he reports mild abdominal pain as well as decreased appetite.

Examination

Patient has a temperature of 99.9°F. The sclera is slightly jaundice. There are no other skin changes. The abdomen is nontender; no hepatosplenomegaly is present.

Laboratory Testing

ALT 1800 IU/mL, AST 1100 IU/mL; anti-hepatitis A virus, anti-HCV, and anti-HDV are negative. HBsAg and IgM anti-HBC are positive. HBV DNA is undetectable.

Treatment

CD is told to continue avoiding alcohol intake and to increase fluid intake to replace volume lost. He is told to avoid acetaminophen. He is educated on transmission of HBV. In addition to encouraging testing of his sexual partners, he is told to use barrier protection during sexual intercourse and to not share toothbrushes, razors, needles, or any other injection equipment. He is told to cover open cuts and scratches and to clean any blood spills with bleach solution. He is advised to not donate blood, organs, or sperm. He is referred to a local liver/gastrointestinal clinic and encouraged to keep his follow-up appointment, because he will need extended monitoring.

Child Case Study 12-2

LH is a 22-year-old woman presenting to the ED in labor. She recently immigrated from sub-Saharan Africa and reports no medical history. With the assistance of an interpreter, it is determined she is roughly 37 weeks pregnant. On initial evaluation, she is noted to have scleral icterus and slight jaundice. LH is transported to the labor and delivery unit where, on arrival, she gives birth to a baby boy, DH.

Examination

DH is a 6-hour-old male infant whose status is uncomplicated after spontaneous vaginal delivery. Initial newborn assessment reveals a healthy-appearing infant, with an Apgar score of 8. He weighs 3000 g, is 17 inches long, and has a head circumference of 12 inches.

Laboratory Testing

Predelivery laboratory tests initiated in the ED for the mother are negative for group B streptococcus and positive for the HBeAg. All other laboratory results are within normal limits. Postbirth laboratory results for DH are within normal limits.

Treatment

DH received 0.5 mL of the hepatitis B immune globulin (HBIG) intramuscularly and 0.5 mL of the hepatitis B vaccination (Recombivax HB) within 12 hours after birth.

At DH's follow-up visit with the pediatrician, there were no reported complications. Repeat laboratory testing did not reveal any signs of HBV. DH completes the hepatitis B vaccinations at his 1- and 6-month pediatrician visits.

References

1. Viral hepatitis: hepatitis B information. Centers for Disease Control and Prevention Web site. https://www.cdc.gov/hepatitis/hbv/. Updated June 13, 2019. Accessed August 2, 2019.

2. Viral hepatitis: Q&As for health professionals. Centers for Disease Control and Prevention Web site. https://www.cdc.gov/hepatitis/hbv/hbvfaq.htm#overview. Updated May 16, 2019. Accessed August 2, 2019.

3. Trépo C, Chan HL, Loc A. Hepatitis B virus infection. *Lancet.* 2014;384(9959):2053-2063.

4. Terrault NA, Lok ASF, McMahon BJ, et al. Update on prevention, diagnosis, and treatment of chronic hepatitis B: AASLD 2018 hepatitis B guidance. *Hepatology.* 2018;67(4):1560-1599.

5. Disease burden from hepatitis A, B, and C in the United States. Centers for Disease Control and Prevention Web site. https://www.cdc.gov/hepatitis/PDFs/disease_burden.pdf. Updated April 18, 2018. Accessed August 2, 2019

6. Viral hepatitis 2016 surveillance: hepatitis B virus. Centers for Disease Control and Prevention Web site. https://www.cdc.gov/hepatitis/statistics/2016surveillance/index.htm. Updated April 16, 2018. Accessed August 8, 2019.

Chapter 13

Hepatitis C

Alice Springer Bristow, DNP, CRNP, FNP-BC, CWCN, CNE
April Love, MSN, RN, RNC-OB, CNE
Elisabeth Pelt, MSN, APRN, WHNP-BC

Disease and Mimics

— Hepatitis C virus (HCV) is an RNA virus of the Flaviviridae family with varying surface proteins, some capable of changing constantly to allow the virus to avoid the immune system's protection.[1,2]

— It is the most common chronic bloodborne infection in the United States. Seven genotypes with more than 67 subtypes have been identified. Genotype 1 is the most common worldwide, including in the United States.[3]

— The greatest risk of transmission comes from injection drug use, which can occur when sharing contaminated needles or other drug paraphernalia. Additional, though less common, means of transmission include noninjection drug use (eg, snorting); chronic hemodialysis; receipt of clotting factor concentrates before 1987; receipt of blood products, immune globulin, organs, or tissue before 1992; household or occupational contact; or unregulated tattoos or piercing practices.[3] Vertical transmission of HCV is the leading cause of HCV infection in children.[4]

— Once exposed, HCV RNA is detectable in the blood within 1 to 3 weeks. Seroconversion from exposure to antibody production (anti-HCV) occurs around 8 to 9 weeks. More than 97% of persons exposed to HCV show detectable anti-HCV within 6 months.[3]

— Unlike hepatitis A and B, no vaccine currently exists for HCV prevention.[3]

— Infections occurring within 6 months of HCV exposure are considered acute, and approximately 15% to 25% of those exposed are able to spontaneously clear the virus from their bodies without treatment.[3,4] Acute infections that do not resolve within 6 months develop into chronic HCV infections.

— Most patients who test positive for HCV are asymptomatic or have nonspecific symptoms. Approximately 20% to 30% of those newly infected will experience fatigue, abdominal pain, nausea, poor appetite, or jaundice within an average of 2 to 12 weeks after exposure.[3]

— Those with chronic HCV infections are likewise asymptomatic or have nonspecific symptoms, such as chronic fatigue and depression.[3] Many will develop chronic liver disease, including cirrhosis and liver cancer. Because of the generally slow progression of chronic liver disease in the HCV-infected population, HCV infection is often not recognized until asymptomatic patients are screened during blood donation or routine examinations.[3]

Epidemiology

An estimated 3.5 million people in the United States live with HCV (including almost one-third of incarcerated individuals). Approximately 50% are unaware they are infected.[5] There has been an increase in acute cases reported since 2012, with the highest rate of incidence in American Indians/Alaska natives.[6] Because of the clinically obscure presentation of HCV, many infections will go undiagnosed and therefore unreported, affecting data collection and potential treatment. Acute cases are estimated to be 13.9 times the number of reported cases in any year.[6] Approximately 75 to 85 individuals out of every 100 with acute infections will develop chronic infections. Of those, 10 to 20 individuals will go on to develop cirrhosis within 20 to 30 years, making HCV the leading cause of liver transplantation.[3,7] A small percentage will develop hepatocellular carcinoma or hepatic decompensation.

Despite an increase in direct-acting antiviral (DAA) therapy, rates of infection remain high, most likely as a result of injection drug use and high-risk sexual behaviors. Approximately 50% of persons who inject drugs (PWID) will become infected.[3] HCV is rarely transmitted through sexual practices except in men who have sex with men (MSM) who are positive for human immunodeficiency virus (HIV).[5] Of the estimated 1.2 million people living with HIV in the United States, an estimated 25% are coinfected with HCV.[3] Approximately 6 of every 100 infants born to HCV-infected mothers contract the virus.[1] The risk of transmission is significantly higher if the mother has a high viral load or is coinfected with HIV. Infants born to women infected with HCV are more likely to be small for gestational age, have low birthweight, be admitted to the neonatal intensive care unit, and require assisted ventilation.[4]

Screening Recommendations

Screening consists of a simple blood test initially assessing for the presence of HCV antibody. **Figure 13-1** outlines the recommended testing sequence for identifying HCV infection.

One-time HCV screening is indicated for persons born from 1945 through 1965, regardless of risk category.[3,5] Birth-cohort testing is based on HCV prevalence (75% of all HCV infections).

Figure 13-1. *Recommended testing sequence for hepatitis C. (Courtesy of CDC, Atlanta, GA.)*

Recommended Testing Sequence for Identifying Current Hepatitis C (HCV) Infection

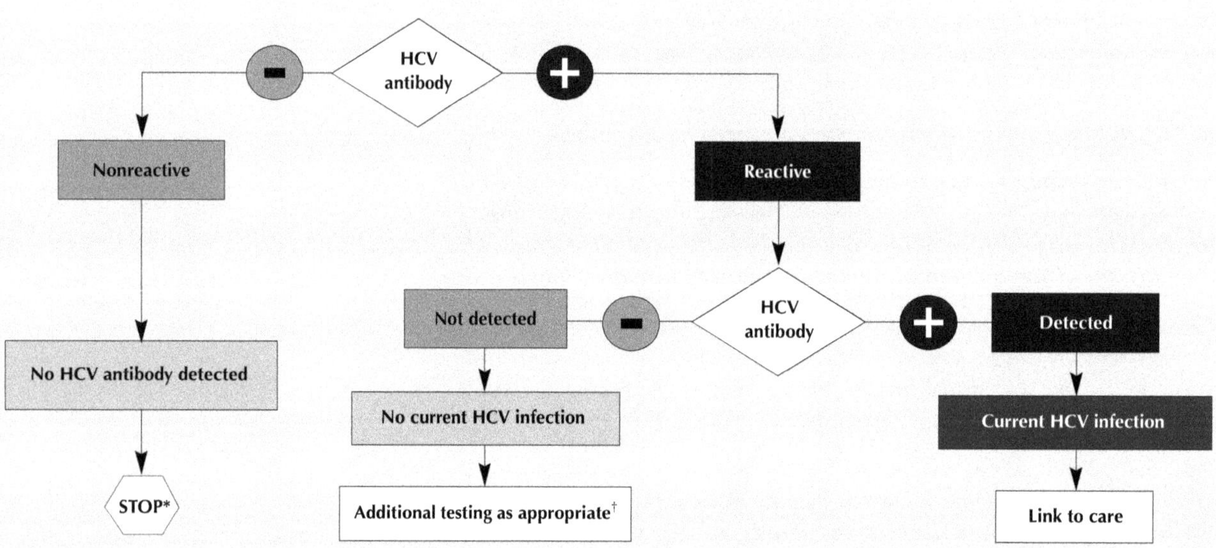

**For persons who might have been exposed to HCV within the past 6 months, testing for HCV RNA or follow-up testing for HCV antibody is recommended. For persons who are immunocompromised, testing for HCV RNA can be considered.*

† To differentiate past, resolved HCV infection from biologic false positivity for HCV antibody, testing with another HCV antibody assay can be considered. Repeat HCV RNA testing if the person tested is suspected to have had HCV exposure within the past 6 months or has clinical evidence of HCV disease, or if there is concern regarding the handling or storage of the test specimen.

Adapted from Centers for Disease Control and Prevention. Testing for HCV infection: an update of guidance for clinicians and laboratorians. MMWR Morb Mortal Wkly Rep. *2013;62(18):362-365.*

Figure 13-1

Others are screened based on behaviors, exposures, or other factors that could induce contraction of the virus, including[5]:

— Injection drug use, current or past, even with single historical event

— Intranasal drug or illicit substance use

— Long-term hemodialysis (current or historical)

— Needlestick exposures in unregulated setting (including tattoos)

— Health care and public safety workers or first responders with sharps (needlestick) or mucosal exposure to HCV-infected persons

— Children of HCV-positive mothers

— Recipients of blood transfusions or organ transplants before 1992

— Incarcerated persons

Other indicators to test include:

— HIV infection

— Unexplained chronic liver disease and elevated alanine aminotransferase (ALT)

— Solid organ donors (deceased and living)

Annual testing for HCV is indicated for[5]:

— PWID

— HIV-infected MSM

Periodic testing should be offered to other individuals with ongoing risk factors. Testing consists of an initial assessment for the presence of HCV antibodies. Follow-up testing includes an HCV nucleic acid amplification test (NAAT) to determine the viral load or presence of the virus in the bloodstream.[5] **Table 13-1** outlines initial testing and follow-up guidelines, and **Table 13-2** outlines HCV testing interpretations.

Table 13-1. Initial Testing and Follow-Up Guidelines
MAIN LABORATORY TESTS
— HCV antibody (anti-HCV) — If positive, follow up with HCV NAAT to detect viremia (see below)
HCV ANTIBODY NEGATIVE
— If negative and not in risk categories, may assume lack of HCV exposure — If negative and possibility of exposure within the past 6 months, consider follow-up testing — If negative and suspected liver disease, test for HCV RNA — If negative and immunocompromised, consider test for HCV RNA
HCV ANTIBODY POSITIVE
— If positive, test for current infection with HCV RNA test — Quantitative HCV RNA needed before initiation of antiviral therapy to assess for viral load (viremia) — HCV genotype and subtype testing and quantitative HCV RNA are recommended to guide treatment decisions regarding most appropriate antiviral pharmacotherapy — Child-Turcotte-Pugh score can be used to grade the severity of liver involvement
Data from https://www.hcvguidelines.org.[5]

Table 13-2. Interpretation of Results of Tests for HCV Infection and Further Actions

Test Outcome	Interpretation	Further Actions
HCV antibody nonreactive	No HCV antibody detected	Sample can be reported as nonreactive for HCV antibody. No further action required. If recent exposure in person tested is suspected, test for HCV RNA.*
HCV antibody reactive	Presumptive HCV infection	A repeatedly reactive result is consistent with current HCV infection, past HCV infection that has resolved, or biologic false positivity for HCV antibody. Test for HCV RNA to identify current infection.
HCV antibody reactive, HCV RNA detected	Current HCV infection	Provide person tested with appropriate counseling and link person tested to care and treatment.†
HCV antibody reactive, HCV RNA not detected	No current HCV infection	No further action required in most cases. If distinction between true positivity and biologic false positivity for HCV antibody is desired, and if sample is repeatedly reactive in the initial test, test with another HCV antibody assay. In certain situations,§ follow-up with HCV RNA testing and appropriate counseling.

**If HCV RNA testing is not feasible and person tested is not immunocompromised, do follow-up testing for HCV antibody to demonstrate seroconversion. If the person tested is immunocompromised, consider testing for HCV RNA.*
†It is recommended before initiating antiviral therapy to retest for HCV RNA in a subsequent blood sample to confirm HCV RNA positivity.
§If the person tested is suspected of having HCV exposure within the past 6 months, or has clinical evidence of HCV disease, or if there is concern regarding the handling or storage of the test specimen.
Reprinted from the Centers for Disease Control and Prevention.

Treatment

Since the HCV was first identified in 1989, treatment has rapidly evolved from the interferons with thrice weekly injections for up to 48 weeks in the 1990s to the use of oral direct-acting antivirals today. Current regimens are simple enough to be implemented through a primary care setting.[8,9] Elimination of viral load through medication has increased from 10% to virtually 100% for most patients. The addition of ribavirin, a synthetic antiviral nucleoside analogue, as an adjunctive therapy has proven useful for patients with more resistant cases.[5] New therapies are expensive but may offer savings in health care costs over the long term.[9]

The goal of treatment is sustained virological response (SVR), which is considered synonymous with "cure" and is of benefit to all patients with chronic HCV. SVR is equivalent to the continued absence of HCV RNA for at least 12 weeks after pharmacotherapy is completed.[5] These patients will exhibit HCV antibodies but will lack HCV RNA per the NAAT. Desired outcomes include decrease of mortality and morbidity such as end-stage liver disease and hepatocellular carcinoma.

Treatment decisions are made on the basis of HCV genotype, presence or absence of baseline NS5A resistance-associated substitutions, and presence or absence of hepatic pathological conditions (specifically cirrhosis). **Table 13-3** outlines treatment recommendations for the most common HCV genotypes. Within 12 weeks before beginning therapy and in addition to HCV-specific tests, the following blood tests are recommended[5]:

— Liver panel

— Complete blood cell count (CBC)

— International normalized ratio (INR)

— Calculated (estimated) glomerular filtration rate (eGFR)

— Hepatitis B virus (HBV), because reactivation of HBV can occur with HCV therapy

Imaging may also be ordered to assess hepatic function.

Table 13-3. Treatment Recommendations[5]

The regimens described are for treatment-naïve patients. For treatment-experienced patients (those who have been treated in the past with pegylated interferon/ribavirin) or who have experienced treatment failure, some of the recommendations still apply, though it is prudent for the prescriber to select the pharmacotherapy carefully after a full history and appropriate pretreatment assessments. Alternative treatments are recommended but are less favorable based on longer duration of treatment, reduced efficacy, limited supportive data, or more complexity in prescribing or management. These are not covered here but may be accessed at hcvguidelines.org.*

Elbasvir/grazoprevir TRADE NAME: **ZEPATIER**	Glecaprevir/pibrentasvir TRADE NAME: **MAVYRET**	Ledipasvir/sofosbuvir TRADE NAME: **HARVONI**	Sofosbuvir/velpatasvir TRADE NAME: **EPCLUSA**
Genotype 1a 12 weeks† without cirrhosis or with compensated cirrhosis	**Genotype 1a** 8 weeks† without cirrhosis and 12 weeks† with compensated cirrhosis	**Genotype 1a** 12 weeks† without cirrhosis or with compensated cirrhosis; if nonblack, HIV negative, and RNA level is <6 million IU/mL, may consider 8-week course	**Genotype 1a** 12 weeks† without cirrhosis or with compensated cirrhosis
Genotype 1b 12 weeks† without cirrhosis or with compensated cirrhosis	**Genotype 1b** 8 weeks† without cirrhosis or 12 weeks† with compensated cirrhosis	**Genotype 1b** 12 weeks† without cirrhosis or with compensated cirrhosis; if nonblack, HIV negative, and RNA level is <6 million IU/mL, may consider 8-week course	**Genotype 1b** 12 weeks† without cirrhosis or with compensated cirrhosis
	Genotype 2 8 weeks† without cirrhosis or 12 weeks† with compensated cirrhosis		**Genotype 2** 12 weeks† without cirrhosis or with compensated cirrhosis
	Genotype 3 8 weeks† without cirrhosis or 12 weeks† with compensated cirrhosis		**Genotype 3** 12 weeks† without cirrhosis or with compensated cirrhosis
Genotype 4 12 weeks† without cirrhosis or with compensated cirrhosis	**Genotype 4** 8 weeks† without cirrhosis or 12 weeks with compensated cirrhosis	**Genotype 4** 12 weeks without cirrhosis or with compensated cirrhosis	**Genotype 4** 12 weeks† without cirrhosis or with compensated cirrhosis
	Genotype 5 or 6 8 weeks† without cirrhosis or 12 weeks† with compensated cirrhosis	**Genotype 5 or 6** 12 weeks without cirrhosis or with compensated cirrhosis	**Genotype 5 or 6** 12 weeks† without cirrhosis or with compensated cirrhosis

(continued)

Table 13-3. Treatment Recommendations[5] *(continued)*

Elbasvir/grazoprevir TRADE NAME: **ZEPATIER**	Glecaprevir/pibrentasvir TRADE NAME: **MAVYRET**	Ledipasvir/sofosbuvir TRADE NAME: **HARVONI**	Sofosbuvir/velpatasvir TRADE NAME: **EPCLUSA**
DOSAGE			
Daily fixed dose combination of elbasvir (50 mg)/grazoprevir (100 mg) for patients without baseline NS5A RASs[a] for elbasvir	Daily fixed-dose combination of glecaprevir (100 mg)/pibrentasvir (40 mg); recommended total daily dose 300 mg glecaprevir and 120 mg pibrentasvir	Daily fixed-dose combination of ledipasvir (90 mg)/ sofosbuvir (400 mg)	Daily fixed-dose combination of sofosbuvir (400 mg)/velpatasvir (100 mg)
One tablet daily taken orally with or without food for 12 weeks duration (except as noted)	Three (100 mg/40 mg) tablets daily taken orally at the same time with or without food for 8 weeks; extend to 12 weeks if compensated cirrhosis present	One tablet daily taken orally with or without food for 8 or 12 weeks	One tablet daily taken orally with or without food. If decompensated cirrhosis (Child-Pugh B or C), add ribavirin for 12-week course of treatment Consider referral to provider with expertise in more complex treatments
Unusual patient populations such as HIV/HCV coinfection and decompensated cirrhosis may require a more complex medication regimen; consider referral to a specialist trained in caring for such patients. Further pertinent recommendations can be found at https://www.hcvguidelines.org/unique-populations.			

For more information on treatment, see the CDC's sexually transmitted disease guidelines at https://www.cdc.gov/hepatitis/hcv/hcvfaq.htm#section4.

**https://www.hcvguidelines.org/.*

†Level of evidence 1A (evidence or general agreement that a given diagnostic evaluation, procedure, or treatment is beneficial, useful, and effective; data are derived from multiple randomized clinical trials, meta-analyses, or equivalent).

Data from https://www.hcvguidelines.org.[5]

During therapy, regular visits or telephone contacts to monitor for nonadherence and side effects are recommended. There should be an inventory of all medications, including over-the-counter and herbal or dietary supplements, to assess for potential drug-drug interactions. Patients on diabetes medications should be counseled about the possibility of symptomatic hypoglycemia, and those on warfarin should be advised about the risk for subtherapeutic anticoagulation levels. Both should be monitored.[10] Creatinine level, eGFR, and hepatic function panel are recommended after 4 weeks of treatment for all regimens. If the patient is taking ribavirin, CBC should be done, as clinically indicated, to assess for drug-related adverse effects. If the patient is taking elbasvir/grazoprevir, hepatic function panel at 8 weeks and 12 weeks during 16-week course of treatment is indicated. Check HCV viral load after 4 weeks of therapy and 12 weeks after completion of therapy, but do not stop therapy if HCV RNA levels are not assessed.[5]

A 10-fold increase in ALT at any time during treatment is an indication to discontinue therapy. An increase less than 10-fold accompanied by systemic symptoms such as nausea, vomiting, jaundice, weakness, or abnormal laboratory readings also indicate discontinuation of therapy.

Once SVR is achieved, patients without an advanced liver pathological condition can be monitored as a general patient population. For patients with advanced liver disease, health care providers may use laboratory testing, ultrasound, and periodic screening for varices to monitor. Health care providers may assess for HCV recurrence if the patient has continued risk factors and behaviors.

For patients who fail to achieve SVR, the health care provider may stop treatment and monitor for liver damage progression with regular laboratory testing and imaging as noted earlier or evaluate for retreatment with available alternative treatments.[10]

Special Considerations

When taking into account special considerations of HCV, it is imperative to review patient populations. With the evolvement of effective DAAs and the improvement of safety profiles in certain special populations, therapy for these populations has changed, resulting in a reduction of patients needing special consideration.[11]

— ***Pregnancy:*** Pregnant women should be tested during initial prenatal assessment for anti-HCV if they have any risk factors.[3] Though antiviral therapies are contraindicated in pregnancy because of teratogenic risks, prenatal screening allows for the introduction of additional interventions in intra- and antepartum that may reduce the risk of transmission from mother to infant during birth.[11,12] This risk is elevated if the mother has a high viral load or is coinfected with HIV.[3] If invasive prenatal diagnostic testing is necessary, women should be thoroughly counseled on the risk of vertical transmission.[4] The Centers for Disease Control and Prevention (CDC) is currently exploring whether further HCV screening among pregnant women is necessary.[3] Providers should avoid internal fetal monitoring, prolonged rupture of membranes, and episiotomies in HCV-positive women.[4] Cesarean section is not recommended if HCV is the only indication.[4] HCV-infected women are not advised to avoid breastfeeding, because no current evidence suggests that HCV is spread through breastmilk.[3,4] Precautions should be considered if HCV-infected women desire to breastfeed and have fissures or bleeding nipples.[3]

— ***Pediatrics:*** The CDC recommends that screening should be completed for infants born to HCV-infected women.[3] It is advised that testing on infants born to HCV-infected women should wait until the infant is 18 months of age because of the coverage of anti-HCV from the mother until this time.[3] If diagnosis is desired before this time, then initial testing for HCV RNA can be obtained at 1 to 2 months of age. However, the HCV RNA testing should also be repeated at a subsequent visit.[3] Studies have shown higher rates of spontaneous clearance and slower viral progression in the pediatric population. The World Health Organization recommends deferring treatment for patients 0 to 12 years of age until more data are available.[11]

— ***HIV:*** Liver damage can occur more rapidly in those coinfected with HIV. As such, all patients living with or at risk for HIV should be screened for HBV and HCV.[3] Patients who are coinfected with HCV and HIV should still receive antiviral therapy for HCV and should be referred to an expert provider who routinely treats this special population.[3]

— ***PWID:*** This is the most common risk factor for HCV in the United States.[11] The barriers to medical care for these individuals must be considered. This group often encounters socioeconomic barriers which may prevent them from seeking health care. It is vital to combat these barriers to provide optimal health care to this key population.[11]

Case Studies

Adult Case Study 13-1

The patient is a 58-year-old woman who presents to the emergency department (ED) for left knee pain secondary to a fall 5 weeks prior. She reports history of stage 2 chronic kidney disease, hypertension (reports that she has not taken her medication in about 3 months), obesity, tobacco use (45 pack-year history), and frequent use of marijuana. She also reports drinking alcohol approximately 5 times per week.

Risk factors include a history of intravenous (IV) drug use ("once or twice and only in the 1970s"), as well as a long-term sexual partner who is reportedly positive for hepatitis (type unknown). Her last medical care was an x-ray examination in the ED after her fall.

Examination

At initial new patient sick visit, screening protocols were discussed and ordered for cervical, breast, and colon cancer. Because of birth cohort screening, the patient is checked for presence of anti-HCV. The physical examination is unremarkable, including no hepatomegaly or abdominal tenderness.

Laboratory Testing

Routine laboratory tests are ordered. Patient has elevated blood urea nitrogen level, a creatinine level of 1.6 mg/dL, a vitamin D level of 19.3 ng/mL, and elevated triglyceride levels at 335 mg/dL. Her eGFR is 41 mL/min.

CBC results are within normal limits. Aspartate aminotransferase (AST) and ALT, alkaline phosphatase, and total bilirubin are all within normal limits. All screens are negative with the exception of anti-HCV.

The patient is contacted and asked to return to the clinic for HCV RNA testing by polymerase chain reaction (PCR) and is found to have 1 570 000 IU/mL, genotype 1a.

INR is 1.1 and FibroSure score is F0-F1, indicating no to minimal fibrosis. Screening for hepatitis A, hepatitis B, and HIV are all negative.

Treatment

Recommended therapy consists of Harvoni* for 12 weeks. Patient is initially denied by Medicare, but appeals. Patient must abstain from alcohol and illicit drug intake for 6 months before initiating treatment. Monthly clinic visits are arranged for this patient to monitor for readiness for therapy, but after the third month, she is lost to follow-up, and avenues of communication, including cell phone and certified mail, are not successful. If the patient had demonstrated consistency in adherence to her scheduled care regimen, she most likely would have been approved for treatment.

*The cost of 12 weeks of Harvoni is about $95 000, and it is estimated it would cost approximately $331 billion to treat every American with chronic HCV. There are wide variations worldwide in the costs of DAAs, as well as differences among states in what insurers, both public and private, will pay.[13] Competition seems to be working favorably in achieving price reductions among some pharmacological agents, but it remains to be seen if equal access to therapy will come in time for at-risk patients to prevent permanent liver damage and the associated increase in morbidity and mortality. It is an issue that both health care providers and health care policymakers must consider for this potentially devastating, yet curable, diagnosis.

Child Case Study 13-2

PT and AT are a 39-year-old man and 38-year-old woman who have been married for 13 years and have 2 children, a boy and girl ages 11 and 9, respectively. After the birth of their second child, they decided not to have any more biological children because of some perinatal complications, but approaching midlife, they began to consider adding to their family through adoption.

Because of the long waits within the United States for infants, they decided to pursue international adoption. After a lengthy and expensive process, they were notified that they were eligible to adopt a 16-month-old infant girl, ST, from Russia.

They were able to learn very little of the child's health history from the Russian adoption source. Recommended screenings were conducted within her country of origin and again shortly after her entry into the United States, all of which were negative for worrisome findings.

The child assimilated into her new family well, but because of a trio of urinary tract infections within the first 6 months with her new family, further diagnostic workups are ordered, including a CBC and complete metabolic panel.

Laboratory Testing

Her ALT is found to be mildly elevated at 76 U/L (normal range is 7 to 56 U/L), with AST at 50 U/L (normal range is 10 to 40 U/L). Understanding the HCV prevalence in her country of origin, the health care provider orders further testing, including anti-HCV. Results of RNA PCR subsequent to a positive anti-HCV reveal a viral load of 130 000 IU/L.

Monitoring

ST's care is referred to a pediatric hepatologist, who monitors her for the next 3 years with laboratory tests done every 6 months. At age 30 months, ST is re-evaluated and the ALT and AST have returned to normal ranges, but viremia remains detectable at 28 000 IU/L. At 36 months of age, viremia has decreased to 10 000 IU/L, with no detectable HCV RNA at ages 42 months, 48 months, or 54 months. At age 5 years, ST is released from the specialist's care and resumes normal annual primary care health screenings and examinations.

Supplemental Information

More than 5000 children, most younger than 5 years of age, were adopted internationally in 2016, representing 91 countries.[14] Birth family history is often not forthcoming. The US State Department requires a medical examination in the child's country of origin to assess for physical and mental disorders and the communicable diseases, such as intestinal parasites, syphilis, hepatitis B, and HIV. Further testing is recommended for international adoptees once they arrive in the United States, including testing for HCV, but there are no official reportable parameters that would guide testing of these children.[14]

Of the world's estimated 115 million HCV-infected persons, 11 million are likely children younger than 15 years, with up to 5 million of these viremic. The largest numbers are in Asia, the Middle East, and Africa, as well as in the United States, particularly in Appalachian regions, where increasing numbers of HCV-positive infants parallel increases in the opioid epidemic.[15] However, with no official screening protocols for children and adolescents, statistics regarding the disease in youth may not be accurate.[16]

Vertical transmission is the main method of transmission in children, and 8% of the world's pregnant women are affected by hepatitis C.[17] Because of the presence of maternal antibodies, testing before a child is 18 months of age is not considered useful, though HCV RNA PCR assay exhibits sensitivity for children older than 1 month. A positive test on 2 different occasions is required to diagnose an infected child.[16]

Infants born with HCV may have abnormal liver enzyme levels within the first year of life, but spontaneous clearance rates exceed the adult population, and about 25% to 50% of infants infected at birth will clear the virus within the first 2 years. Some have reportedly cleared the virus without treatment by age 7.[18] Up to 20% of children can develop a more aggressive form of HCV, but advanced pathological liver conditions are generally uncommon until adulthood.[18] Children who continue to carry a viral load are considered chronically infected and should be monitored for growth and development, genotype, and liver function. Treatment is not recommended for children younger than 3 years.[18]

Families of children with chronic HCV should be educated on risk for transmission and safe behaviors, such as avoiding sharing toothbrushes, razors, and nail clippers. There is no need to restrict activities for children with a diagnosis of HCV, nor are there laws requiring parents to share the medical history of an HCV-positive child. It is assumed that coaches and school nurses have been trained in infection control processes that would be implemented in the case of a cut or wound, thereby releasing the family from forced disclosure of HCV status.[18]

No universal screening recommendations exist, but certain pediatric populations warrant extra vigilance when it comes to HCV infection.[15] These include the following:

- Children whose mothers are positive for HCV or have a history of IV drug use
- Children with HIV
- Victims of sexual assault
- History of multiple sex partners
- History of illicit IV drug use
- Children with clinical signs of hepatitis, including elevations in ALT or AST
- Children who are international adoptees or refugees, particularly if the children come into the United States from an area with high prevalence (Africa, China, Russia, Eastern Europe, and Southern and Southeast Asia)

References

1. Sokal E, Nannini P. Hepatitis C virus in children: the global picture. *Arch Dis Child.* 2017;102(7):668-671.
2. Torgan C. Hepatitis C virus structure. National Institutes of Health Web site. https://www.nih.gov/news-events/nih-research-matters/hepatitis-c-virus-structure. Published March 3, 2014. Accessed July 21, 2019.
3. Viral hepatitis: hepatitis C information. Centers for Disease Control and Prevention Web site. https://www.cdc.gov/hepatitis/hcv/index.htm. Updated June 13, 2019. Accessed July 12, 2019.
4. Society for Maternal-Fetal Medicine; Hughes BL, Page CM, Kuller JA. Hepatitis C in pregnancy: screening, treatment, and management. *Am J Obstet Gynecol.* 2017;217(5):B2-B12.
5. Recommendations for testing, managing, and treating hepatitis C. HCV Guidelines Web site. http://www.hcvguidelines.org. Accessed August 3, 2019.
6. Viral hepatitis surveillance – United States, 2016. Center for Disease Control and Prevention Web site. https://www.cdc.gov/hepatitis/statistics/2016surveillance/pdfs/2016HepSurveillanceRpt.pdf. Updated April 16, 2018. Accessed July 12, 2019.
7. Bhamidimarri KR, Satapathy SK, Martin P. Hepatitis C virus and liver transplantation. *Gastroenterol Hepatol (N Y).* 2017;13(4):214-220.
8. Interferons and ribavirin. The Hepatitis C Trust Web site. http://www.hepctrust.org.uk/information/treatment/current-treatments/interferons-and-ribavirin. Accessed August 3, 2019.
9. Burstow NJ, Mohamed Z, Gomaa AI, et al. Hepatitis C treatment: where are we now? *Int J Gen Med.* 2017;10:39-52.
10. The American Association for the Study of Liver Diseases, The Infectious Diseases Society of America. HCV guidance: recommendations for testing, managing, and treating hepatitis C. HCV Guidelines Web site. https://www.hcvguidelines.org/evaluate. Updated May 24, 2018. Accessed August 19, 2019.
11. Ramers CB, Trooskin SB. Hepatitis C virus in the modern direct-acting antiviral era: where have all the special populations gone? *Clin Liv Dis (Hoboken).* 2018;12(5):143-149.
12. Final recommendation statement: hepatitis C virus infection in adolescents and adults: screening. US Preventive Services Task Force Web site. https://www.uspreventiveservicestaskforce.org/uspstf/document/RecommendationStatementFinal/hepatitis-c-screening. Updated March 2, 2020. Accessed May 27, 2020.
13. Toich L. Will hepatitis C virus medication costs drop in the years ahead? Pharmacy Times Web site. https://www.pharmacytimes.com/resource-centers/hepatitis/will-hepatitis-c-virus-medicaton-costs-drop-in-the-years-ahead. Published February 8, 2017. Accessed August 8, 2019.
14. Staat MA. International adoption: infectious disease aspects. UpToDate Web site. https://www.uptodate.com/contents/international-adoption-infectious-disease-aspects. Updated August 7, 2019. Accessed September 9, 2019.
15. Jonas MM. Hepatitis C virus infection in children. UpToDate Web site. https://www.uptodate.com/contents/hepatitis-c-virus-infection-in-children. Updated July 8, 2019. Accessed September 9, 2019.
16. Espinosa C, Jhaveri R, Barritt AS 4th. Unique challenges of hepatitis C in infants, children, and adolescents. *Clin Ther.* 2018;40(8):1299-1307.
17. Dibba P, Cholankeril R, Li AA, et al. Hepatitis C in pregnancy. *Diseases.* 2018;6(2):e31.
18. Narkewicz MR. Hepatitis C in children. American Liver Foundation Web site. https://liverfoundation.org/hepatitis-c-in-children/. Updated April 24, 2020. Accessed May 27, 2020.

Chapter 14

Molluscum Contagiosum

Angelia Trujillo, DNP, MSN, WHNP-BC
Kathy Bell, MS, RN, SANE-A, SANE-P, DF-AFN
Trinity Ingram-Jones, DNP, MSN, APRN, CPNP, PCNS, AFN-BC, SANE-A, SANE-P, DF-AFN

Disease and Mimics

— Molluscum contagiosum is an infection caused by the molluscum contagiosum virus (MCV).[1]

— The infection usually results in a benign, mild skin disease characterized by small, raised lesions. The lesions are usually white, pink, or flesh-colored with a dimple or pit in the center, and they often have a pearly appearance. Lesions can range from the size of a pinhead to the size of a pencil eraser and may become itchy, sore, or swollen (**Figures 14-1** through **14-3**).[1]

— This double-stranded DNA virus has 4 subtypes. MCV-1 is mostly seen in children. MCV-2 is mainly responsible for lesions in people living with human immunodeficiency virus (HIV). MCV-3 and MCV-4 are present in Asia and Australia.[2]

— Histologically, molluscum contagiosum lesions have classic features under a microscope.[3] The lesion appears as a cup-shaped indentation of the epidermis in the dermis. The proliferated rete ridges descend downward and encircle the dermis. The epidermis is usually thickened, and Henderson-Paterson bodies are seen within the epidermis. These bodies enclose the virus particles.[3]

— The virus that causes molluscum contagiosum spreads from direct person-to-person physical contact and through contaminated fomites. Fomites are inanimate objects that can become contaminated with the virus. In the instance of molluscum contagiosum, this can include linens such as clothing and towels, bathing sponges, pool equipment, and toys. Although the virus might be spread by sharing swimming pools, baths, saunas, or other wet and warm environments, this has not been proven. Researchers who have investigated this idea think it is more likely the virus is spread by sharing towels and other items around a pool or sauna than through water.

— Someone with molluscum contagiosum can spread it to other parts of their body by touching or scratching a lesion and then touching their body somewhere else. This is called autoinoculation. Shaving and electrolysis can also spread mollusca to other parts of the body. Molluscum can spread from 1 person to the other by sexual contact. Many, but not all, cases of molluscum contagiosum in adults are caused by sexual contact.[1]

— Molluscum contagiosum typically resolves within 6 to 12 months but can take as long as 4 years.[1]

— Molluscum lesions can occur anywhere on the body, including the face, neck, arms, legs, abdomen, and genital area, but rarely occur on the palms of the hands or soles of the feet. They can appear alone or in groups.[1]

— Little has been verified with regard to the incubation period of molluscum contagiosum; however, it is estimated to be between 2 weeks and 6 months. Most cases occur in children older than 1 year, with only 1 known case reported in an infant (at 7 days postpartum).

— Atopic dermatitis may be a risk factor for contracting molluscum contagiosum as a result of the barrier breaks and immune cell dysfunction in atopic skin. In addition, these patients may be more likely to autoinoculate (excoriation of primary lesions and spread to areas of normal skin) new areas of skin because of the underlying pruritus from their atopy.

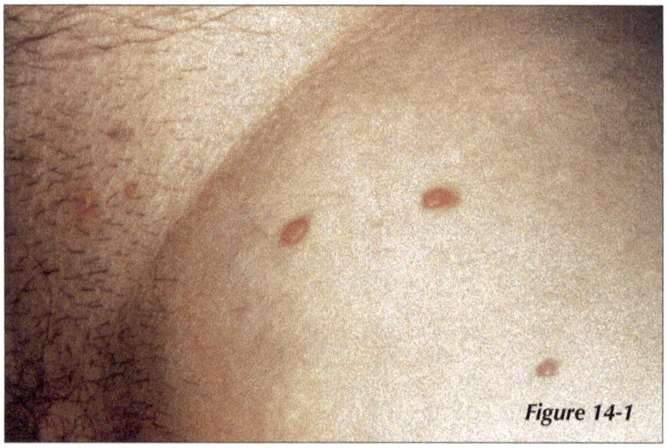

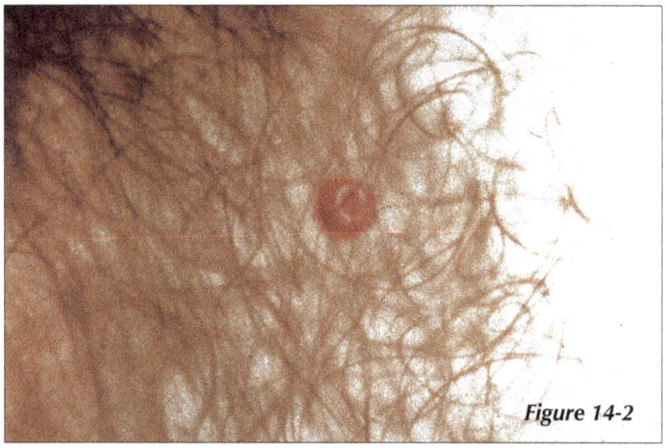

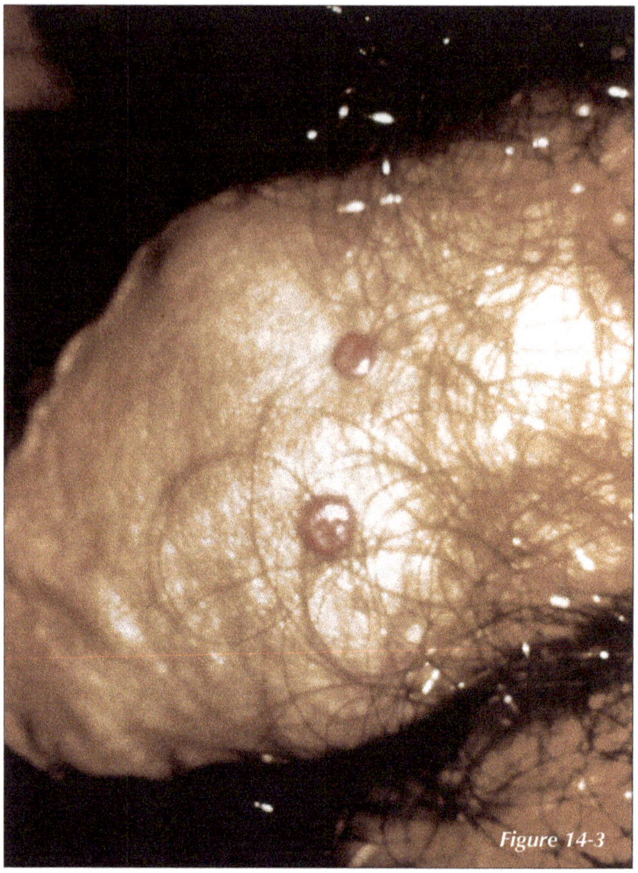

Figure 14-1. *Molluscum contagiosum, vulva and thighs. (Courtesy of CDC, Atlanta, GA.)*

Figure 14-2. *Molluscum contagiosum. (Courtesy of CDC, Atlanta, GA.)*

Figure 14-3. *Molluscum contagiosum, penis. (Courtesy of CDC, Atlanta, GA.)*

Epidemiology

Although it is not limited to children, molluscum contagiosum is most common in children 1 to 10 years of age.[1] It is also diagnosed in sexually active teens and adults.[2] Lesions are classified in 3 ways: commonly seen skin lesions on the faces and limbs of children; sexually transmitted lesions on the abdomen, inner thighs, and genitals of sexually active adults; and the diffuse and recalcitrant eruptions on patients with immunosuppressive disorders (eg, AIDS).[1]

People with weakened immune systems are at a higher risk for getting molluscum contagiosum, and their growths may look different, be larger, and be more difficult to treat. Atopic dermatitis may also be a risk factor as a result of frequent breaks in the skin. For this reason, patients with atopic dermatitis are also more likely to spread the infection to other parts of their body. People who live in warm, humid climates with crowded living conditions are also at a higher risk.[1]

There is evidence that molluscum contagiosum infections have been on the rise in the United States since 1966, but these infections are not routinely monitored because they are rarely serious and usually disappear without treatment.[1]

Treatment Guidelines

In healthy patients, molluscum contagiosum infection is self-limited, and treatment is often unnecessary. Pruritis associated with underlying atopic disease increases the spread of lesions and the risk of secondary infection, particularly among members of the pediatric population, which may prompt the need for treatment. Lesions in the genital area may also prompt the need or desire for treatment, particularly among members of the adult patient population.[1] The most common concern of this diagnosis is of a cosmetic nature. The diagnosis is typically made by looking at the skin. Occasionally, scraping or a biopsy examination is done to confirm the diagnosis.[2] It is characterized by small pearly papules with a central depression whose core may be expressed, producing a white, cheesy material. The lesions average 2 to 5 mm in size and are usually painless.

Cryotherapy, curettage, or laser therapy can be used to physically remove molluscum lesions. Though these options are quick remedies for existing lesions, local anesthesia is often required, and patients may experience postprocedural pain, irritation, and scarring.[1]

Used for the gradual removal of lesions, oral therapy is the preferred treatment option for pediatric patients and those concerned with physical scarring. Oral cimetidine is safe, painless, and well tolerated, but lesions on the face do not respond to this treatment option as effectively as lesions found elsewhere on the body.[1] Oral therapy is less painful and associated with less scarring than physical removal of molluscum.

Topical podophyllotoxin cream (0.5%) is a reliable at-home therapy but is not recommended for use by pregnant women because of presumed toxicity to the fetus. The therapeutic effect of this treatment option is localized, and each lesion must be treated individually. Iodine and salicylic acid, potassium hydroxide, tretinoin, cantharidin, and imiquimod are treatment options that require a prescription. Imiquimod has not proven effective in treating molluscum lesions in children, and because of possible adverse effects, it is not recommended for use in the pediatric population.[1]

Special Considerations

The best way to avoid getting molluscum contagiosum is by following good hygiene habits. The virus lives only in the skin, and once the lesions are gone, the virus is gone and cannot be spread to others.

— ***Immunocompromised:*** Patients with immunocompromising conditions, including those infected with HIV, typically have more widespread and prolonged eruptions, which are often recalcitrant to therapy.[3] Patients with HIV/AIDS and other immunocompromising conditions (eg, solid organ transplant recipients) can develop "giant" lesions (≥15 mm in diameter), larger numbers of lesions, and lesions that are more resistant to standard therapy.

— ***Differential diagnosis:*** The following diseases should be considered in the differential diagnosis of molluscum contagiosum: cryptococcosis, basal cell carcinoma, keratoacanthoma, histoplasmosis, coccidioidomycosis, and verruca vulgaris. For genital lesions, condyloma acuminata and vaginal syringoma should be considered.

— ***Atopic dermatitis:*** Patients with atopic dermatitis also have more widespread and prolonged eruptions, which are often recalcitrant to therapy.[3,4] Atopic dermatitis may also be a risk factor because of frequent breaks in the skin. For this reason, a patient with atopic dermatitis is also more likely to spread the infection to other parts of their body.

Case Studies

Adult Case Study 14-1

FZ is a 32-year-old male construction worker and body builder who presents to the urgent care clinic requesting sexually transmitted infection (STI) testing. He reports "bumps" over his abdomen, upper thighs, and pubic area for the past 4 months. He reports he has been abstinent for the last year and had negative STI testing 2 years ago. He reports that there about 30 "pink, pimple-like bumps that itch." He has tried scratching them off and shaving and they "keep spreading."

Examination

Multiple 1- to 3-mm raised, white, yellow, and skin-colored nodules over lower abdomen, mons pubis, and upper thighs. Approximately half of the nodules have a centralized depression.

Laboratory Testing

Herpes simplex virus (HSV) polymerase chain reaction (PCR) swab of 4 to 5 lesions across pubis, abdomen, and upper thighs is negative for HSV-1 and HSV-2. The patient declines other testing for STIs.

Treatment

After a review of treatment options—including (1) no treatment, because molluscum contagiosum often will self-resolve; (2) in-office procedures to physically remove or destroy the lesions (curettage, cryotherapy, laser podophyllin resin, trichloroacetic acid, and cantharidin); and (3) at-home treatment options, including topical creams or oral therapy—FZ opts to use topical podophyllotoxin cream (0.5%). He is directed to apply the cream to lesions twice daily for 3 days a week and repeat weekly for up to 4 weeks until lesions are resolved.

Child Case Study 14-2

JT is a 7-year-old girl brought to her pediatrician's office by her mother for lesions around her mouth and on her stomach that started approximately 1 month ago. JT denies discomfort, itching, fever, and redness to sites. The child is homeschooled, up to date on immunizations, and has no chronic health conditions. The mother reports that JT was away at her grandparents' farm for the summer.

Examination

On examination, there are 3 raised, smooth, 2- to 3-mm round papules with white, depressed centers on the right cheek and 3 similar papules noted on the waistband area. Papules are soft and nontender without ulceration, redness, or signs of infection noted.

Laboratory Testing

Viral HSV type-specific PCR swab of lesion is obtained and is negative for HSV-1 and HSV-2. Based on clinical findings, the diagnosis of molluscum contagiosum is made.

Treatment

A discussion regarding treatment options includes (1) no treatment, because molluscum contagiosum often will self-resolve; (2) in-office procedures to physically remove or destroy the lesions (curettage, cryotherapy, laser podophyllin resin, trichloroacetic acid, and cantharidin); and (3) at-home treatment options, including topical creams or oral therapy. Parent opted to complete at-home topical treatment with podophyllotoxin cream (0.5%) applied twice daily to papules for 3 days per week and repeated weekly for 1 month. Patient is to return to the clinic for reevaluation at 1 month. The parent is directed to aid child in avoiding self-inoculation by scratching.

References

1. Molluscum contagiosum. Centers for Disease Control and Prevention Web site. https://www.cdc.gov/poxvirus/molluscum-contagiosum/index.html. Updated May 11, 2015. Accessed August 11, 2019.

2. Schaffer JV, Berger EM. Molluscum contagiousum. *JAMA Dermatol.* 2016; 152(9):1072.

3. Badri T, Gandhi GR. *Molluscum Contagiosum*. Treasure Island, GL: StatPearls Publishing; 2019.

4. Kimberlin DW. *Red Book: 2018-2021 Report of the Committee on Infectious Diseases.* 31st ed. Elk Grove, IL: American Academy of Pediatrics; 2018.

Section IV

Ectoparasitic Diseases

Chapter 15

Scabies

Pamela H. Bryant, DNP, CRNP, CPNP-AC/PC
Lauren Mays, DNP, CRNP, FNP-BC
Alice Springer Bristow, DNP, CRNP, FNP-BC, CWCN, CNE

Disease and Mimics

— Scabies is caused by an infestation of the skin by the microscopic human itch mite Sarcoptes scabiei var. hominis (**Figure 15-1**).[1] They present as thin, gray or white, serpiginous, thread-like lines. Scabies mites burrow into the upper layer of the skin, where they live and lay eggs.[2]

— The mites are spread by direct, prolonged skin-to-skin contact with a person who has scabies. An infested person can spread scabies even if they are asymptomatic.

— In a person who has not had scabies before, initial symptoms appear within 2 to 6 weeks after exposure. An individual who has previously been infested will usually exhibit symptoms in 1 to 4 days.[3]

— Scabies can spread easily in crowded areas where there is close body contact and skin-to-skin contact can easily be made.[3] Childcare facilities, extended-care facilities, prisons, and nursing homes are examples of common sites for scabies outbreaks.[3]

— Crusted scabies, formerly known as Norwegian scabies, is characterized by a large number of mites with widespread, crusted, hyperkeratotic lesions.[2] This type of scabies usually occurs in individuals with developmental disabilities or who are immunocompromised.[2] This type of scabies is extremely contagious and can easily spread through direct skin-to-skin contact with infected people or their clothing, bedding, or furniture.[3]

— Dogs and other animals can be infested with a different type of scabies mite that does not replicate in humans.[2] When an animal scabies mite burrows into the human skin, it may cause temporary itching, but no treatment is required; this type of scabies mite cannot survive on humans for long.[3]

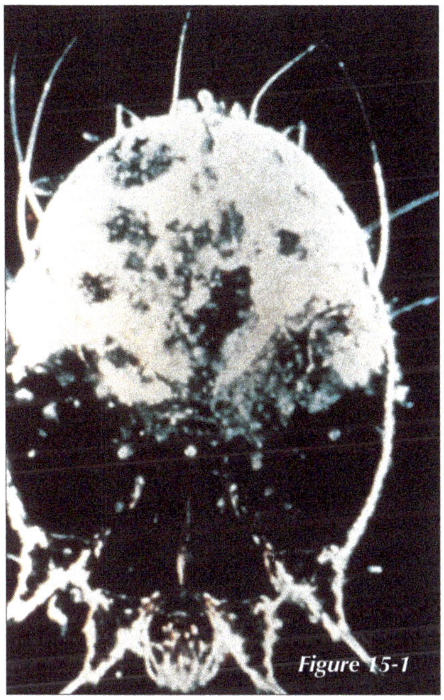

Figure 15-1. *Scabies mite. (Courtesy of CDC, Atlanta, GA)*

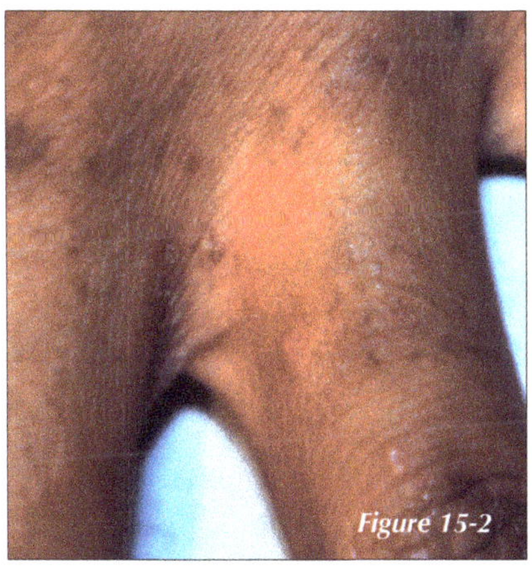

Figure 15-2. *The dorsal surface of a human hand focused on the interdigital web space between the index and middle fingers. Presence of papules caused by an infestation of scabies. (Courtesy of CDC, Atlanta, GA)*

Epidemiology

Humans are usually the source of infestation, with transmission occurring through prolonged close, personal contact.[2] Scabies is characterized by intense itching (pruritus) and erythematous flare-ups that may consist of papules, nodules, vesicles, or bullae caused by the mites burrowing into the upper layers of the dermis.[2] The itching is most intense at nighttime.[2] In older children and adults the sites that are commonly affected are areas between the fingers and toes (**Figure 15-2**), flexor aspects of wrists, extensor surfaces of elbows, anterior axillary folds, waistline, thighs, navel, genitalia (**Figure 15-3**), areola, abdomen, intergluteal cleft, and buttocks.[2] Children younger than age 2 years usually have an eruption that is vesicular and manifests on the scalp, face, palms of hands, and soles of feet, whereas these areas are spared in older children and adults.[2] Adults with scabies often acquire it from sexual contact.[2]

Diagnosis is made by clinical examination and confirmed by identification of mite eggs or mite fecal matter (scybala).[2]

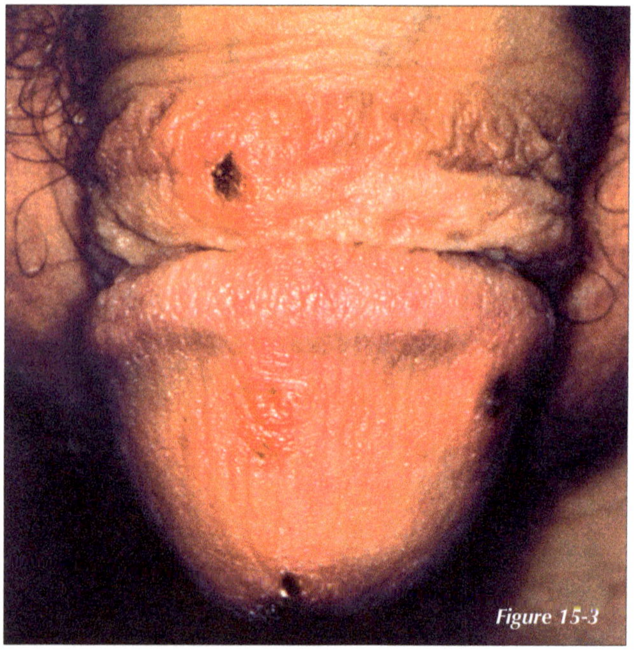

Figure 15-3. *Close view of the genitalia of a male patient reveals the presence of erosive, inflamed lesions caused by an infestation of scabies. The lesions included the skin on the glans penis and the preputial skin. (Courtesy of CDC, Atlanta, GA)*

Treatment Guidelines

In adults and children, scabicides are used to treat human scabies. The scabicide cream is applied to all areas of the body, which includes the entire head and neck area down to the feet.[3] Treatment can usually take 4 to 8 weeks.[3] All persons involved should be treated at the same time to prevent reinfestation. Bedding and clothing used by the infested person should be decontaminated by washing in hot water and drying in a hot dryer, by dry cleaning, or by sealing in a plastic bag for at least 72 hours before the treatment.[3]

Topical permethrin 5% cream is the drug of choice to treat scabies.[2] It is particularly good for infants and young children (not younger than age 2 months).[2] In infants and young children, treatment of the head and neck is required because scabies usually affects the face, scalp, and neck.[2] Two or more applications, each a week apart, may be necessary to eliminate all the mites. Sulfur (5% to 10%) ointment is safe for topical use in children, including infants younger than 2 months of age. In individuals with crusted scabies, oral (ivermectin) and topical (permethrin cream 5% or benzyl benzoate 25%) medications are used.[4,5]

Depending on the severity of the infection, ivermectin should be taken in 3 doses (approximately days 1, 2, and 8), 5 doses (approximately days 1, 2, 8, 9, and 15), or 7 doses (approximately days 1, 2, 8, 9, 15, 22, and 29). Topical permethrin should be administered every 2 to 3 days for 1 to 2 weeks to treat crusted scabies. Benzyl benzoate 25% (with or without tea tree oil) may be used as an alternative topical agent to permethrin; benzyl benzoate (10% or 12.5%) may be used in children. A topical keratolytic cream may also be used to help reduce the crusting of the skin and aid in the absorption of the topical permethrin or benzyl benzoate. Clean clothing should be worn after treatment.

Those who have had skin-to-skin contact with an infested individual should also be treated. All members of a household must be treated at the same time. Individuals with crusted scabies require quick and aggressive medical treatment for their infestation to prevent outbreaks of scabies. Contaminated clothing should be washed in hot water or dry cleaned. Scabies mites do not survive outside the body for more than 2 to 3 days. Retreatment may be required.[1]

Special Considerations

— ***Pregnancy:*** Permethrin (FDA Pregnancy Category B) is the preferred therapy for pregnant and lactating women.[6]

— ***Infants and children:*** Infants and children aged 2 months to 10 years should be treated with permethrin 5% cream applied as a single application from head to toe, left on the skin for 8 to 14 hours, and then rinsed off. Reapply in 7 days if mites reappear.[6] For infants younger than 2 months, topical sulfur is the treatment of choice.[6] Lindane should not be used in children younger than 10 years because of risks of systemic toxicity, such as seizures and death.[6]

— ***HIV:*** Scabies is the most common parasitic infection among patients with human immunodeficiency virus (HIV), often resulting in hyperinfestation.[7] Physical presentation includes a diffuse, extremely pruritic, red or crusted lesion and may also include psoriatic-type lesions.[7] Secondary infections can occur in immunocompromised patients from bacteria entering the fissures of the skin. Common infections include impetigo, ecthyma, paronychia, and furunculosis.[8] Secondary infections should be treated with appropriate antibiotics.[6]

Case Studies

Adult Case Study 15-1

A 36-year-old female patient presents to the clinic with a chief complaint of "itching all over." She reports the symptoms first began approximately 2 weeks ago and states the itching is worse at night. She has tried over-the-counter diphenhydramine (Benadryl) with no relief. She denies any new medications and has no known drug allergies.

Examination

On physical examination, the provider notes erythematous vesicles with linear burrows in the flexor aspects of the wrists, elbows, and interdigital web spaces of the hands bilaterally. Papules are noted on the genitalia and areola of both breasts.

Laboratory Testing

A skin scraping sample is taken by placing a drop of mineral oil directly over multiple burrows on the patient's skin and gently scraping parallel and laterally across the skin with the side of a scalpel blade. The skin sample is examined under a light microscope, and the diagnosis of scabies is confirmed with the identification of mites and larvae present on the slide.

Treatment

Permethrin 5% topical lotion is the treatment of choice. The patient is told to apply the lotion liberally from head to toe, ideally before bedtime, and to leave the lotion on the skin for 8 to 14 hours and then rinse thoroughly. The patient is told she may reapply in 7 days if live mites reappear and to return to the clinic if the treatment is unsuccessful.

Adult Case Study 15-2

A 19-year-old women who is "sore all over" presented without an appointment to the urgent care center. She reported that she has had sores for about a year, and they "wax and wane" throughout the year but are worse in the winter. However, she complains that the new sores began about 2 weeks ago and "make lines on my hands and it's moving up my arms" and "they don't feel like the other sores." She reports that they "itch" and occasionally have pus. She admits drug use, specifically methamphetamine (meth) for about 5 years, and says she lives in an abandoned home. She goes into drugstores and squeezes petroleum jelly (Vaseline) and other open lotions on the sores to get relief, but to little avail. She came in because she is tired of scratching, particularly at night. She denies any medications and has no known drug or food allergies. She says she is "not ready to give up the meth just yet."

Examination

On physical examination, the provider objectively notes erythematous vesicles with linear burrows in the flexor aspects of the wrists, elbows, and interdigital web spaces of the hands bilaterally and observes the patient scratching these areas. Papules in various stages of healing cover the entire body except in areas unreachable to the patient's hands, and the provider observes the patient picking at the sores. Bitten nails have sores in the parenchyma, except for the right fifth digit. The skin is in various stages of healing.

Laboratory Testing

A skin scraping sample is taken by placing a drop of mineral oil directly over multiple burrows on the patient's skin and scraping parallel and laterally across the skin gently with the side of a scalpel blade. The skin sample is examined under a light microscope, and the diagnosis of scabies is confirmed with the identification of mites and larvae present on the slide. Additionally, a complete blood cell count reveals an elevated C-reactive protein (CRP) level, a measurement of inflammation. Her CRP is 90 mg/dL, and her liver enzymes are high, so the advanced practice nurse advises her of the need for a comprehensive workup. The patient declines her services and leaves after receiving topical medication from the clinic pharmacy.

Treatment

Permethrin 5% is the treatment of choice. The patient is told to apply the lotion liberally from head to toe, ideally before bedtime, and to leave it on the skin for 8 to 14 hours and then rinse thoroughly. The patient may reapply in 7 days if the "itching with lines" reappears and is encouraged to return to address the inflammatory markers in her blood when she is ready.

Child Case Study 15-3

A 6-month-old girl is brought to the primary care clinic with "bugs in her eyes." They appeared 2 days ago, and the infant continues to scratch at her eyes, so the mother is worried about her hurting herself. The mother denies that she or her partner have "bugs," but the baby does sleep in their bed.

Examination

On inspection and application of clear tape to the eyelashes, the microscopic evaluation reveals scabies.

Treatment

The adults are provided with permethrin 5%, a topical lotion for the treatment of scabies. The mother and her partner are instructed to apply the lotion, leaving the medication on the skin for 8 to 14 hours, followed by a thorough rinse. At the end of that time, the mother and the partner may reapply the lotion, particularly if live mites reappear. The mother is also instructed to not apply the lotion to the infant or the infant's eyes. Rather, the mother is instructed to apply petroleum jelly to the brows and lashes for at least 7 days,[9] continuing to apply as long as mites are visible.

References

1. Parasites: treatment. Centers for Disease and Prevention Web site. https://www.cdc.gov/parasites/scabies/treatment.html. Updated October 31, 2018. Accessed July 23, 2019.
2. American Academy of Pediatrics. Sexually transmitted diseases. In: Kimberlin DW, ed. *Redbook: 2018 Report of the Committee on Infectious Diseases*. 31st ed. Elk Grove, IL: American Academy of Pediatrics; 2018:718-721.
3. Workowski KA, Bolan GA; Centers for Disease Control and Prevention. Sexually transmitted diseases treatment guidelines, 2015. *MMWR Recomm Rep*. 2015;64(RR-3):1-137.
4. Currie B, Davis J. Crusted (Norwegian) scabies grading scale and treatment plan: Royal Darwin Hospital infectious diseases department protocol. Centers for Disease Control and Prevention Web site. https://www.cdc.gov/parasites/resources/pdf/CrustedScabiesNT.pdf. Accessed May 23, 2019.
5. Sharma R, Singal A. Topical permethrin and oral ivermectin in the management of scabies: a prospective, randomized, double blind, controlled study. *Indian J Dermatol Venereol Leprol*. 2011;77(5):581-586.
6. Goldstein BG, Goldstein AO. Scabies: epidemiology, clinical features, and diagnosis. UpToDate Web site. https://www.uptodate.com/contents/scabies-epidemiology-clinical-features-and-diagnosis. Updated August 2, 2019. Accessed August 9, 2019.
7. Goldstein BG, Goldstein AO. Scabies: management. UpToDate Web site. https://www.uptodate.com/contents/scabies-management. Updated July 27, 2018. Accessed August 8, 2019.
8. Lopez FA, Sanders CV. Fever and rash in HIV-infected patients. UpToDate Web site. https://www.uptodate.com/contents/fever-and-rash-in-hiv-infected-patients. Updated March 25, 2019. Accessed August 9, 2019.
9. Canadian Paediatric Society. Scabies management. *Paediatr Child Health*. 2001;6(10):775-777.

Chapter 16

Pediculosis Pubis

Lauren Mays, DNP, CRNP, FNP-BC
Pamela H. Bryant, DNP, CRNP, CPNP-AC/PC

Disease and Mimics

— Pediculosis pubis may be sexually transmitted through close contact.

— Pruritis of the anogenital area is a common symptom of pubic lice.[1]

— It is caused by the pubic crab louse *Pthirus pubis* (*P. pubis*), which is an oval-shaped insect approximately 1 to 4 mm in length.[2]

— The parasite lives on the skin, usually where hair is present, and feeds on the host's blood (**Figure 16-1**).[2]

— The parasite is found most commonly in the pubic region, but infestation can involve the eyelashes, eyebrows, beard, axilla, perianal area, and, rarely, the scalp.[1,2]

— The female pubic louse (**Figure 16-2**) lays about 3 eggs per day, which attach to the shaft of the hair as nits and hatch within 8 to 10 days.[1]

— The presence of bluish or slate-colored macules (maculae ceruleae) on the chest, abdomen, or thighs is a sign of heavy pubic lice infestation.[1]

Figure 16-1. *A close view of the skin of a patient who presented with an infestation of crab lice,* P. pubis*, causing the condition known as pediculosis pubis. (Courtesy of CDC, Atlanta, GA.)*

Figure 16-2. *Female crab louse. (Courtesy of CDC, Atlanta, GA.)*

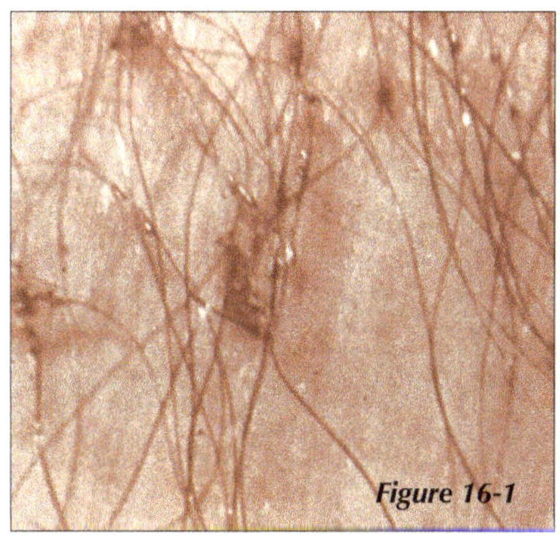

Epidemiology

Pubic lice infestation is more prominent in adults and is usually contracted sexually.[1] Pubic lice found on a child's eyelashes or eyebrows may be indicative of sexual abuse, although other modes of transmission are possible.[1] Pediculosis pubis is an infection primarily seen in adolescent and adult males and females and is not typically seen in prepubertal children because of the absence of pubic hair. Adult pubic lice can survive away from a host for up to 48 hours, and their eggs can remain viable for up to 10 days under suitable environmental conditions.[1]

Symptoms usually occur in both females and males approximately 1 to 2 weeks after initial contact. Patients primarily complain of severe itching throughout all areas of the external genitalia, particularly in areas where there is hair growth. Additionally, the child or a family member may report having actually seen a crab louse in the genital area. Although rare, infestation on eyelashes and eyebrows can occur in both prepubertal children and adolescents.

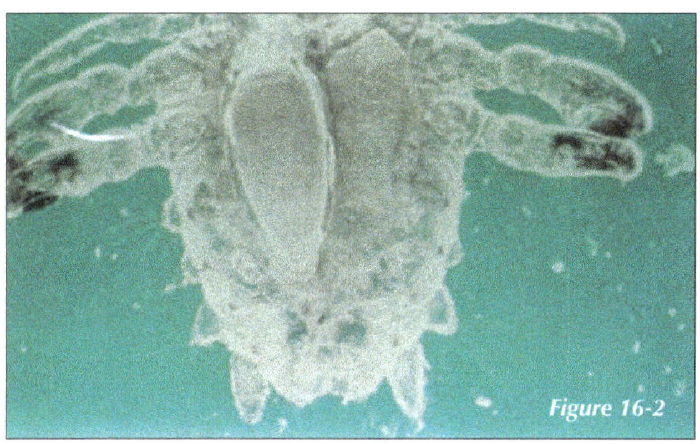

During inspection of the external genitalia of female and male patients, clinicians may first notice small yellow-white nits attached to the base of the pubic hair shafts. The eyelashes and eyebrows are also inspected for nits and the crab louse. If such an observation is made, the health care provider should collect the nit as evidence and send the evidence to the laboratory. The nits may also be viewed more closely by microscope. If sexual abuse is suspected in prepubertal children, it is possible to type both the suspect's and victim's DNA in the louse. Diagnosis of child sexual abuse is made by considering both the clinical history and clinical findings.

Treatment Guidelines

Treatment of choice includes topical pediculicides, such as permethrin (1% cream rinse) and pyrethrin/piperonyl butoxide (0.33%/4% shampoo), plus the removal of nits.[3,4] Instruct patients to apply the pediculicide on clean, dry skin to all areas of suspected involvement. Leave the solution on for 10 minutes and then wash thoroughly. Remove nits with a fine-tooth comb, tweezers, or fingernails.[3,4]

Follow-up should occur 1 week after treatment, if symptoms persist. A second treatment is often needed 10 days after initial application.[4] Advise patients to repeat the steps of the initial treatment. Avoid using these medications on the face or around the eyes.

Alternative therapy for pediculosis pubis includes malathion lotion (0.5%) applied to the affected areas. Patients should leave this lotion on for 8 to 12 hours and then rinse thoroughly.[4] Common complaints regarding this therapy include the odor of the ointment, lengthened treatment time, and hazards of application.[4] Hazards include burning and stinging of the skin and flammability. Do not smoke while using this product or expose the treated area to open flames or electric heat sources (such as hairdryer or styling tools).[5]

Patients with infestation should encourage their sexual partners to be examined, and partners should be treated if an infestation is present.[4] Advise your patient to avoid sexual contact until infestation is cleared. Members of the household do not have to be treated if no infestation is present.[4] Encourage patients to launder any clothing and bedding they have used during infestation in hot water.[4]

Special Considerations

— ***Pregnancy:*** Pregnant and lactating women should be treated with permethrin (Food and Drug Administration Category B).[6] It is not known if this medication is distributed in the breast milk; therefore, it is recommended to pump and discard the milk after administration of this medication.[6]

— ***HIV:*** Treatment guidelines remain the same for persons infected with human immunodeficiency virus (HIV).

— ***Treatment failure:*** Failure to eradicate the infestation is typically based on noncompliance to therapy or reexposure. Ensure proper education and compliance with treatment guidelines.

Case Studies

Adult Case Study 16-1

A 33-year-old man presents to clinic with complaints of extreme itching around his groin and upper thighs. He denies any uretheral discharge or dysuria. He reports this has been going on for approximately 10 days, and it has gotten so bad he is unable to sleep at night. He reports he has multiple sexual partners and uses barrier protection during intercourse.

Examination

On physical examination, excoriations and sores are noted on the skin of the pubic area and upper thighs with crawling lice and nits visible on inspection.

Diagnostic criteria is based on clinical history and physical examination, and given these findings, this patient is diagnosed with pediculosis pubis.

Treatment

Treatment recommendations include permethrin 1% cream rinse applied on clean, dry skin to the affected areas of the pubic area and upper thighs. Leave the ointment on for 10 minutes and then thoroughly rinse. After rinsing, use a fine-tooth comb or tweezers to remove any remaining nits. Educate this patient on the importance of notifying sexual partners from the last month so they may be evaluated and treated, as well as laundering all clothing and bedding used since symptoms were present.

Follow up with the patient in 1 week for reevaluation, and inform the patient of the possibility of a second treatment if lice or nits persist.

Child Case Study 16-2

A 17-year-old boy presents with a complaint of persistent itching in his pubic region that he says occurs mostly at night. This has been going on for about 1 week. He reports that his mother has not tried any new laundry detergent nor is he on any medications. His vital signs are within normal limits, and there is no history of a sexually transmitted infection. On further questioning, he admits he had sex with 2 different girls recently but says he used a condom. His physical examination reveals Tanner stage V. No redness or swelling is noted.

Examination

On further inspection, a scant amount of pin-sized blood spots on his underwear are noted. He also has grayish-white pubic lice visible on his pubic region. No discharge is noted from his penis. His lower abdomen, inner thighs, buttocks, scalp, eyebrows, and lashes are clean and have no visible signs of lice.

Treatment

Treatment recommendations include permethrin 1% cream rinse applied on clean, dry skin to the affected areas of the pubic area. Leave the ointment on for 10 minutes and then thoroughly rinse. After rinsing, use a fine-tooth comb or tweezers to remove any remaining nits.

Educate this patient on the importance of notifying sexual partners from the last month so they may be evaluated and treated, as well as laundering all clothing and bedding used since symptoms were present.

Follow up with the patient in 1 week for reevaluation, and inform the patient of the possibility of a second treatment if lice or nits persist.

References

1. American Academy of Pediatrics. Sexually transmitted diseases. In: Kimberlin DW, ed. *Redbook: 2018 Report of the Committee on Infectious Diseases.* 31st ed. Elk Grove, IL: American Academy of Pediatrics; 2018:613-614.
2. Parasites: pubic "crab" lice. Centers for Disease Control and Prevention Web site. https://www.cdc.gov/parasites/lice/pubic/. Updated September 24, 2013. Accessed September 10, 2019.
3. 2015 sexually transmitted diseases treatment guidelines: ectoparasitic infections. Centers for Disease Control and Prevention Web site. https://www.cdc.gov/std/tg2015/ectoparasitic.htm. Updated June 4, 2015. Accessed September 10, 2019.
4. Goldstein AO, Goldstein BG. Pediculosis pubis and pediculosis ciliaris. UpToDate Web Site. https://www.uptodate.com/contents/pediculosis-pubis-and-pediculosis-ciliaris. Updated October 25, 2018. Accessed September 10, 2019.
5. Malathion (Rx). Medscape Web site. https://reference.medscape.com/drug/ovide-malathion-topical-343502#0. Accessed September 10, 2019.
6. Permethrin (Rx, OTC). Medscape Web site. https://reference.medscape.com/drug/nix-elimite-permethrin-topical-343503#6. Accessed September 10, 2019.

Chapter 17

Trichomoniasis

Pamela H. Bryant, DNP, CRNP, CPNP-AC/PC
Lauren Mays, DNP, CRNP, FNP-BC
Alice Springer Bristow, DNP, CRNP, FNP-BC, CWCN, CNE
Elizabeth Coleman, MSN, CRNP, CPNP-PC
Patricia M. Speck, DNSc, CRNP, FNP-BC, DF-IAFN, FAAFS, DF-AFN, FAAN

Disease and Mimics

- *Trichomonas vaginalis* is a flagellate protozoan that causes trichomoniasis. Trichomoniasis, bacterial vaginosis (BV), *Chlamydia*, and gonorrhea are common sexually transmitted infections (STIs) transmitted after sexual assault.[1] For individuals with human immunodeficiency virus (HIV), an increased risk of pelvic inflammatory disease (PID) is associated with concurrent trichomoniasis or BV.[2]
- Adult women characteristically have a diffuse, malodorous, yellow-green, or frothy discharge and vulvovaginal irritation. On examination, females may also have a "strawberry cervix."[3]
- Most males are asymptomatic but may have symptoms of urethritis, epididymitis, or prostatitis. Untreated infections can progress to salpingitis or prostatitis in males.
- Perinatal infections are usually found in urine samples of infants and can persist for up to 1 year if untreated. After infancy, finding *T. vaginalis* in prepubertal and non–sexually active girls strongly suggests sexual abuse.[4] No cases of fomite transmission have been reported.
- *T. vaginalis* is a motile protozoan (**Figure 17-1**), but subjective analysis of a wet mount microscope slide is relatively insensitive. Nucleic acid amplification testing (NAAT) is encouraged if *Trichomonas* is not identified on a wet mount.[3]
- Adult patients with clinical presentations that are consistent with *Trichomonas* infections typically receive standard treatment based on that suspicion. *T. hominis*, a commensal species, is a bowel organism that can be misdiagnosed as *T. vaginalis* but can be differentiated by an experienced laboratory technician by measuring the length of the undulating membrane. *T. tenax* is a related species associated with oral gingivitis.
- Differential diagnosis includes BV, candida vulvovaginitis, gonorrhea, *Chlamydia*, vaginal atrophy/atrophic vaginitis, irritants, allergens, and retained foreign bodies.[5]

Figure 17-1. *The flagellated protozoan* Trichomonas vaginalis.

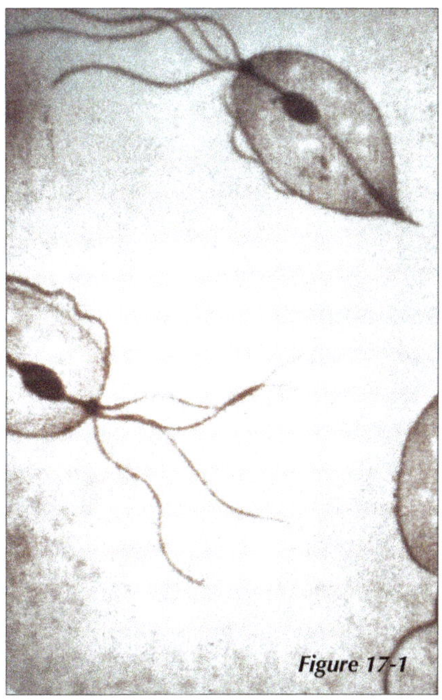

Epidemiology

The most prevalent nonviral STI in the United States is trichomoniasis.[3] The incidence of *T. vaginalis* in the United States is around 2.3 million (3.1%) among women between ages 14 and 49 years.[1,6] The prevalence among black women is 13% compared with 1.8% of non-Hispanic white women.[3] It is easily passed between sexual partners during penile-vaginal sex.[3] Correctly and regularly using condoms during penile-vaginal sexual encounters is the best way to prevent the transmission of *T. vaginalis*.[3]

Treatment Guidelines

Therapy for *T. vaginalis* should begin immediately after diagnosis. Treatment can be expected to alleviate symptoms and possibly lower the spread of *T. vaginalis*.[3,7] Current partners are presumed to be infected and should be referred for treatment or, in most states, may be treated without clinical evaluation through expedited partner therapy.[8] Both partners should abstain from sexual activity until treatment is complete and any symptoms have resolved.

Because the parasite infests several sites within the genital area, systemic treatment is warranted.[9,10] The only known pharmacological therapy is the class of drugs known as 5-nitroimidazole drugs, whose mechanism of action is bactericidal, likely causing the dismantling of DNA structure.[9] Within this class, metronidazole and tinidazole are both approved by the Food and Drug Administration (FDA), with comparable efficacy in 2-g doses.[3] These medications are generally well tolerated with mild, usually gastrointestinal (GI), side effects. Larger doses tend to have increased side effects, leading to cessation of therapy or lack of compliance (**Table 17-1**).[9]

The recommended treatment regimen is as follows[3,7,10]:

— Metronidazole 2 g orally in a single dose *OR*

— Metronidazole 500 mg orally twice daily for 7 days *OR*

— Tinidazole 2 g orally in a single dose

Because of high rates of reinfection, it is recommended that the patient be retested 3 months after completion of therapy.[3,7]

Table 17-1. Comparison of Trichomoniasis Recommended Therapies

Recommended Medication

	Metronidazole	Tinidazole
Dosage[3]	2 g PO in single dose	2 g PO in single dose
Cure rate[3,10]	84% to 98%[3]	92% to 100%[3]
Cons		More expensive[3]
Pros		Higher serum level; fewer GI side effects[3] Equivalent or superior in resolution of symptoms and infection[3,7]
Half-life	7.3 hours[3]	12.5 hours[3]
Pregnancy	Pregnancy Class B; CDC recommends infected symptomatic pregnant women receive 2 g PO in a single dose. Breastfeeding should be withheld during treatment and for 12 to 24 hours after treatment. Asymptomatic pregnant women may wish to defer treatment until after 37 weeks gestation.[3]	Pregnancy class C; not recommended for pregnant women; withhold breastfeeding during treatment and for 3 days after final dose.[3]
Alcohol: In all cases, patients receiving 1 of these drugs should abstain from alcohol to prevent a disulfiram-like reaction.	Abstain from alcohol during treatment and for 24 hours after treatment.[3]	Abstain from alcohol during treatment and for 72 hours after treatment.[3]
Antimicrobial resistance	4% to 10% of cases[3]	1% of cases[3]

(continued)

Table 17-1. Comparison of Trichomoniasis Recommended Therapies ***(continued)***

Special Cases

	Metronidazole	Tinidazole
Women with HIV	500 mg twice daily for 7 days[3] Retest in 3 months[3,7,11]	
Refractory cases[3]	Metronidazole 500 mg PO twice daily for 7 days. If repeated treatment fails, consider metronidazole or tinidazole 2 g PO for 5 or 7 days.[3,7] If there are continued treatment failures with 1-week regimens, consider susceptibility testing. Higher doses of tinidazole at 2 to 3 g for 14 days in combination with intravaginal tinidazole has been used but should be managed in consultation with an immunologist or gynecologist who is trained to care for complex infections.	

PO, per os (orally).
Data from Centers for Disease Control and Prevention (CDC). 2015 sexually transmitted disease treatment guidelines. MMWR Morb Mortal Wkly Rep. 2015;64(3):1-81; CDC. Trichomoniasis: treatment and care. https://www.cdc.gov/std/trichomonas/treatment.htm. Updated January 4, 2017. Accessed July 31, 2019; and Smith DS. Trichomoniasis treatment & management. https://emedicine.medscape.com/article/230617-treatment#showall. Updated December 6, 2018. Accessed July 31, 2019.

Though single-dose therapy increases compliance, under certain circumstances, longer duration of treatment may be in order.[12] Persistent symptoms can indicate either a reinfection or treatment failure. If reinfection cannot be confirmed, it is recommended that the patient and any partners be treated with metronidazole 500 mg orally twice daily for 7 days. If this is not effective, providers may initiate metronidazole or tinidazole at 2 g orally for 5 or 7 days.[7]

Longer duration of treatment is associated with decreased compliance,[12] though recent research suggests that cure rates improve with longer duration of treatment, even for routine cases.[13] If nonadherence and reinfection from a subsequent sexual encounter can be excluded, the parasite can be tested for susceptibility, or the patient can be referred to an infectious disease expert. In addition, the Centers for Disease Control and Prevention (CDC) assists with management of difficult cases. For more information visit the CDC website (https://www.cdc.gov/laboratory/specimen-submission/detail.html?CDCTestCode=CDC-10239).

Finally, these medications may be administered parenterally, but metronidazole topical gel is considered ineffective against *T. vaginalis.* Other treatment modalities, such as herbal remedies, boric acid intravaginal capsule (somewhat effective), topical antimicrobials, and photodynamic light therapy, have been investigated, but most are minimally effective at best.[14-16] In light of increasing rates of resistance to metronidazole, further research is warranted to find alternate forms of therapy. Refer to **Table 17-2** for diagnostic assays and characteristics for *Trichomonas vaginitis.*

Special Considerations

— ***Pregnancy/neonates:*** Effects of trichomoniasis during pregnancy include preterm labor, premature rupture of membranes, low birth weight of the infant, and transfer of the infection to the infant during childbirth.[6] Benefits outweigh the risks in treating both symptomatic and asymptomatic patients during pregnancy to avoid these adverse obstetrical outcomes.[6] Metronidazole (US FDA Pregnancy Category B) 2 g orally as a single dose is the mainstay of treatment. Therapy can be modified to metronidazole 500 mg orally twice daily for 7 days for patients who suffer from nausea and vomiting during pregnancy.[6] Metronidazole is secreted in the breast milk; therefore, pumping and expelling the breast milk for 12 to 24 hours after treatment is recommended.[3]

Table 17-2. Diagnostic Tests for *Trichomonas Vaginalis*

DIAGNOSTIC TEST	METHOD	SAMPLE	COMMENTS
Wet mount	Microscopic visualization	Vaginal or urethral secretions	Inexpensive and operator dependent; results within minutes of collection
Culture	Culture	Vaginal or urethral secretion, urine (f), semen	Expensive; gold standard before NAAT
Rapid Test	EIA	Vaginal swabs, saline solution for prep	CLIA waived
DNA	NAAT	Vaginal swabs, endocervical specimen, urine	CLIA waived

CLIA, Clinical Laboratory Improvement Amendments; EIA, enzyme immunoassay; NAAT, nucleic acid amplification test. Modified from Association of Public Health Laboratories. Advances in laboratory detection of Trichomonas vaginalis *(updated). https://www.aphl.org/aboutAPHL/publications/Documents/ID_2016November-Laboratory-Detection-of-Trichomonas-update.pdf. November 2016. Accessed December 3, 2019.*

— ***HIV infection:*** The CDC recommends annual screening for *T. vaginalis* in all HIV-infected women.[3] HIV-infected patients diagnosed with trichomoniasis are at increased risk of developing PID and should be treated with longer therapy than patients without HIV.[3,6] The recommended treatment is metronidazole 500 mg orally twice daily for 7 days in this population. The CDC recommends retesting HIV-infected women 3 months after completion of therapy.[3]

— ***Other considerations:*** Patients with an immunoglobulin E (IgE)–mediated allergy to 5-nitroimidazoles should be referred for desensitization, because alternative drugs are less effective at eradicating the infection.[3,6] All sexual partners should be treated. All patients should avoid alcohol for 24 hours after metronidazole therapy.

Case Studies

Adult Case Study 17-1

A 67-year-old woman has experienced bleeding after intercourse for several years. She denies itching and discharge symptoms. The couple denies having other sexual partners since their marriage 35 years ago, and the patient denies all symptoms until the postcoital bleeding started.

Examination

The physical presentation is normal, except for the cervix. On inspection, the cervix is beefy red and friable.

Laboratory Testing

A Papanicolaou (Pap) sample is sent to the laboratory for analysis. Laboratory analysis of Pap sample indicates normal cervical cells with *T. vaginalis*. Urine collected from husband is also positive for *T. vaginalis*.

Treatment

The differential diagnosis includes cervical cancer because the patient is menopausal. It is not uncommon to find asymptomatic *T. vaginalis* in nursing home patients, who are treated with metronidazole 500 mg orally twice daily for 14 days,[7] because the infection is not routine and there is a potential for noncompliance.

Child Case Study 17-2

A 17-year-old boy presents with mild dysuria for 1 week. The patient has no fever, adequate fluid intake, and no history of urinary tract infection or STI. Dipstick analysis shows a slight elevation of leukocytes in urine but is otherwise normal. On further questioning, the patient admits to having multiple sexual partners in the past 2 months and had sex without a condom a few weeks ago. This encounter was with a female partner who recently mentioned having a yellow-green discharge to the patient.

Examination

Physical examination shows no abnormalities. No swelling, redness, or lesions are visible on the penis, scrotum, rectum, or surrounding areas. Additionally, no discharge is seen from the penis.

Laboratory Testing

NAAT for *T. vaginalis* on a urethral swab, urine sample, or semen sample is the preferred testing method. If this is not possible, an immediate wet mount of the sample(s) could suffice as a backup option. Consider testing for other STIs as well, including HIV.

Treatment

If the test is positive for *T. vaginalis*, treatment should be metronidazole 2 g orally in a single dose, tinidazole 2 g orally in a single dose, or metronidazole 500 mg orally twice a day for 7 days. Additionally, all sexual partners should be brought to the clinic for examination and treatment as well. Female partners should be retested 3 months after completion of treatment.

Patients are counselled to abstain from alcohol until 24 hours after treatment with metronidazole and 72 hours after treatment with tinidazole. Patients should abstain from sex until the treatment of the patient and all partners is completed and patient is no longer exhibiting symptoms.

Clinical Pearls

Although this patient was having mild symptoms, many patients with trichomoniasis never have symptoms, especially males. This is why a thorough health history is very important, especially in child and adolescent populations, because an STI might not be the first differential that comes to mind.

References

1. *Trichomonas* fact sheet. Centers for Disease and Prevention Web site. https://cdc.gov/std/trichomonas/stdfact-trichomoniasis.htm. Updated January 31, 2017. Accessed July 5, 2019.

2. American Academy of Pediatrics. Sexually transmitted diseases. In: Kimberlin DW, ed. *Red Book: 2018 Report of the Committee on Infectious Diseases*. 31st ed. Elk Grove, IL: American Academy of Pediatrics; 2018:896-904.

3. Centers for Disease Control and Prevention. 2015 sexually transmitted disease treatment guidelines. *MMWR Morb Mortal Wkly Rep*. 2015;64(3):1-81.

4. Kellogg N; American Academy of Pediatrics Committee on Child Abuse and Neglect. The evaluation of sexual abuse in children. *Pediatrics*. 2005;116(2):506-512.

5. Sutton M, Sternberg M, Koumans EH, McQuillan G, Berman S, Markowitz L. The prevalence of *Trichomonas vaginalis* infection among reproductive-age women in the United States, 2001-2004. *Clin Infect Dis*. 2007;45(10):1319-1326.

6. Sobel JD. Trichomoniasis. UpToDate Web site. https://www.uptodate.com/contents/trichomoniasis. Updated February 10, 2019. Accessed July 31, 2019.

7. Trichomoniasis: treatment and care. Centers for Disease Control and Prevention Web site. https://www.cdc.gov/std/trichomonas/treatment.htm. Updated January 4, 2017. Accessed July 31, 2019.

8. Sexually Transmitted Diseases (STDs): legal status of EPT. Centers for Disease Control and Prevention Web site. https://www.cdc.gov/std/ept/legal/default.htm. Updated June 25, 2019. Accessed July 31, 2019.

9. Cudmore SL, Delgaty KL, Hayward-McClelland SF, Petrin DP, Garber GE. Treatment of infections caused by metronidazole-resistant *Trichomonas vaginalis*. *Clin Microbiol Rev*. 2004;17(4):783-793.

10. Smith DS. Trichomoniasis treatment & management. Medscape Web site. https://emedicine.medscape.com/article/230617-treatment#showall. Updated December 6, 2018. Accessed July 31, 2019.

11. Howe K, Kissinger PJ. Single-dose compared with multidose metronidazole for the treatment of trichomoniasis in women: a meta-analysis. *Sex Transm Dis*. 2017;44(1):29-34.

12. Muzny CA, Richter S, Kissinger P. Is it time to stop using single-dose oral metronidazole for the treatment of trichomoniasis in women? *Sex Transm Dis*. 2019;46(5):e57-e59.

13. Kissinger P, Muzny CA, Mena LA, et al. Single-dose versus 7-day-dose metronidazole for the treatment of trichomoniasis in women: an open-label, randomised controlled trial. *Lancet Infect Dis*. 2018;18(11):1251-1259.

14. Chacon M, Fonseca THS, Oliveira S, et al. Chlorinated metronidazole as a promising alternative for treating trichomoniasis. *Parasitol Res*. 2018;117(5):1333-1340.

15. Cock IE, Selesho MI, Van Vuuren SF. A review of the traditional use of southern African medicinal plants for the treatment of selected parasite infections affecting humans. *J Ethnopharmacol*. 2018;220:250-264.

16. Fonseca T, Gomes JMS, Alacoque M, Vannier-Santos MA, Gomes MA, Busatti HGNO. Transmission electron microscopy revealing the mechanism of action of photodynamic therapy on *Trichomonas vaginalis*. *Acta Trop*. 2019;190:112-118.

Section V

YEAST

Chapter 18

Candidiasis and Balanitis

Angelia Trujillo, DNP, MSN, WHNP-BC
Nicole Marnell, DNP, APRN, CPNP-PC
Trinity Ingram-Jones, DNP, MSN, APRN, CPNP, PCNS, AFN-BC, SANE-A, SANE-P, DF-AFN
Alice Springer Bristow, DNP, CRNP, FNP-BC, CWCN, CNE

Candidiasis

Disease and Mimics

— Vulvovaginal candidiasis (VVC) is usually caused by *Candida albicans*, but it can also be caused by other *Candida* species or yeasts.[1] Yeast is a commensal vaginal flora that colonizes in up to 20% of reproductive-age women.[2] An alteration in the vaginal environment can cause over-proliferation of yeast, often leading to a symptomatic ailment.[2]

— VVC is not a reportable disease and is not considered to be a sexually transmitted infection (STI) because those who are not sexually active can be affected. However, it can occasionally be sexually transmitted, particularly in women with a high frequency of sexual intercourse.[3]

— Because it is rarely transmitted through sexual contact, partner intervention is not usually recommended.[4,5]

— Typical symptoms include pruritus, vaginal soreness, dyspareunia, external dysuria, and abnormal vaginal discharge (thick, white, curd-like). However, none of these symptoms are specific to VVC.[1] Vulvar involvement also includes pruritus, external dysuria, edema, and erythema.[1]

— A diagnosis of *Candida vaginitis* is suggested by the presence of external dysuria and vulvar pruritus, pain, swelling, and redness. Signs include vulvar edema, fissures, excoriations, and thick, curdy vaginal discharge (**Figures 18-1** and **18-2**).[1]

Figures 18-1 and 18-2. Candida vaginitis. *(Courtesy of Diana Faugno, MSN, RN, CPN, SANE-A, SANE-P, FAAFS, DF-IAFN, DF-AFN.)*

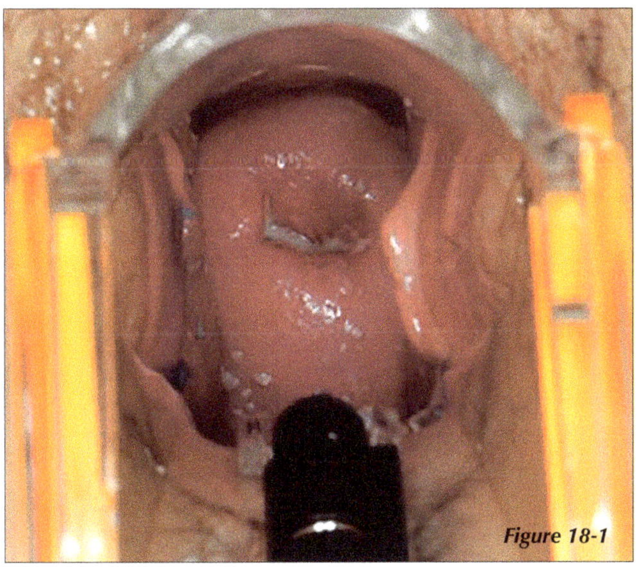

Figure 18-1

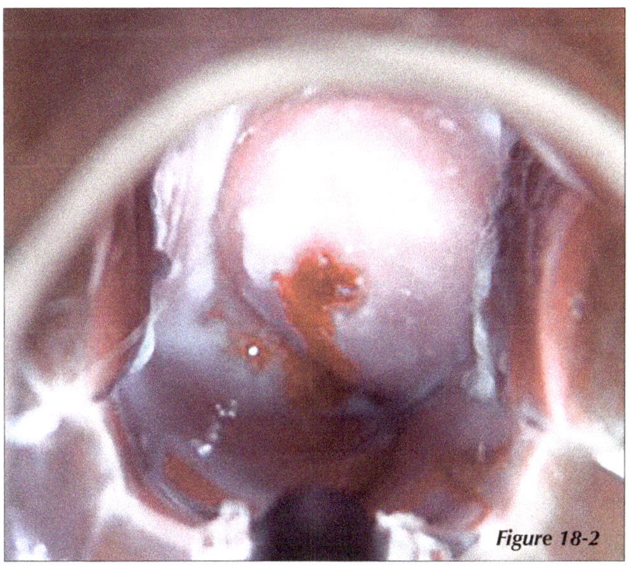

Figure 18-2

— A diagnosis can be made with either a wet preparation or Gram stain of vaginal discharge. If a wet mount is negative but signs and symptoms persist, a vaginal culture for *Candida* should be considered. *Candida* identification by culture in the absence of symptoms is not an indication for treatment, because approximately 10% to 20% of women harbor *Candida* or other yeasts in the vagina.[1]

— VVC can be classified as *complicated* or *uncomplicated*. VVC is uncomplicated when outbreaks are sporadic or infrequent, mild to moderate, likely caused by *Candida albicans*, and occur in a non-immunocompromised woman. VVC is considered complicated when outbreaks are recurrent and severe; when they are caused by non-*albicans* candidiasis; and when they occur in women with diabetes, immunocompromising conditions (eg, human immunodeficiency virus [HIV]), or who are undergoing immunosuppressive therapy.[1]

— Vaginal cultures should be taken from women with complicated VVC to confirm diagnosis and identify unusual species.[1]

— Recurrent vulvovaginal candidiasis (RVVC) is defined as 4 or more episodes of symptomatic VVC within 1 year. It affects less than 5% of women.[1]

Epidemiology

An estimated 75% of women will have at least 1 episode of VVC in their lifetime, and 40% to 45% will have 2 or more episodes.[1] Approximately 10% to 20% of VVC cases are complicated and require special diagnostic and therapeutic considerations.[1] VVC is the second most common cause of vaginitis after bacterial vaginosis, with a higher incidence in women of reproductive age.[3] An accurate accounting of the incidence and prevalence of VVC is challenging because treatment is generally empirical and over-the-counter remedies allow for self-diagnosis and treatment.[4] VVC costs an annual adjusted $2.84 billion in the United States alone.[4]

Treatment Guidelines

Uncomplicated VVC

Uncomplicated VVC is effectively treated with short-course topical formulations. Topically applied azole drugs are more effective than nystatin. According to the Centers for Disease Control and Prevention (CDC),[1] 80% to 90% of patients who complete therapy with these topical or oral agents will experience symptom relief and have negative follow-up cultures (**Table 18-1**).

Table 18-1. Summary of Treatment Guidelines for Uncomplicated VVC

Over-the-Counter Intravaginal Agents	Prescription Intravaginal Agents	Oral Agent
Clotrimazole 1% cream 5 g intravaginally daily for 7 to 14 days ***OR*** Clotrimazole 2% cream 5 g intravaginally daily for 3 days ***OR*** Miconazole 2% cream 5 g intravaginally daily for 7 days ***OR*** Miconazole 4% cream 5 g intravaginally daily for 3 days ***OR*** Miconazole 100 mg vaginal suppository, 1 suppository daily for 7 days ***OR*** Miconazole 200 mg vaginal suppository, 1 suppository for 3 days ***OR*** Miconazole 1200 mg vaginal suppository, 1 suppository for 1 day ***OR*** Tioconazole 6.5% ointment 5 g intravaginally in a single application	Butoconazole 2% cream (single-dose bioadhesive product), 5 g intravaginally in a single application ***OR*** Terconazole 0.4% cream 5 g intravaginally daily for 7 days ***OR*** Terconazole 0.8% cream 5 g intravaginally daily for 3 days ***OR*** Terconazole 80 mg vaginal suppository, 1 suppository daily for 3 days	Fluconazole 150 mg PO in a single dose

PO, per os (orally).
For more information on treatment, see the CDC's sexually transmitted disease guidelines at https://www.cdc.gov/std/tg2015/candidiasis.htm.[1]

Recurrent Vulvovaginal Candidiasis

Individual episodes of RVVC respond well to short-duration oral or topical azole therapy. A longer duration of initial therapy may be used to attempt mycologic remission before initiating a maintenance antifungal regimen. The CDC recommends treatment with topical therapy for 7 to 14 days or oral therapy with a 100-mg, 150-mg, or 200-mg dose of fluconazole every 3 days for a total of 3 doses (day 1, 4, and 7) for this purpose.[1]

Suppressive maintenance therapies are effective in reducing the incidence of RVVC. Weekly dosing of oral fluconazole (ie, 100-mg, 150-mg, 200-mg doses) for 6 months is the first-line maintenance regimen. Intermittent topical treatments can be considered if the first-line regimen is not feasible. After maintenance therapy is discontinued, 30% to 50% of patients will experience current disease. Those who remain symptomatic and culture-positive after maintenance therapy should be managed in consultation with a specialist.

Severe VVC

Characterized by extensive vulvar erythema, edema, excoriation, and fissure formation, severe VVC is associated with lower clinical response rates in patients treated with short courses of topical or oral therapy. The CDC recommends a 7- to 14-day course of topical azole or 150 mg of oral fluconazole in 2 sequential doses (second dose 72 hours after initial dose).[1]

Non-*Albicans* VVC

Successful treatment of non-*albicans* VVC is difficult, and at least 50% of patients with positive cultures for non-*albicans Candida* will be asymptomatic or minimally symptomatic. For these reasons, clinicians should make every effort to exclude other causes of vaginal symptoms in these patients. According to the CDC, optimal treatment of non-*albicans* VVC is not known.[1] The suggested first-line therapy is 7 to 14 days with a non-fluconazole oral or topical azole regimen. Recommended treatment of recurrent infection is daily administration of a 600-mg boric acid gelatin capsule intravaginally for 2 weeks. Treatment with this regimen is associated with a 70% clinical and mycological eradication rate, but if symptoms recur, referral to a specialist is advised.

Balanitis

Disease and Mimics

— Balanitis is a fairly common inflammation affecting the glans penis.[7]

— Posthitis affects the foreskin, whereas balanoposthitis includes both the foreskin and the glans (**Figure 18-3**). The latter only occurs in uncircumcised males.[7]

— Presenting symptoms are pain; tenderness; pruritus; erythematous excoriations; unpleasant odor; and a thick, cheesy white discharge. Inflammation may lead to a foreskin that cannot retract (phimosis). Trapping of the foreskin behind the glans penis is called paraphimosis and is an indication for urgent intervention.[7]

— The most common cause of balanitis is yeast overgrowth (*Candida albicans*) facilitated by the warm, moist genital environment.[7]

— The primary risk factor is poor hygiene in the uncircumcised male. Other conditions increasing the risk for this disorder include morbid obesity, condom catheters, chemical hypersensitivity, chronic edema (eg, congestive heart failure), and diabetes and immunosuppression, both of which can increase symptom severity. Skin conditions such as eczema, psoriasis, and lichen planus can elicit symptoms, warranting consultation with a dermatologist or other specialist.[7]

— Balanitis is not an STI itself, but it may be caused by bacteria and viruses that are transmitted through intimate contact.[7]

Figure 18-3. Penis of male patient, which had become swollen and erythematous as a result of a balanoposthitis. *(Courtesy of CDC, Atlanta, GA.)*

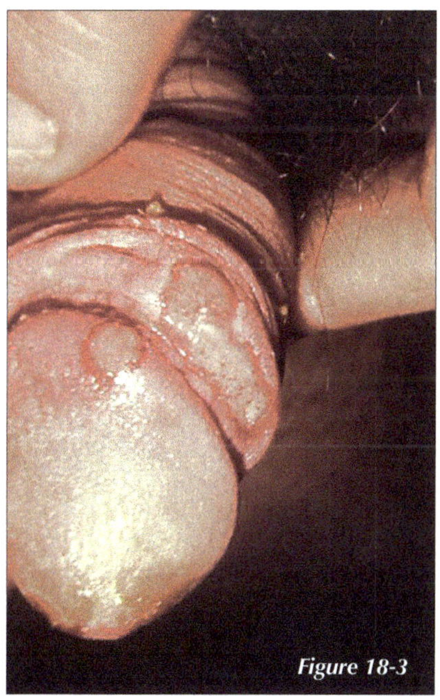

— Three types of balanitis exist:

— ***Zoon's balanitis:*** Inflammation of glans penis and foreskin affecting middle-aged and older uncircumcised men.[7]

— ***Circinate balanitis:*** Commonly associated with reactive arthritis; characterized by excoriations, pustular lesions, and ring-shaped erythema.[7]

— ***Pseudoepitheliomatous keratotic and micaceous balanitis:*** Less common condition with wart-like growths on the glans penis considered to be precancerous in some cases.[7]

Epidemiology

Balanitis occurs in approximately 1 in 4 boys and 1 in 30 uncircumcised men.[7] Uncircumcised men and boys younger than 4 years of age are at the greatest risk. At age 5, the foreskin becomes easier to retract, and the risk for balanitis decreases.[7] Circumcised males have a 68% lower prevalence of balanitis.[7] Males with balanitis have a 3.8-fold increase in the risk for penile cancer.[7]

Treatment Guidelines

Uncomplicated balanitis can be effectively treated with clotrimazole cream 1% or miconazole cream 2% applied topically for 5 to 7 days. Fluconazole 150 mg (1 tablet) orally may also be considered. If significant inflammation is present, the topical clotrimazole 1% cream or miconazole 2% cream can be mixed with hydrocortisone 1%. It is essential to treat sexual partners to reduce the risk of reinfection, eliminate a reservoir, and also provide advice on genital hygiene.[8] More complicated cases of balantis, such as circinate balantis, should be referred to a specialist. Cases that do not resolve with this treatment regimen may represent an aerobic or anaerobic infection or trichomoniasis.[8] Testing via culture for either of these is recommended before further treatment.

Special Considerations for Candidiasis and Balanitis

VVC does not cause an increase in mortality but can increase morbidity because the disorder and its associated symptoms are a source of both mental and physical discomfort.[3] In addition, untreated VVC may increase the risk for infertility, menstrual and pregnancy complications, and pelvic inflammatory disease.[3]

Penile candidiasis is most common among uncircumcised men and should be included in the differential diagnosis of any penile glans inflammation.[6] Long-term outcomes of balanitis include painful inflammation, phimosis, paraphimosis, strictures of the meatus, and progression of premalignant to malignant lesions.[6] Research data suggest that circumcision reduces the risk for balanitis.[6]

— ***Compromised host:*** Patients with underlying immunodeficiency, poorly controlled diabetes, or immunocompromising conditions and those receiving immunosuppression therapy do not respond well to short-term therapies. These patients should be prescribed prolonged, conventional treatment regimens of 7 to 14 days duration, in addition to correcting modifiable conditions.[1]

— ***Pregnancy:*** VVC often occurs during pregnancy. Only topical azole therapies of 7-day duration are recommended for use in pregnant patients.[1]

— ***HIV infection:*** Though vaginal *Candida* colonization rates are higher among patients infected with HIV, recommended therapy for uncomplicated and complicated VVC is the same for these patients. Although long-term, weekly prophylactic therapy with 200 mg of oral fluconazole has been effective in reducing colonization and symptomatic VVC among HIV-positive patients, this regimen is not recommended in the absence of complicated VVC.[1]

Case Studies

Adult Case Study 18-1

ST is a 30-year-old male engineer who presents to his family practice clinic requesting STI testing. He reports redness; itching; pain; and white, thick "stuff" that he states he can "wipe away" that has been present under his foreskin for the past 5 days. He reports a new partner 2 months ago. Prior STI testing was completed by both partners before they started their relationship. ST is negative for *Chlamydia*, gonorrhea, *Trichomonas*, syphilis, hepatitis C, and HIV. He denies pain with urination.

Examination

Glans penis is reddened and has white papules and plaques present under foreskin. No erosions or fissures are present, and there are no alterations to intertriginal or gluteal creases. If oral sex is part of the history, encourage oral examination as well.

Laboratory Testing

Potassium hydroxide (KOH) wet mount examination of white material obtained from glans is positive for pseudohyphae. Culture may also be completed to identify *Candida* elements. Herpes simplex virus (HSV) type-specific culture is obtained from the glans and tonsillar pillars. The patient is HSV-1 and HSV-2 negative.

Treatment

The patient is prescribed topical azole cream (clotrimazole 1% or miconazole 2%) twice daily for 5 to 7 days or fluconazole 150 mg orally taken in 2 doses, 3 days apart. Discussion regarding genital hygiene is a priority of care for this individual. It is also essential that the patient's partner is evaluated and treated for yeast vaginitis to reduce partner infection or reinfection. Failure of resolution of balanitis after treatment may indicate the need for cultures to rule out *Trichomonas* or other aerobic or anaerobic infections. If these cultures are negative, a biopsy would be indicated because balanitis may be a complication of lichen, psoriasis, or neoplasia.

Child Case Study 18-2

AD is a 12-year-old girl who is brought to the pediatric clinic by her mother for concerns about vaginal pruritus and abnormal vaginal discharge, described as clumpy and white, for 3 days. There is no report of fever or sexual activity. AD completed a 10-day course of oral antibiotics 3 days ago for acute otitis media. Menarche occurred 6 months ago. She has no history of chronic conditions. Immunizations are up to date.

Examination

Thick, white, nonodorous vaginal discharge is present on the vulva on inspection. No lesions are present. Mild vulvar edema and excoriations are noted.

Laboratory Testing

A KOH (wet prep) sample of the vaginal discharge shows yeast hyphae. Culture confirms VVC.[4]

Treatment

AD is prescribed terconazole 0.4% cream 5 g intravaginally for 7 days.[1]

References

1. 2015 sexually transmitted diseases treatment guidelines: vulvovaginal candidiasis. Centers for Disease Control and Prevention Web site. https://www.cdc.gov/std/tg2015/candidiasis.htm. Updated June 4, 2015. Accessed July 15, 2019.

2. Rice A, Elwerdany M, Hadoura E, Mahmood T. Vaginal discharge. *Obstet Gynaecol Reprod Med.* 2016;26(11):317-323.

3. Gonçalves B, Ferreira C, Alves CT, Henriques M, Azeredo J, Silva S. Vulvovaginal candidiasis: epidemiology, microbiology and risk factors. *Crit Rev Microbiol.* 2016;42(6):905-927.

4. Blostein F, Levin-Sparenberg E, Wagner J, Foxman B. Recurrent vulvovaginal candidiasis. *Ann Epidemiol.* 2017;27(9):575-582.
5. Fong IW. The value of treating the sexual partners of women with recurrent vaginal candidiasis with ketoconazole. *Genitourin Med.* 1992;68(3):174-176.
6. Edwards L. *Genital Dermatology Atlas.* 2nd ed. Philadelphia, PA: Lippincott Williams & Wilkins; 2011.
7. Wray AA, Khetarpal S. *Balanitis.* Treasure Island, FL: StatPearls Publishing; 2019.
8. Pandya I, Shinojia M, Vadukul D, Marfatia Y. Approach to balanitis/balanoposthitis: current Guidelines. *Indian J Sex Transm Dis AIDS.* 2014:35(2):155-157.

Section VI

Spirochete

Chapter 19

Syphilis

Lauren Traveller, DNP, APRN, FNP-C
Robert Vargas, BS
Rachell A. Ekroos, PhD, APRN-BC, AFN-BC, FAAN

Disease and Mimics

— Syphilis is a bacterial infection caused by *Treponema pallidum* (**Figure 19-1**). Although primarily spread through direct contact with a lesion, a small fraction of cases occur through blood transmissions such as sharing needles or direct blood transfusions.[1]

— Syphilis is a chronic bacterial infection. If left untreated, it can progress through several stages leading to irreversible neurological and cardiovascular complications.

— Clinical staging for syphilis is based on symptoms and includes primary, secondary, latent, and tertiary stages.[2]

— Syphilis is known as the "great pretender" because of its progressive nature causing myriad symptoms and giving it the ability to masquerade as many other conditions.[3]

— Diagnosis of syphilis can be made via dark-field microscopy or through serological tests (**Figure 19-2**).

— Congenital syphilis occurs through the transplacental transmission of *T. pallidum* from an infected mother to the developing fetus during pregnancy (**Figures 19-3** through **19-6**).

— Because of the potential for false negatives with serological testing, a reactive nontreponemal test requires a treponemal test for an accurate diagnosis.[4]

— Treatments typically involve the use of benzathine penicillin G.[4]

— There is an increased risk of acquiring human immunodeficiency virus (HIV) with a syphilis diagnosis, particularly among men who have sex with men (MSM).[5]

Figure 19-1. *Syphilis;* Treponema pallidum. *(Courtesy of CDC, Atlanta, GA.)*

Figure 19-2. *Syphilis;* Treponema pallidum *on dark field. (Courtesy of CDC, Atlanta, GA.)*

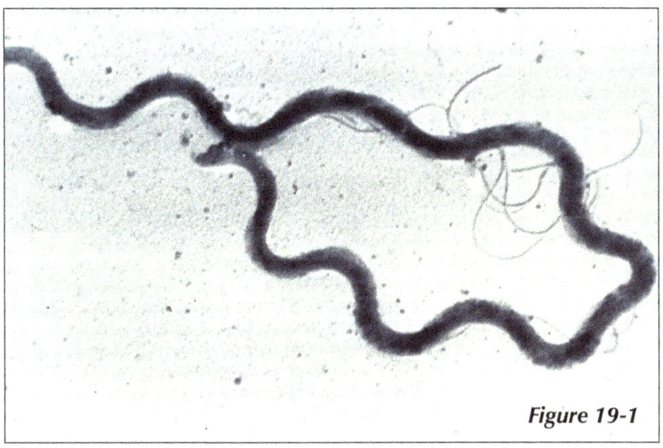

Figure 19-1

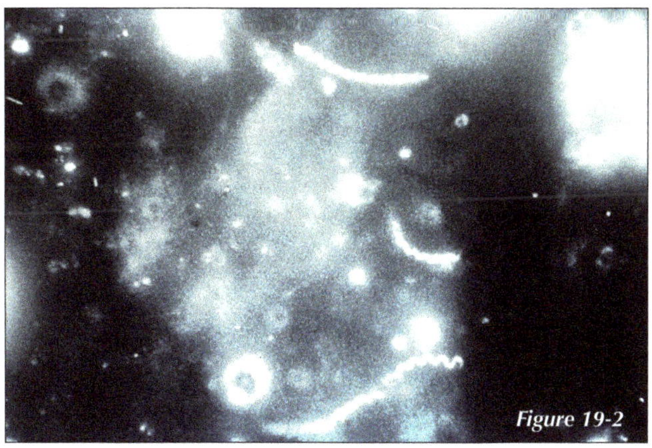

Figure 19-2

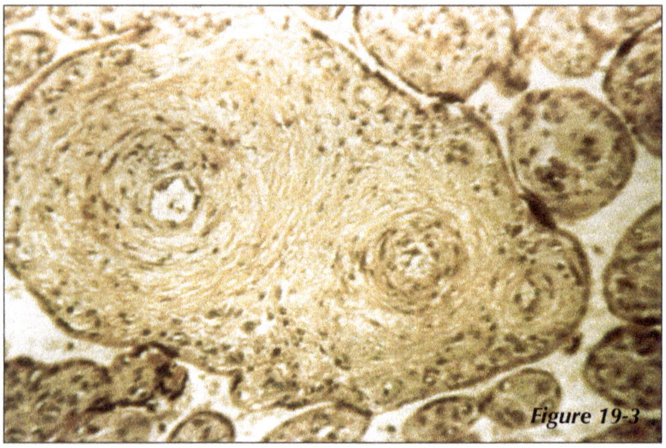

Figure 19-3. *Congenital syphilis; increased size of villi secondary to vasculitis and increased connective tissue. (Courtesy of CDC, Atlanta, GA.)*

Figure 19-4. *Congenital syphilis; mucous patches. (Courtesy of CDC, Atlanta, GA.)*

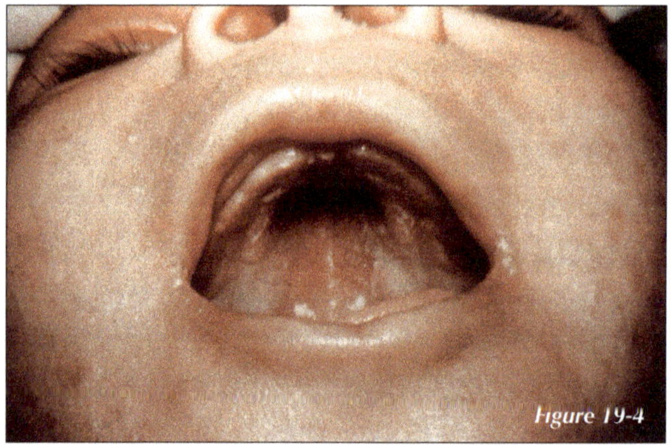

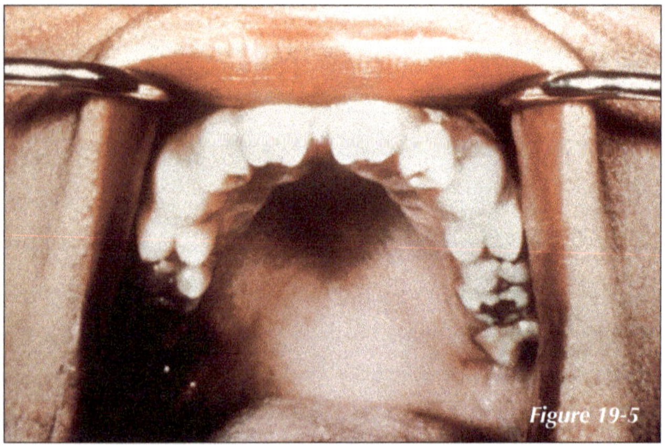

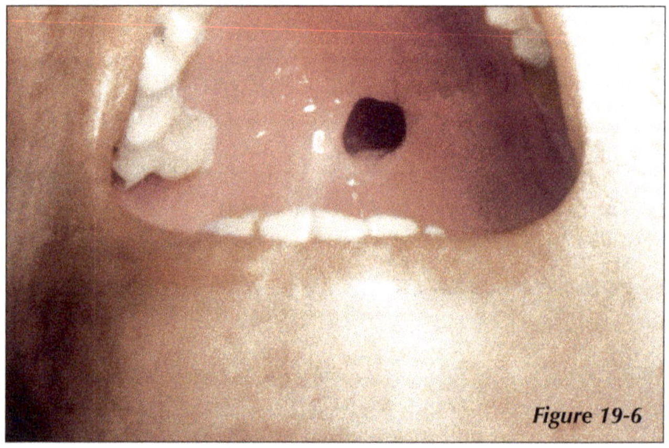

Figure 19-5. *Congenital syphilis; Hutchinson's teeth. (Courtesy of CDC, Atlanta, GA.)*

Figure 19-6. *Congenital syphilis; perforation of palate. (Courtesy of CDC, Atlanta, GA.)*

Epidemiology

New cases of syphilis have continued to increase within the United States. The highest rates of reported primary and secondary syphilis are among men aged 25 to 29 years. A racial disparity exists, with the highest prevalence among African Americans.[5]

Symptoms of syphilis vary by stage and among individuals. Presentation of symptoms often starts about 3 weeks (range 9 to 90 days) after *T. pallidum* infection. The initial stage, primary syphilis, typically presents as a painless indurated lesion with raised margins called a ***chancre*** (**Figures 19-7** through **19-11**). Syphilitic chancres are approximately 0.5 to 1.5 cm in diameter and can occur on the external anogenital structures such as the penis, scrotum, labia, introitus, and anus; in the rectum; and in or around the mouth.[2,3] Some patients may report a painful lesion if the chancre appears in a location where secondary injury may occur, such as from an abrasion (eg, friction abrasion from a raised seam in clothing) or a laceration (eg, overstretching of tissue and creating a tear near or on the chancre). Chancres typically resolve within 3 to 6 weeks regardless of treatment status. Because of the typical painless quality of syphilitic chancres, patients often are unaware of the lesion or, if they notice, are not aware of the health significance.

If left untreated, the bacteria will proliferate and migrate via the lymphatic system into the bloodstream. Subsequent secondary syphilis (**Figures 19-12** through **19-14**) can present between 7 to 12 weeks after infection with generalized symptoms such

Figure 19-7. Primary syphilis chancre. (Courtesy of CDC, Atlanta, GA.

Figure 19-8. Primary syphilis chancre. (Courtesy of CDC, Atlanta, GA.)

Figure 19-9. Primary syphilis chancre. (Courtesy of CDC, Atlanta, GA.)

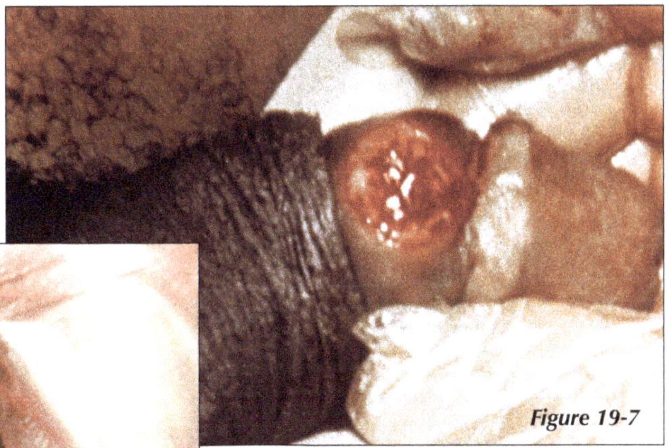

Figure 19-7

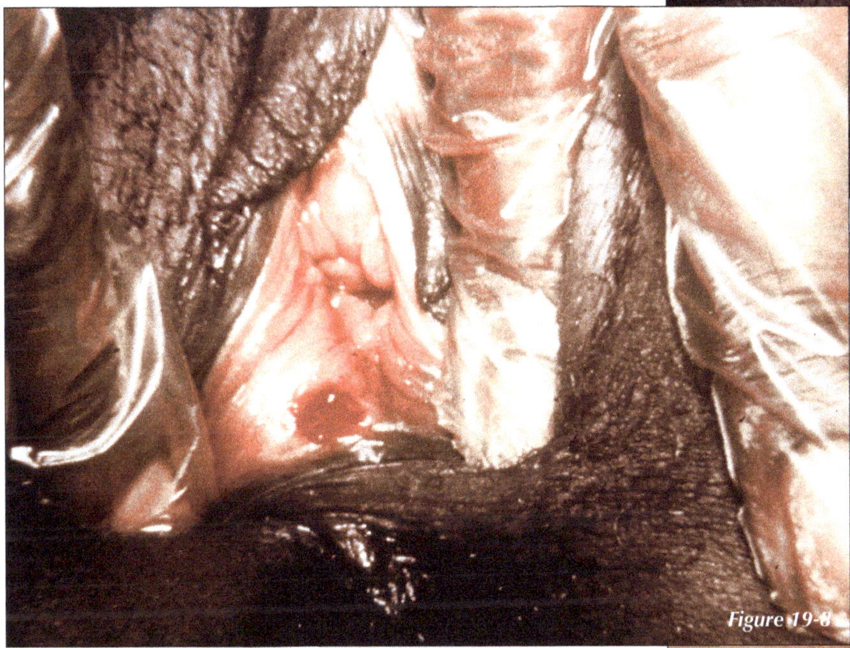

Figure 19-8

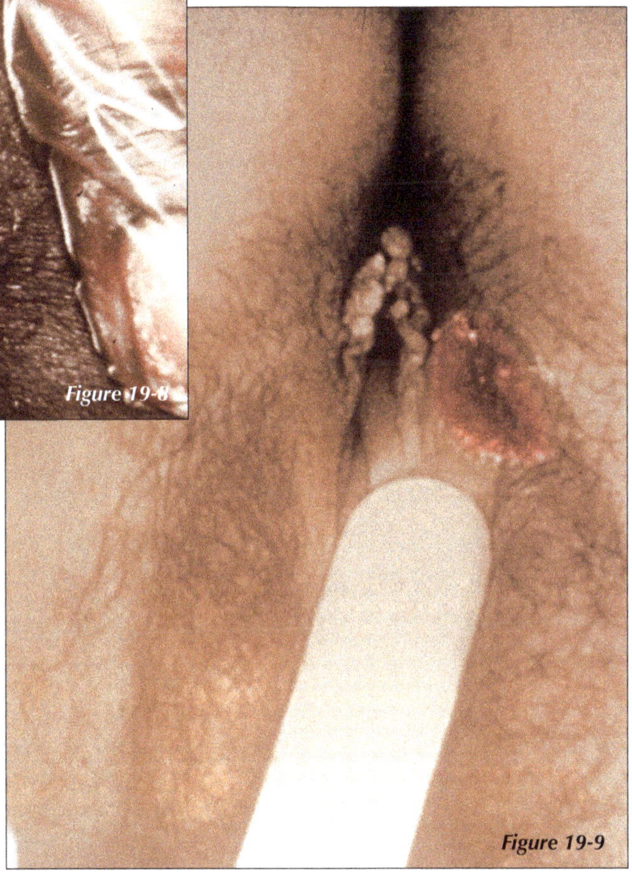

Figure 19-9

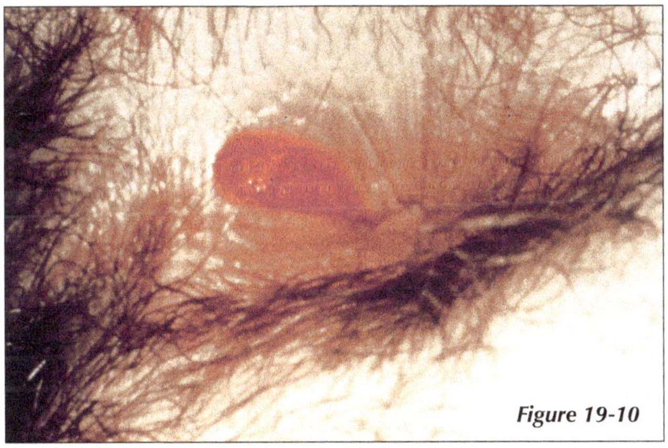

Figure 19-10

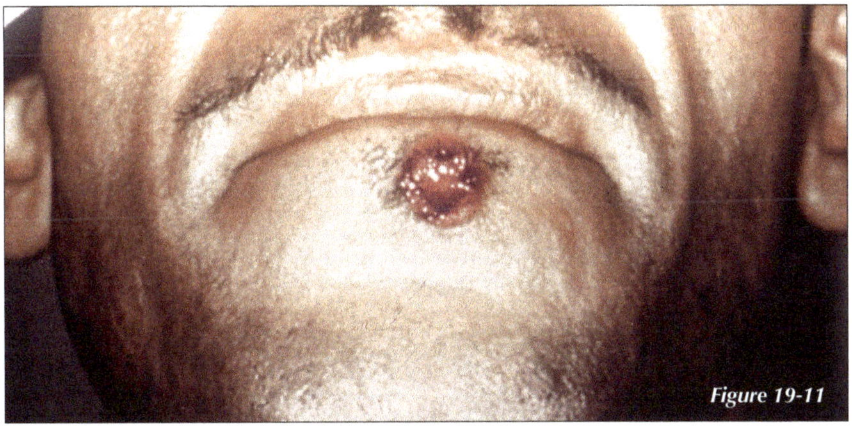

Figure 19-11

Figure 19-10. Primary syphilis chancre of anus. (Courtesy of CDC, Atlanta, GA.)

Figure 19-11. Primary syphilis chancre. (Courtesy of CDC, Atlanta, GA.)

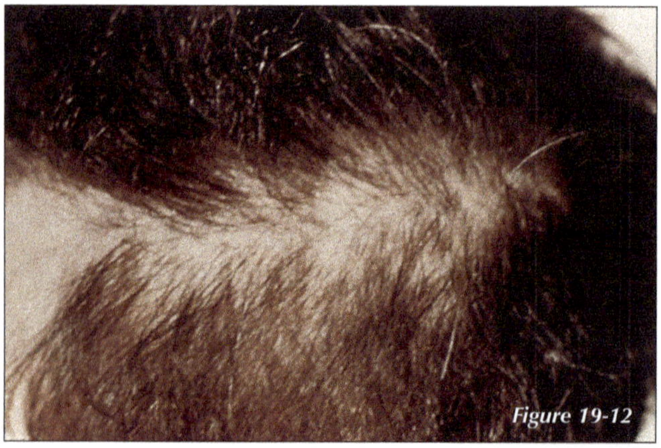

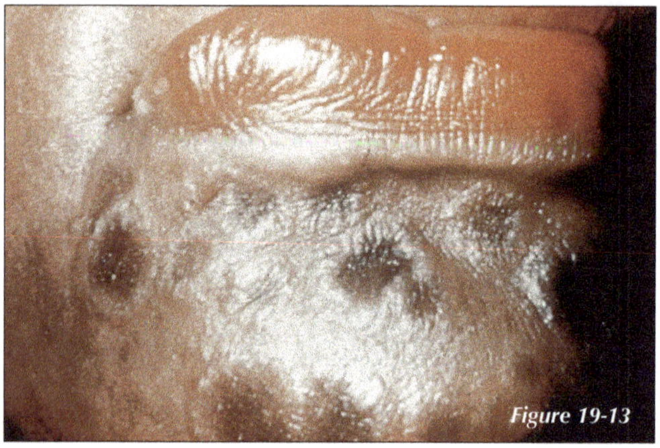

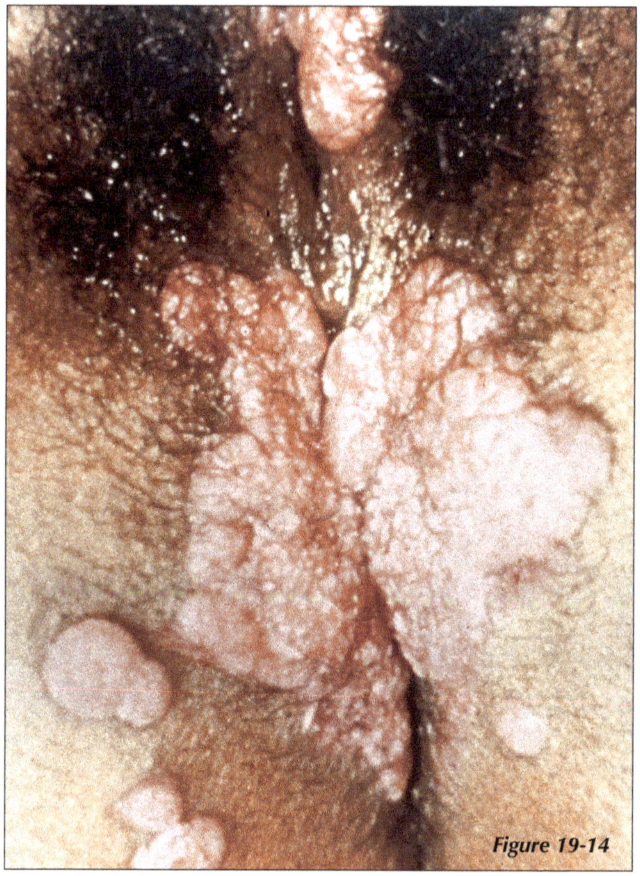

Figure 19-12. *Secondary syphilis; alopecia. (Courtesy of CDC, Atlanta, GA.)*

Figure 19-13. *Secondary syphilis. (Courtesy of CDC, Atlanta, GA.)*

Figure 19-14. *Secondary syphilis; condylomata lata. (Courtesy of CDC, Atlanta, GA.)*

as fever, fatigue, weight loss, and swollen lymph glands.[6] A classic feature seen in secondary syphilis is a nonpruritic, macular rash (distinct spots) on the palms of the hands, soles of the feet, or torso that may go unnoticed depending on skin color and condition.[2,3] Additional symptoms of secondary syphilis can include patchy hair loss, headaches, and muscle aches.[3] Any of these symptoms may reoccur but will subside within a period of 4 to 12 months even without treatment.

Lack of clinical signs and symptoms are the primary characterization of latent syphilis. When a negative screening test within the past 12 months is confirmed, it is considered to be an early latent infection; otherwise, it is a considered a late latent infection (greater than 12 months since infection).[2] Latent syphilis can last years.[3] During this asymptomatic stage, patients may become alerted to the infection because of an annual sexually transmitted infection (STI) screening, screening as a result of another illness or pregnancy, notification by a sexual contact who was diagnosed, or notification by a disease investigator from the local health department.

Further lack of treatment can result in the development of tertiary syphilis as a result of the surviving treponemes in various tissues. Tertiary syphilis only occurs in about 28% of untreated patients. If it develops, tertiary syphilis will typically present between 10 and 30 years after the initial infection.[3] Cutaneous manifestations include subcutaneous nodules (gummas) that invade the dermis in various regions of the body.[2] Subsequent necrosis of the nodule can lead to ulcerations that affect underlying muscle and bone. Several organs within the cardiac and nervous systems may also be affected in addition to the cutaneous manifestations.

Tertiary syphilis can also present as neurosyphilis, involving treponemal invasion of the central nervous system.[2,7] Neurosyphilis includes several clinical manifestations such as syphilitic meningitis, meningovascular syphilis, general paresis, and tabes dorsalis. Some patients present asymptomatically; others may only report headaches or signs of meningitis or present with symptoms such as visual impairment, gait disturbances, paresthesia, and epilepsy.[7] Cardiovascular syphilis can present with aortitis that can subsequently lead to aortic root dilation, aneurysm formation, and aortic insufficiency.[8] Patients with neurosyphilis symptoms (visual disturbances, meningitis, altered mental status) warrant further cerebrospinal fluid (CSF) examination that includes a CSF cell count and reactive CSF–Venereal Disease Research Laboratory (VDRL) test.[4]

Because of the potential for transplacental transmission of syphilis, congenital syphilis is a concern for any mother who has reactive serological tests. There has been an increased incidence of congenital syphilis in the United States every year since 2012.[5,9] Congenital syphilis infection and presentation vary depending on the staging of the mother's disease, fetal gestation, and the immunological response of the fetus.[10] Potential complications for the developing fetus include failure to thrive, cutaneous lesions, permanent deformities, spontaneous abortions, stillbirth, and perinatal death. Any infant born to a woman with reactive serological tests should receive a thorough physical examination to assess for any evidence of syphilis.[3,9] Infants and children older than 1 month with primary or secondary syphilis or reactive serological tests should receive a sexual abuse evaluation.[4]

Diagnosis of syphilis consists of a series of several tests and techniques to confirm a positive diagnosis. Although not commonly used, dark-field microscopy is the only definitive method for immediate diagnosis and treatment of early syphilis from a direct sample. The most commonly used laboratory tests for syphilis are treponemal and nontreponemal tests. Treponemal tests include the *T. pallidum* hemagglutination assay, the fluorescent treponema antibody absorption test, and the enzyme or chemiluminescence immunoassays that detect specific antibodies against *T. pallidum*. Nontreponemal tests include the VDRL test and rapid plasma reagin (RPR) tests. The RPR tests are useful in screening for syphilis and providing a quantitative titer for measuring disease activity to guide treatment response.

When using the nontreponemal options for initial syphilis screening, a high rate of false positives can occur with many medical conditions. Therefore, a reactive nontreponemal test requires a subsequent treponemal test to achieve an accurate diagnosis. For this reason, a reverse screening algorithm (**Figure 19-15**) adopted by many laboratories assists in avoiding false positives and in identifying syphilis in previously treated patients or those with untreated late latent syphilis. This reverse screening method starts with a treponemal test followed by a standard nontreponemal test with titer if the treponemal test is reactive.[4]

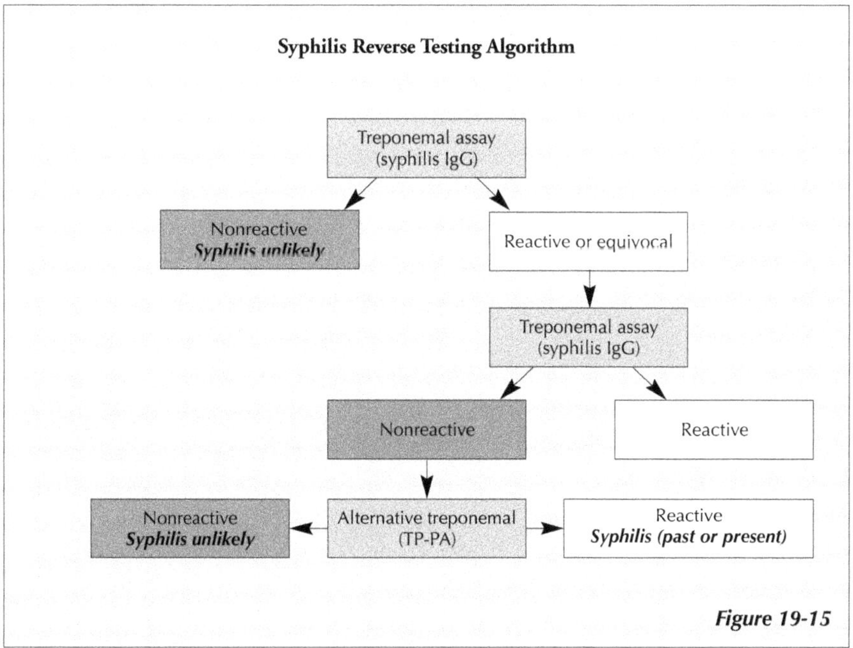

Figure 19-15. *Syphilis reverse testing algorithm.*

Treatment Guidelines

Parenteral administration of penicillin G is the preferred treatment for syphilis regardless of disease stage. Using benzathine penicillin G (Bicillin L-A) is important because combination benzathine penicillin, procaine penicillin, and oral penicillin are not appropriate for treatment when benzathine penicillin G is indicated.[4] Dosage and preparation vary depending on the stage and clinical manifestation. Patients should follow up clinically and serologically at intervals of 6, 12, 18, and 24 months after treatment.[4] **Table 19-1** provides a summary of the current treatment guidelines for the different stages of syphilis.

Table 19-1. Summary of Treatment Guidelines for Syphilis[4]

Stage	Population	Penicillin G
Primary and secondary syphilis	Adults ≥ 18 years of age	Benzathine penicillin G 2.4 million units IM in a single dose
	Infants and children < 18 years of age	Benzathine penicillin G 50 000 units/kg IM, up to the adult dose of 2.4 million units in a single dose
Early latent syphilis	Adults ≥ 18 years of age	Benzathine penicillin G 2.4 million units IM in a single dose
	Infants and children < 18 years of age	Benzathine penicillin G 50 000 units/kg IM, up to the adult dose of 2.4 million units in a single dose
Late latent syphilis or latent syphilis of unknown duration	Adults ≥ 18 years of age	Benzathine penicillin G 7.2 million units total, administered as 3 doses of 2.4 million units IM each at 1-week intervals
	Infants and children < 18 years of age	Benzathine penicillin G 50 000 units/kg IM, up to the adult dose of 2.4 million units, administered as 3 doses at 1-week intervals (total 150 000 units/kg up to the total adult dose of 7.2 million units)
Tertiary syphilis with normal CSF examination		Benzathine penicillin G 7.2 million units total, administered as 3 doses of 2.4 million units IM each at 1-week intervals
Neurosyphilis & ocular syphilis		Aqueous crystalline penicillin G 18 to 24 million units per day, administered as 3 to 4 million units IV every 4 hours or continuous infusion, for 10 to 14 days ***OR*** Procaine penicillin G 2.4 million units IM once daily ***PLUS*** Probenecid 500 mg orally four times a day, both for 10 to 14 days
Proven congenital syphilis*	Infants aged < 30 days	Aqueous crystalline penicillin G 100 000 to 150 000 units/kg/day, administered as 50 000 units/kg/dose IV every 12 hours during the first 7 days of life and every 8 hours after that for a total of 10 days ***OR*** Procaine penicillin G 50 000 units/kg/dose IM in a single daily dose for 10 days
	Infants and children ≥ 1 month	Aqueous crystalline penicillin G 200 000 to 300 000 units/kg/day IV, administered as 50 000 units/kg every 4 to 6 hours for 10 days

IM, intramuscularly; IV, intravenously.
**Proven congenital syphilis involves any neonate with an abnormal physical examination consistent with congenital syphilis, a serum quantitative nontreponemal serological titer that is fourfold higher than the mother's titer, or a positive dark-field test or polymerase chain reaction (PCR) testing of lesions.[4]*
For more information on treatment guidelines, see the CDC's sexually transmitted disease guidelines at https://www.cdc.gov/std/syphilis/treatment.htm. In addition, the CDC has produced a pocket guide for providers, which can be found at https://www.cdc.gov/std/syphilis/Syphilis-Pocket-Guide-FINAL-508.pdf.

Special Considerations

— *Pregnancy:* All women should undergo serological screening for syphilis early during pregnancy. The only effective treatment for syphilis during pregnancy is benzathine penicillin G, using the regimen appropriate for the stage of infection.[10] Research has demonstrated beneficial evidence of administration of the second dose of benzathine penicillin 2.4 million units intramuscularly (IM) 1 week after the initial dose for pregnant women with primary, secondary, or early latent syphilis.[11] If there is a history of a penicillin allergy, desensitization measures are needed because there are no proven alternatives for treatment of syphilis during pregnancy.[10]

— *HIV infection:* Persons with HIV who test positive for syphilis are recommended the same treatment regimen as those without HIV. All patients with HIV and syphilis should receive a neurological examination because of increased risk of neurological complications. There have been reports of higher rates of serological failure; therefore, careful follow-up is critical to prevent further disease progression. Follow-up should occur 3, 6, 9, 12, and 24 months after treatment.[4]

— *Neonates:* Neonates born to a mother with a reactive serological test should undergo testing for syphilis in addition to HIV testing and a thorough examination assessing for evidence of congenital syphilis (eg, nonimmune hydrops, jaundice, hepatosplenomegaly, rhinitis, skin rash, pseudoparalysis of an extremity). Neonates with a normal physical examination who have quantitative titers equal to or less than fourfold the maternal titer can still be given benzathine treatment if congenital syphilis is possible. Follow-up examinations should be planned every 2 to 3 months and include serological testing until the test becomes nonreactive.[9]

— *Allergies:* Alternative treatment options have limited data to support their use over penicillin. These alternative treatments for those with penicillin allergy include doxycycline 100 mg orally twice daily for 14 days or tetracycline 500 mg 4 times daily for 14 days.[12] If unable to ensure compliance, desensitization measures and subsequent benzathine penicillin treatment are recommended.[4]

— *Coinfection:* There is a correlation between the incidence of HIV and syphilis,[5] particularly among MSM, accounting for more than 50% of primary and secondary syphilis cases overall.[3,5] It is recommended that all persons who have primary and secondary syphilis be tested for HIV infection and have subsequent retesting after 3 months if the first HIV test was negative to confirm status.[4]

Case Studies

Adult Case Study 19-1

SB is a 27-year-old man who presents to the local STI clinic for testing because he heard a recent sexual partner was rumored to have an STI. He is in a new relationship and wants to make sure he is not infected. SB has been sexually active with multiple male partners, both known and unknown, in recent months. He reports receptive anal sexual practices and oral sex (both receiving and giving). SB denies symptoms at this time and has a history of *Chlamydia* treated at the time of diagnosis and syphilis treated with "1 shot." He has no significant medical history and no drug allergies.

Examintation

Physical and anogenital examination show a nonpruritic macular rash faintly visible on bilateral soles of feet.

Laboratory Testing

Urine nucleic acid amplification testing (NAAT) for *Chlamydia* and gonorrhea is negative; pharyngeal NAAT for *Chlamydia* and gonorrhea is negative; rectal NAAT for *Chlamydia* and gonorrhea is negative; HIV antibody testing is negative; *T. pallidum* total antibody screen (IgM and IgG) is reactive with a positive reflex RPR titer (1:128).

Treatment

SB returns to the clinic for treatment and is administered benzathine penicillin G (Bicillin L-A) 2.4 million units IM single dose. Patient education discussions include consistent condom use, safe sexual practices, and sexual health. SB discloses having unprotected sexual contact with a new partner between being tested and receiving the results, so the health care provider discusses the need for partner testing and abstinence until results are known. Condoms are provided. Local public health district is notified per mandatory reporting requirements, and SB is notified regarding disease investigation follow-up procedures. Patient is advised to follow-up in 6 months for serological evaluation.

Child Case Study 19-2

EM is a 1-day-old girl born in the hospital and who remains hospitalized. Her mother reports no prenatal care before admission to the labor and delivery unit at a local hospital. Full STI panel testing results for the mother show a positive serum nontreponemal test. EM's testing is completed after receipt of the mother's results.

Examination

A complete physical and anogenital examination is performed. The findings are negative. The infant is in the low-birth-weight risk category. A lumbar puncture is completed. Long-bone radiographs are completed, and the health care provider is awaiting results.

Laboratory Testing

Complete blood cell count with differential is within normal limits. CSF analysis for VDRL, cell count, and protein is negative. HIV antibody testing is negative. *T. pallidum* particle agglutination assay is reactive. RPR is less than fourfold maternal titer.

Treatment

EM is admitted to the pediatric unit and administered aqueous crystalline penicillin G 100 000 to 150 000 units/kg per day, given as 50 000 units/kg/dose IV every 12 hours during the first 7 days of life and every 8 hours after that for a total of 10 days. The local public health district is notified per mandatory reporting requirements, and the mother is notified regarding disease investigation follow-up procedures.

References

1. Hook EW 3rd. Syphilis. *Lancet.* 2017;389(10078):1550-1557.
2. Schöfer H. Early and late syphilis. In: Gross G, Tyring SK, eds. *Sexually Transmitted Infections and Sexually Transmitted Diseases.* Berlin, Germany: Springer-Verlag Berlin Heidelberg; 2011:151-161.
3. Sexually transmitted diseases (STDs): syphilis—CDC fact sheet (detailed).Centers for Disease Control and Prevention Web site. https://www.cdc.gov/std/syphilis/stdfact-syphilis-detailed.htm. Updated January 30, 2017. Accessed July 25, 2019.
4. 2015 sexually transmitted dieases treatment guidelines: syphilis. Centers for Disease Control and Prevention Web site. https://www.cdc.gov/std/tg2015/syphilis.htm. Updated June 4, 2015. Accessed August 10, 2019.
5. Sexually transmitted diseases surveillance 2017: syphilis. Centers for Disease Control and Prevention Web site. https://www.cdc.gov/std/stats17/syphilis.htm. Updated July 24, 2018. Accessed July 23, 2019.
6. Baughn RE, Musher DM. Secondary syphilitic lesions. *Clin Microbiol Rev.* 2005;18(1):205-216.
7. Prange HW. Neurosyphilis. In: Gross G, Tyring SK, eds. *Sexually Transmitted Infections and Sexually Transmitted Diseases.* Berlin, Germany: Springer-Verlag Berlin Heidelberg; 2011:163-171.
8. Jackman JD Jr, Radolf JD. Cardiovascular syphilis. *Am J Med.* 1989;87(4):425-433.

9. 2015 sexually transmitted diseases treatment guidelines: congential syphilis. Centers for Disease Control and Prevention Web site. https://www.cdc.gov/std/tg2015/congenital.htm. Updated June 4, 2015. Accessed July 25, 2019.

10. 2015 sexaully transmitted diseases treatment guidelines: syphilis during pregnancy. Centers for Disease Control and Prevention Web site. https://www.cdc.gov/std/tg2015/syphilis-pregnancy.htm. Updated June 4, 2015. Accessed July 25, 2019.

11. Wendel GD Jr, Sheffield JS, Hollier LM, Hill JB, Ramsey PS, Sánchez PJ. Treatment of syphilis in pregnancy and prevention of congenital syphilis. *Clin Infect Dis*. 2002;35(suppl 2):S200-S209.

12. Wong T, Singh AE, De P. Primary syphilis: serological treatment response to doxycycline/tetracycline versus benzathine penicillin. *Am J Med*. 2008;121(10):903-908.

Section VII

Test Questions

Objectives

In a problem-oriented analysis (ie, subjective/objective/assessment/plan [SOAP]), the learner will read, evaluate, and analyze cases; formulate a clinical diagnosis with history and symptoms provided by the patient; and provide an objective clinical assessment to determine the reasonable testing necessary for the definitive differential diagnosis.

After completing the exercises presented in this chapter, the learner will be able to:

1. Correctly identify the anogenital anatomy of a patient.
2. Identify and document injuries, age-related normal variants, or medical conditions based on review of case photographs.
3. For the registered nurse (RN) and other medical professionals: follow directions and answers questions.
4. Determine whether or not the case history warrants evidence collection. If yes, list 3 items of evidence to collect, the method for collection, and the reason for the collection.
5. For the RN, advanced practice registered nurse (APRN), and all medical practitioners:
   - Assess the patient, create a nursing diagnosis, create a plan of care that includes a protocol for testing, and demonstrate implementation of the plan of care, as well as adherence to quality with patient-centered and trauma-informed methods in the plan of care.
     - Assessment description
     - Nursing diagnosis http://www.nandanursingdiagnosislist.org/
     - Protocol to implement in the plan of care including testing recommendations
     - Patient education (patient centered and trauma informed)
     - Follow-up recommendations
6. For the advanced practice provider and physician (APP):
   - Create a differential diagnosis and provide treatment options based on the patient's history, laboratory test results, and clinical presentations.
     - Clinical presentation (subjective history)
     - Possible clinical diagnoses (list all possible diagnoses)
     - Laboratory testing for differential
     - Differential diagnosis
   - Prescribe medications to eradicate disease and provide comfort for the patient.
     - Medical treatment(s)
     - Patient instructions for care
   - Follow-up recommendations (test-of-cure timing)
7. Determine and justify whether or not the disease for the case is reportable. If yes, identify the procedure in your community.

Case Study 1

Subjective History

A 43-year-old woman presents with malodorous yellow-green vaginal discharge that has been present for 3 days. She also complains of moderate vaginal irritation while engaging in sexual intercourse. She has had 2 sexual partners within the last month and did not use a condom during either sexual encounter. The last sexual encounter was 7 days ago. The patient regularly practices douching before and after intercourse. She has not taken any over-the-counter medications, has not used any over-the-counter vaginal applications, and is currently not on any prescription medications. She has no known drug allergies.

Activity 1-1. Identifying Missing Subjective Information

The acronym OLDCARTS (Onset, Location, Duration, Character, Aggravating/relieving, Radiation, Timing, Severity) is used to identify the information necessary to continue with your assessment. For the purposes of this activity, identify the absent OLDCARTS information.

____

____

Activity 1-2. Anatomical Identification

Correctly identify the anogenital anatomy of a patient (**Activity Figure 1-2**).

A. ____________________________________

B. ____________________________________

C. ____________________________________

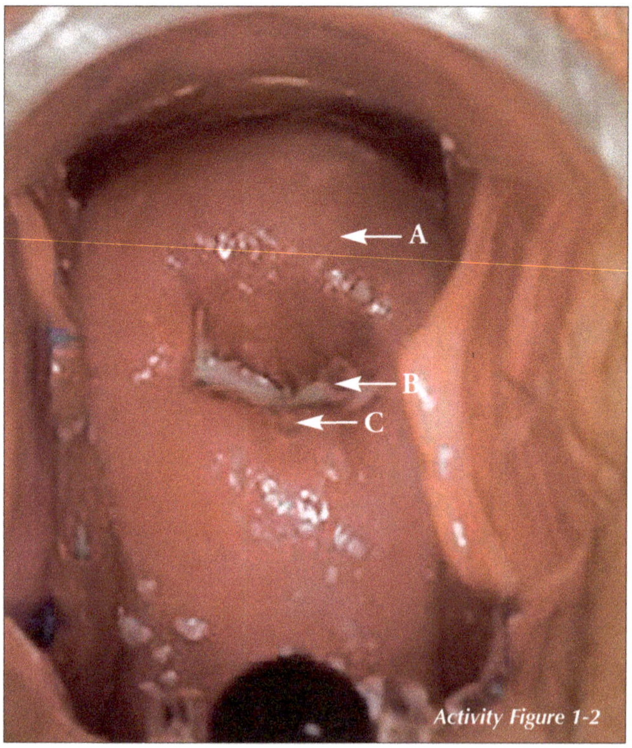

Activity Figure 1-2

Objective History

The cervix is slightly erythematous with small punctate hemorrhages resembling a "strawberry cervix." Otherwise, the examination is normal.

The RN orders the office urine dipstick. The urine dipstick results indicate a moderate increase in leukocytes and trace blood present in the urine specimen. No other abnormalities are observed on the dipstick results.

Activity 1-3. Physical Examination Findings

Identify and document injuries, age-related normal variants, and medical conditions based on a review of the case photographs (**Activity Figure 1-3**).

____

____

____

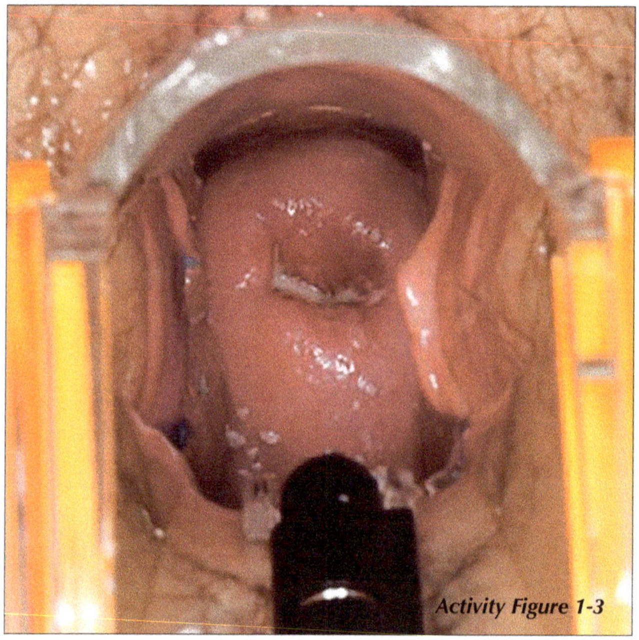

Activity Figure 1-3

Activity 1-4. Clinical Laboratory Improvement Amendments (CLIA)

Laboratory Examination

Using the history and the initial urine findings, list the items from the protocol that can be implemented to assist APPs and physicians in the clinical diagnosis.

____

____

____

____

Activity 1-5. Clinical Laboratory Testing

For APPs and physicians, using the history and the initial urinary findings, list the laboratory tests to assist in the definitive differential diagnosis.

Clinical Assessment

Activity 1-6. Forensic Evidence Collection

Determine whether or not the case history warrants medical forensic evidence collection. If so, list 3 items of evidence that should be collected, the method for collection, and the reason for collection.

Activity 1-7. Nursing Plan of Care Procedure

Assess for and create a nursing diagnosis. Create a plan of care that includes a protocol for testing, demonstrates implementation of the plan of care, and adheres to quality with patient-centered and trauma-informed methods in the plan of care.

Activity 1-8. APP and Physician Differential Diagnosis

For APPs and physicians, complete the previous activities, and create a differential diagnosis based on the patient's history, laboratories, and clinical presentations. Of the possible differential diagnosis, what is the infection?

Treatment, Reporting, and Follow-up Plan of Care

Activity 1-9. Treatment

Provide treatment options and prescribe medications to eradicate disease and provide comfort for the patient.

Activity 1-10. Reporting

Determine if the differential diagnosis of the disease is reportable. If yes, identify the entity in your community to which to report.

Activity 1-11. Follow-Up Recommendations in Plan of Care

Provide follow-up recommendations and patient education to include in the plan of care.

Case Study 2

Subjective - Initial Visit

A 9-year-old girl complains to her mother that "it really hurts to pee." On the second day of the complaints, the mother takes the child to a clinic. The child discloses to the doctor and nurse at the clinic that her stepfather comes into her room at night and "puts his finger in me." She states she can feel his fingernail inside of her. She also states that she "ties my PJs up very tight, but he always takes them down." She says that the stepfather has "used his finger to poke my 'va-jay-jay' (digitally penetrated her vagina) and 'boo-hole' (anus) lots of times." The RN is unable to do a complete examination of the child's anogenital area because complaints of pain prevent separating the labia majora.

Activity 2-1. Identifying Missing Subjective Information

The acronym OLDCARTS (Onset, Location, Duration, Character, Aggravating/relieving, Radiation, Timing, Severity) is used to identify the information necessary to continue with your assessment. For the purposes of this activity, identify the absent OLDCARTS information.

____

____

____

Activity 2-2. Anatomical Identification

Correctly identify the anogenital anatomy of a patient (**Activity Figure 2-2**).

A. ______________________________________

B. ______________________________________

C. ______________________________________

D. ______________________________________

E. ______________________________________

F. ______________________________________

Objective Findings

The patient's temperature is 101.2°F, taken orally. Her heart rate is 90 and respiratory rate is 22. The RN attempts to take a sample for urinalysis, but the child is unable to void on command. The child is unable to tolerate any touching and resists examination because of pain in the area.

The laboratory loses the nucleic acid amplification test (NAAT), and it is never logged into custody (not reported to provider). Scraping of lesions is completed for culture, which is sent to another laboratory. Culture is positive for herpes simplex virus 2 (HSV-2).

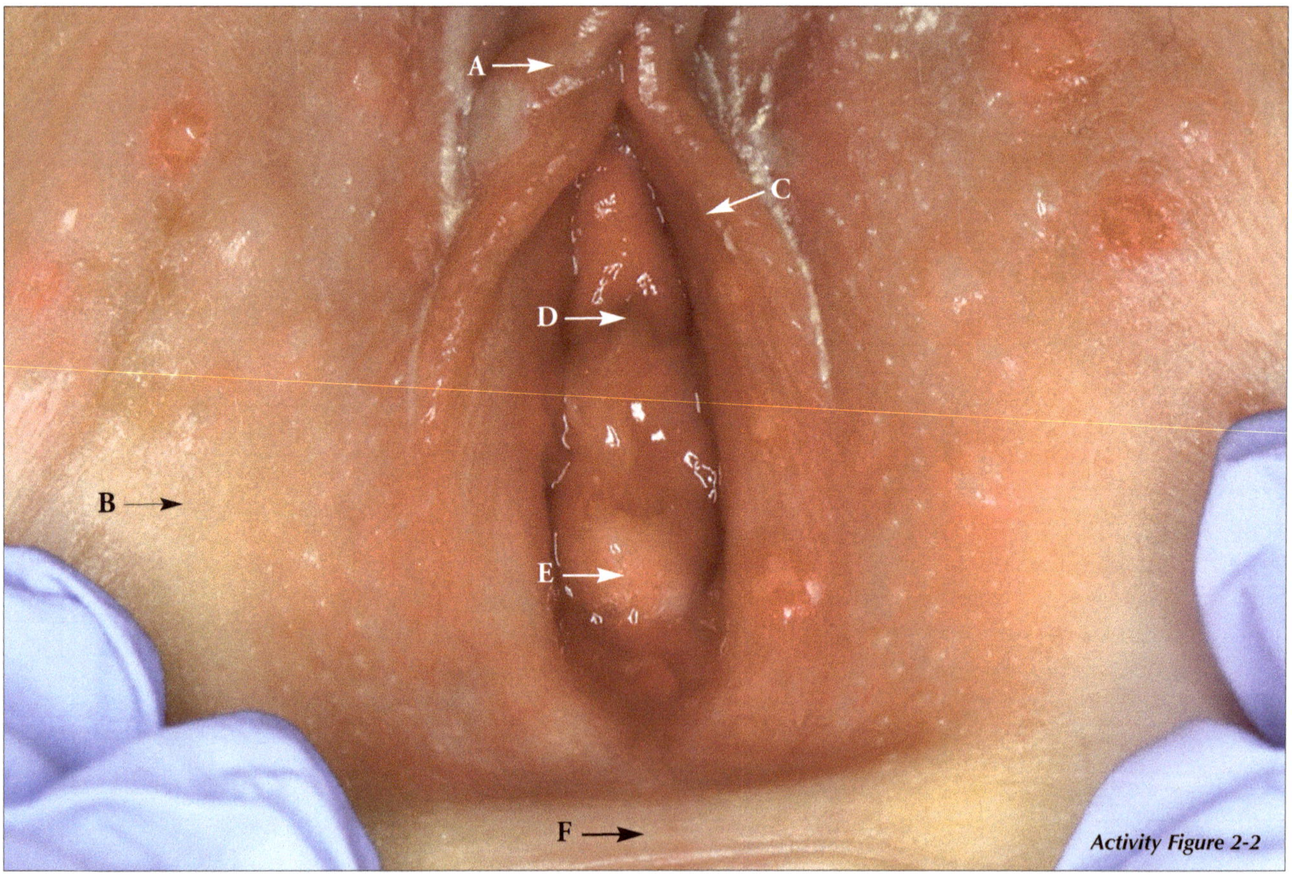

Activity Figure 2-2

Activity 2-3. Physical Examination Findings

Identify and document injuries, age-related normal variants, or medical conditions based on a review of the case photographs (**Activity Figure 2-3**).

____

____

____

A.______________________________

B.______________________________

C.______________________________

Activity 2-4. Clinical Laboratory Improvement Amendments (CLIA) Laboratory Examination

Using the history and the initial urinary findings, list the items to implement in the protocol to assist APPs and physicians in the clinical diagnosis.

____

____

____

____

Activity 2-5. Clinical Laboratory Testing

For APPs and physicians: using the history and the initial urinary findings, list the laboratory tests to assist in the definitive differential diagnosis.

____

____

____

____

____

____

Clinical Assessment

Activity 2-6. Forensic Evidence Collection

Determine whether the case history warrants medical forensic evidence collection. If so, list 3 items of evidence that should be collected, method for collection, and reason for collection.

____

____

____

____

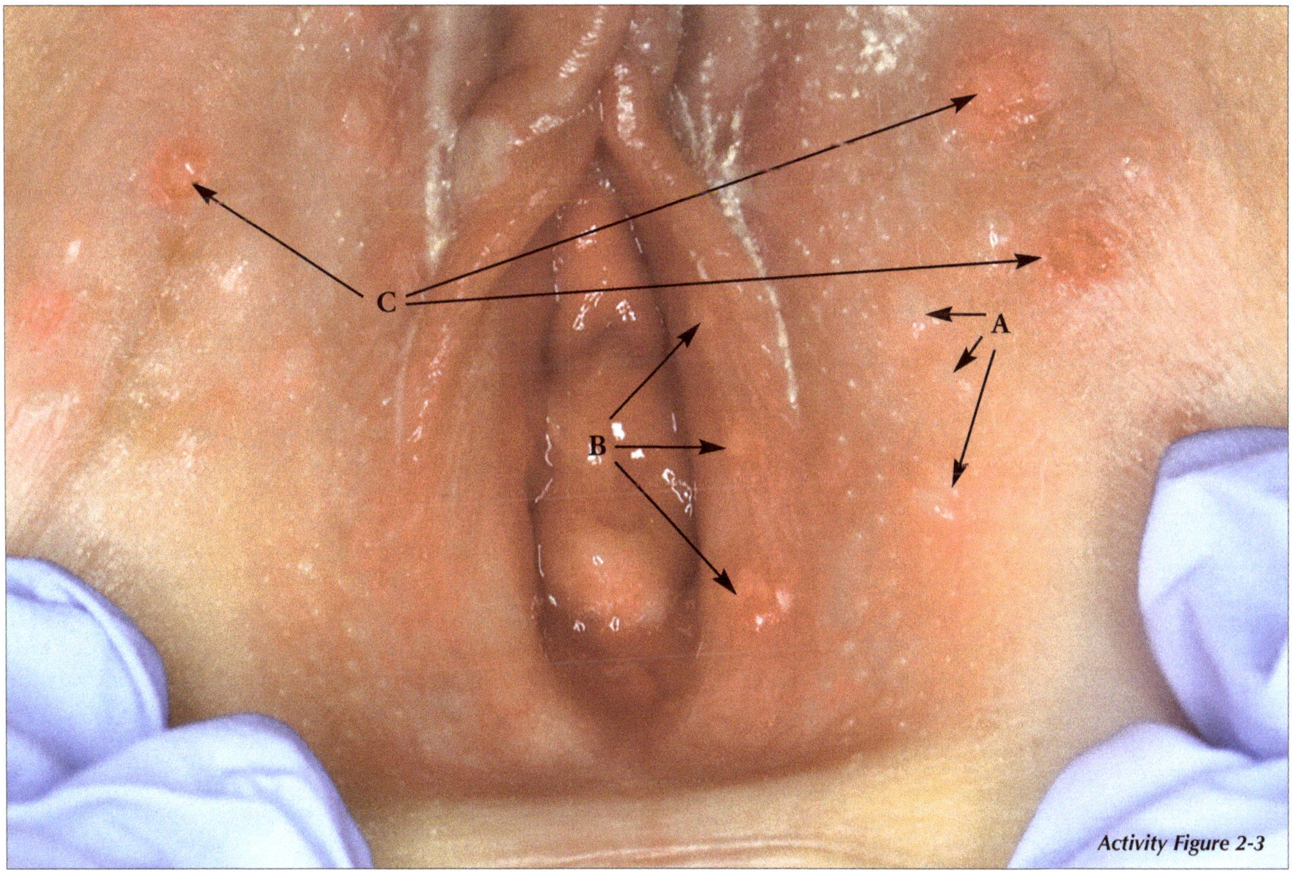

Activity Figure 2-3

Case Study 2 *(continued)*

Activity 2-7. Nursing Plan of Care Procedure

Assess and create a nursing diagnosis. Create a plan of care that includes a protocol for testing, demonstrates implementation of the plan of care, and adheres to quality with patient-centered and trauma-informed methods in the plan of care.

Activity 2-8. APP and Physician Differential Diagnosis

For APPs and physicians: complete the previous activities and create a differential diagnosis based on the patient's history, laboratories, and clinical presentations. Of the possible differential diagnosis, what is the infection?

Treatment, Reporting, and Follow-Up Plan of Care

Activity 2-9. Treatment

Provide treatment options and prescribe medications to eradicate disease and provide comfort for the patient.

Activity 2-10. Reporting

Determine if the differential diagnosis of the disease is reportable. If yes, identify the entity in your community to which to report.

Activity 2-11. Follow-Up Recommendations in Plan of Care

Provide follow-up recommendations and patient education to include in the plan of care.

Subjective - Second Visit

The mother is instructed to bring the child back in 72 to 96 hours for recheck. The child had 20 hours of medication when seen for recheck by the APP.

Activity 2-12. Identifying Missing Subjective Information

The acronym OLDCARTS (Onset, Location, Duration, Character, Aggravating/relieving, Radiation, Timing, Severity) is used to identify the information necessary to continue with your assessment. For the purposes of this activity, identify the absent OLDCARTS information.

Objective Findings

The lesions are healing, and the child is able to tolerate an examination. No acute injury is noted to the anogenital area.

Activity 2-13. Physical Examination Findings

Identify and document injuries, age-related normal variants, or medical conditions based on a review of the case photographs (Activity **Figure 2-13**).

____

____

____

A. ______________________________________

B. ______________________________________

C. ______________________________________

D. ______________________________________

Activity 2-14. Clinical Laboratory Improvement Amendments (CLIA) Laboratory Examination

Using the history and the initial urinary findings, list the items to implement in the protocol to assist APPs and physicians in the clinical diagnosis.

____

____

Activity 2-15. Clinical Laboratory Testing

For APPs and physicians: Using the history and the initial urinary findings, list the laboratory tests to assist in the definitive differential diagnosis.

____

____

Clinical Assessment

Activity 2-16. Forensic Evidence Collection

Determine whether the case history warrants medical forensic evidence collection. If so, list 3 items of evidence that should be collected, method for collection, and reason for collection.

____

____

Activity 2-17. Nursing Plan of Care Procedure

Assess and create a nursing diagnosis. Create a plan of care that includes a protocol for testing, demonstrates implementation of the plan of care, and adheres to quality with patient-centered and trauma-informed methods in the plan of care.

____

____

____

____

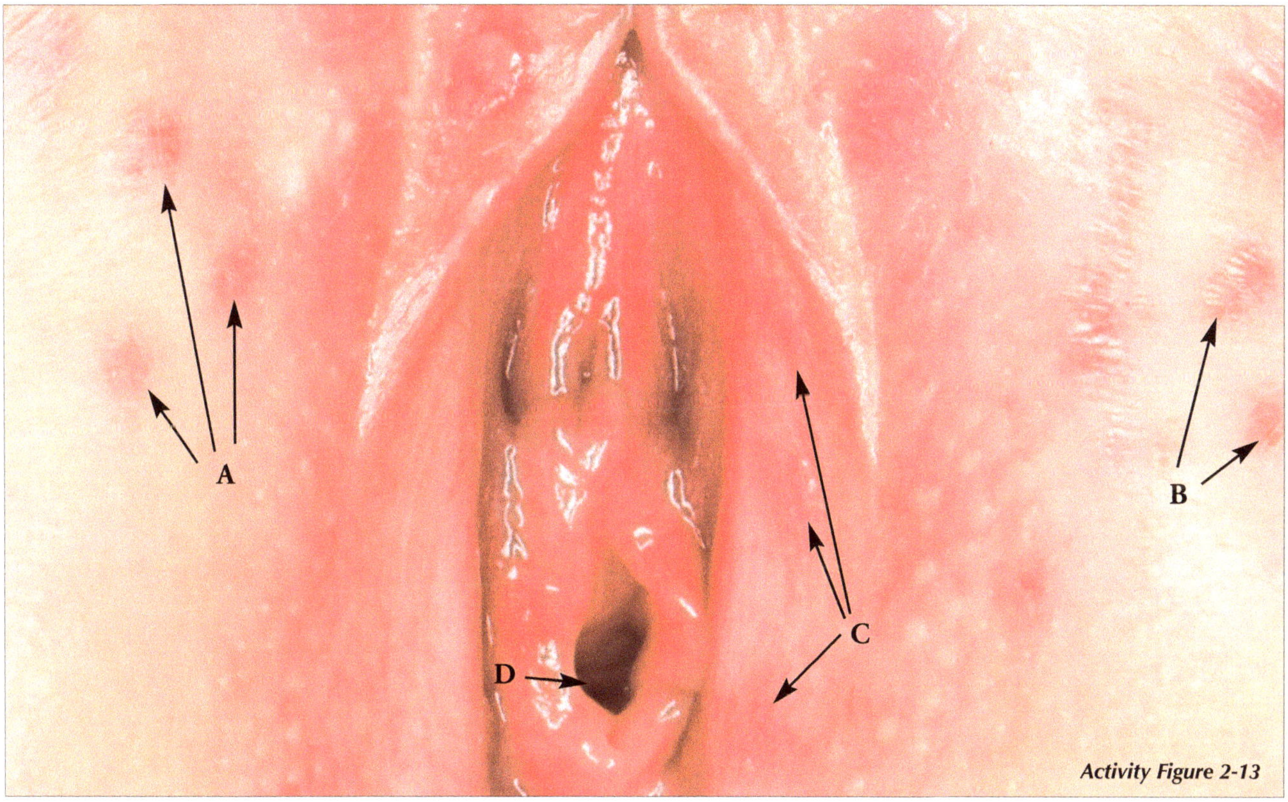

Activity Figure 2-13

CASE STUDY 2 *(CONTINUED)*

Activity 2-18. APP and Physician Differential Diagnosis

For APPs and physicians: Complete the previous activities and create a differential diagnosis based on the patient's history, laboratories, and clinical presentations. Of the possible differential diagnosis, what is the infection?

____

____

TREATMENT, REPORTING, AND FOLLOW-UP PLAN OF CARE

Activity 2-19. Treatment

Provide treatment options and prescribe medications to eradicate disease and provide comfort for the patient.

____

____

____

____

____

____

Activity 2-20. Reporting

Determine if the differential diagnosis of the disease is reportable. If yes, identify the entity in your community to which to report.

____

____

Activity 2-21. Follow-Up Recommendations in Plan of Care

Provide follow-up recommendations and patient education to include in the plan of care.

____

____

____

____

____

____

____

____

____

SUBJECTIVE - FOLLOW-UP VISIT

The child is seen again 1 month after the initial outbreak.

Activity 2-22. Identifying Missing Subjective Information

The acronym OLDCARTS (Onset, Location, Duration, Character, Aggravating/relieving, Radiation, Timing, Severity) is used to identify the information necessary to continue with your assessment. For the purposes of this activity, identify the absent OLDCARTS information.

____

OBJECTIVE FINDINGS

No lesions are noted.

Activity 2-23. Physical Examination Findings

Identify and document injuries, age-related normal variants, or medical conditions based on a review of the case photographs (**Activity Figure 2-23**).

____

____

____

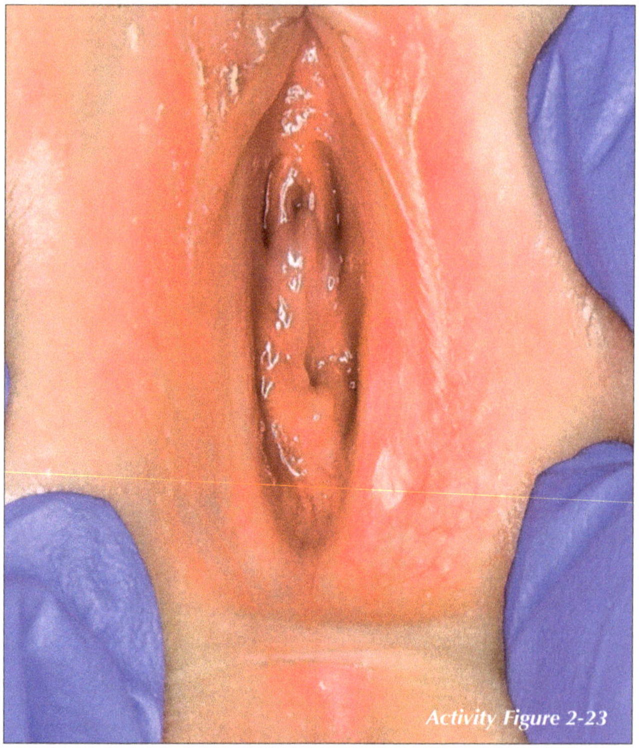

Activity Figure 2-23

Activity 2-24. Clinical Laboratory Improvement Amendments (CLIA) Laboratory Examination

Using the history and the initial urinary findings, list the items to implement in the protocol to assist APPs and physicians in the clinical diagnosis.

Activity 2-25. Clinical Laboratory Testing

For APPs and physicians: Using the history and the initial urinary findings, list the laboratory tests to assist in the definitive differential diagnosis.

Clinical Assessment

Activity 2-26. Forensic Evidence Collection

Determine whether the case history warrants medical forensic evidence collection. If so, list 3 items of evidence that should be collected, method for collection, and reason for collection.

Activity 2-27. Nursing Plan of Care Procedure

Assess and create a nursing diagnosis. Create a plan of care that includes a protocol for testing, demonstrates implementation of the plan of care, and adheres to quality with patient-centered and trauma-informed methods in the plan of care.

Activity 2-28. APP and Physician Differential Diagnosis

For APPs and physicians: Complete the previous activities and create a differential diagnosis based on the patient's history, laboratories, and clinical presentations. Of the possible differential diagnosis, what is the infection?

Treatment, Reporting, and Follow-Up Plan of Care

Activity 2-29. Treatment

Provide treatment options and prescribe medications to eradicate disease and provide comfort for the patient.

Activity 2-30. Reporting

Determine if the differential diagnosis of the disease is reportable. If yes, identify the entity in your community to which to report.

Activity 2-31. Follow-Up Recommendations in Plan of Care

Provide follow-up recommendations and patient education to include in the plan of care.

Case Study 3

Subjective

A 17-year-old boy presents with a complaint of persistent itching in his pubic region, mostly at night. He says it started about 1 week ago. He does not think his mother tried any new laundry detergents and he is not on any medications. His vital signs are within normal limits, and he reports no history of a sexually transmitted infection (STI). On further questioning, he admits to having slept with 2 different girls recently, but he used a condom both times.

Activity 3-1. Identifying Missing Subjective Information

The acronym OLDCARTS (Onset, Location, Duration, Character, Aggravating/relieving, Radiation, Timing, Severity) is used to identify the information necessary to continue with your assessment. For the purposes of this activity, identify the absent OLDCARTS information.

____

____

Activity 3-2. Anatomical Identification

Correctly identify the anogenital anatomy of a patient (**Activity Figure 3-2**).

A.______________________________________

B.______________________________________

C. ______________________________________

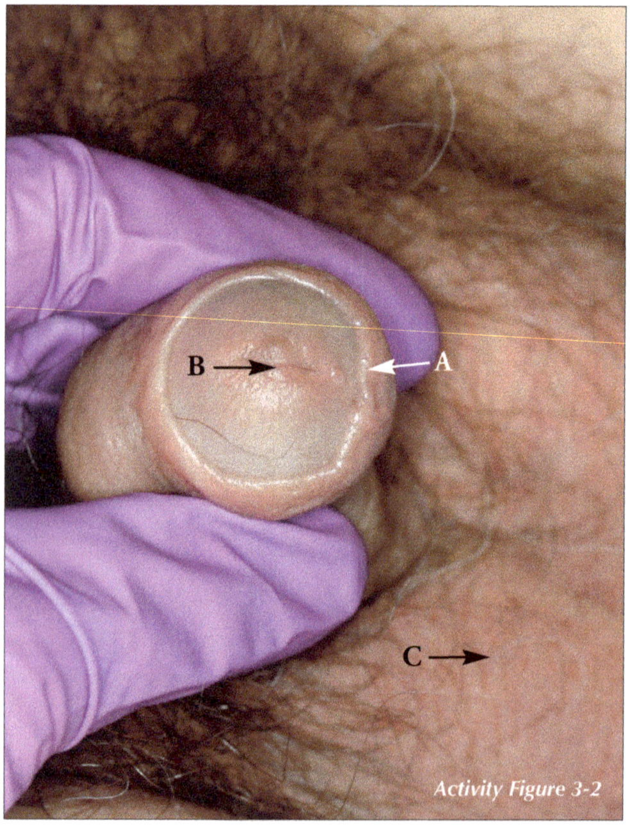

Activity Figure 3-2

Objective Physical Findings

A focused examination of genital area reveals Tanner stage V. Diffuse redness and follicular swelling is visible. On further inspection, diffuse petechiae and follicular eruptions are noted. Blood on the patient's underwear is noted. Significant pubic lice (approximately 100, tan, grayish-white in color) are visible on the hair in his inguinal pubic regions bilaterally. His penis is without discharge and there is no palpable inguinal lymph swelling or pain. His lower abdomen, inner thighs, buttocks, scalp, eyebrows, and lashes are without visible signs of lice.

Activity 3-3. Physical Examination Findings

Identify and document injuries, age-related normal variants, or medical conditions based on a review of the case photographs (**Activity Figure 3-3**).

A.______________________________________

B.______________________________________

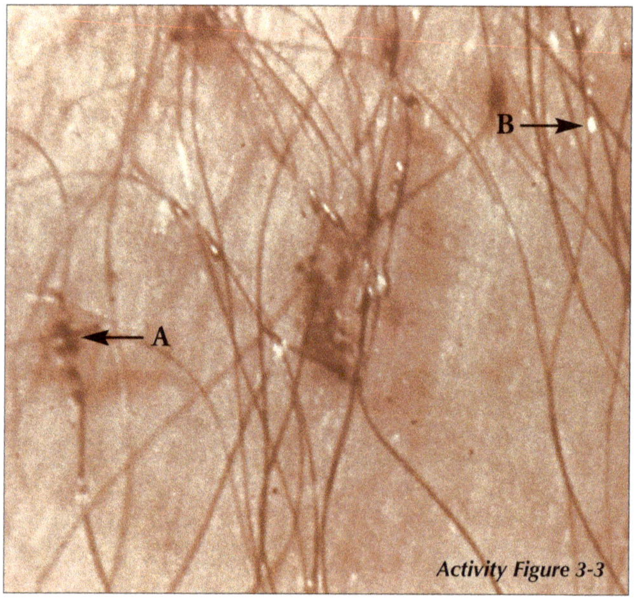

Activity Figure 3-3

Activity 3-4. Clinical Laboratory Improvement Amendments (CLIA) Laboratory Examination

Using the history and the initial objective findings, list the items in the protocol to implement to assist APPs and physicians in the clinical diagnosis.

____

____

Activity 3-5. Clinical Laboratory Testing

For APPs and physicians, using the history and the initial findings, list the laboratory tests to assist in the definitive differential diagnosis.

Clinical Assessment

Activity 3-6. Forensic Evidence Collection

Determine whether the case history warrants medical forensic evidence collection. If so, list 3 items of evidence that should be collected, the method for collection, and the reason for collection.

Activity 3-7. Nursing Plan of Care Procedure

Assess for and create a nursing diagnosis. Create a plan of care that includes a protocol for testing, demonstrates implementation of the plan of care, and adheres to quality with patient-centered and trauma-informed methods in the plan of care.

Activity 3-8. APP and Physician Differential Diagnosis

For APPs and physicians: Complete the previous activities and create a differential diagnosis based on the patient's history, laboratories, and clinical presentations. Of the possible differential diagnosis, what is the infection?

Treatment, Reporting, and Follow-Up Plan of Care

Activity 3-9. Treatment

Provide treatment options and prescribe medications to eradicate disease and provide comfort for the patient.

Activity 3-10. Reporting

Determine if the differential diagnosis of the disease is reportable. If yes, identify the entity in your community to which to report.

Activity 3-11. Follow-Up Recommendations in Plan of Care

Provide follow-up recommendations and patient education to include in the plan of care.

Case Study 4

Subjective

AD is a 12-year-old girl who is brought to the pediatric clinic by her mother for concerns about vaginal pruritus and abnormal vaginal discharge, described as clumpy and white, for 3 days. There is no report of fever or sexual activity. AD completed a 10-day course of oral antibiotics 3 days ago for acute otitis media. Menarche occurred 6 months ago. She has no history of chronic conditions. Immunizations are up to date.

Activity 4-1. Identifying Missing Subjective Information

The acronym OLDCARTS (Onset, Location, Duration, Character, Aggravating/relieving, Radiation, Timing, Severity) is used to identify the information necessary to continue with your assessment. For the purposes of this activity, identify the absent OLDCARTS information.

____

Activity 4-2. Anatomical Identification

Correctly identify the anogenital anatomy of a patient (**Activity Figure 4-2**).

A. ______________________________

B. ______________________________

C. ______________________________

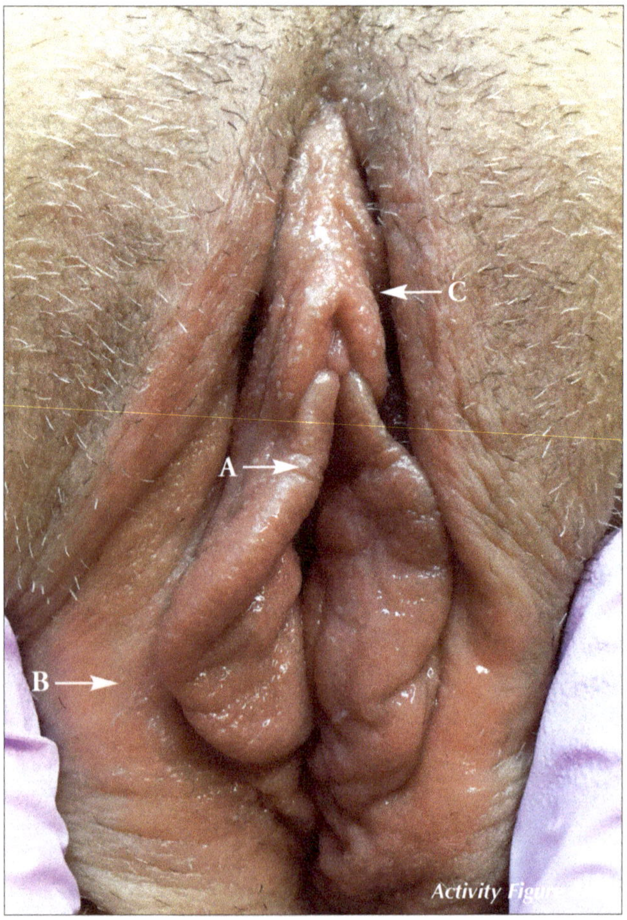

Activity Figure

Objective History and Findings

Thick, white, vaginal discharge with "yeast" (baking bread) odor is present on vulva on inspection. No lesions are present. Mild vulvar edema and excoriations are identified.

A potassium hydroxide (KOH) wet prep sample of the vaginal discharge showed yeast hyphae and buds. Culture confirmed vulvovaginal candidiasis.

Activity 4-3. Physical Examination Findings

Identify and document injuries, age-related normal variants, and medical conditions based on a review of the case photographs (**Activity Figure 4-3**).

____

____

____

____

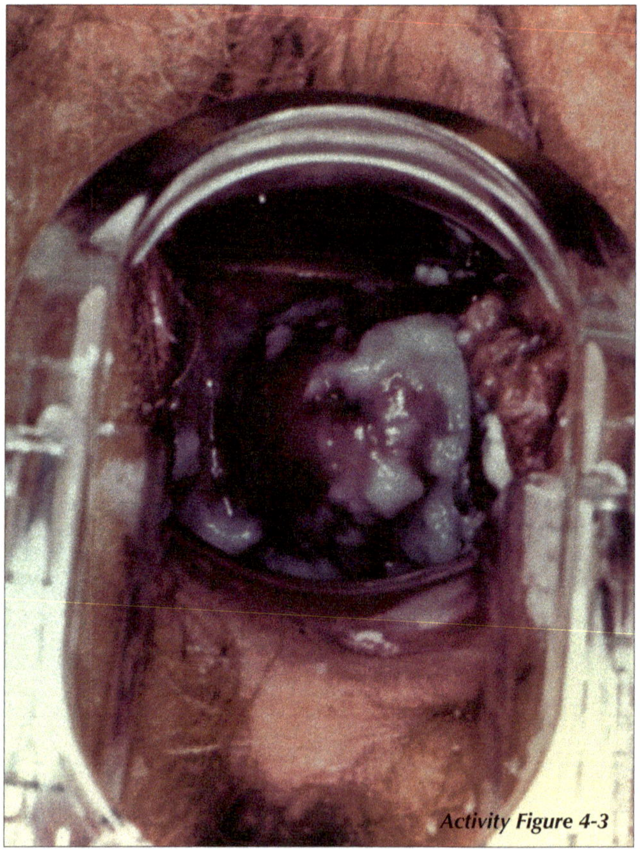

Activity Figure 4-3

Activity 4-4. Clinical Laboratory Improvement Amendments (CLIA) Laboratory Examination
Using the history and the initial urinary findings, list the items in the protocol to implement to assist APPs and physicians in the clinical diagnosis.

Activity 4-5. Clinical Laboratory Testing
For APPs and physicians, using the history and the initial urinary findings, list the laboratory tests to assist in the definitive differential diagnosis.

CLINICAL ASSESSMENT

Activity 4-6. Forensic Evidence Collection
Determine whether the case history warrants medical forensic evidence collection. If so, list 3 items of evidence that should be collected, method for collection, and reason for collection.

Activity 4-7. Nursing Plan of Care Procedure
Assess for and create a nursing diagnosis. Create a plan of care that includes a protocol for testing, demonstrates implementation of the plan of care, and adheres to quality with patient-centered and trauma-informed methods in the plan of care.

Activity 4-8. APP and Physician Differential Diagnosis
For APPs and physicians, complete the previous activities and create a differential diagnosis based on the patient's history, laboratories, and clinical presentations. Of the possible differential diagnosis, what is the infection?

TREATMENT, REPORTING, AND FOLLOW-UP PLAN OF CARE

Activity 4-9. Treatment
Provide treatment options and prescribe medications to eradicate disease and provide comfort for the patient.

Activity 4-10. Reporting
Determine if the differential diagnosis of the disease is reportable. If yes, identify the entity in your community to which to report.

Activity 4-11. Follow-Up Recommendations in Plan of Care
Provide follow-up recommendations and patient education to include in the plan of care.

Case Study 5

Subjective History

PM is an 18-year-old male who works part-time at the neighborhood daycare center, helping clean the premises. Previously in good health, he is taking no medications and has not traveled outside the United States. He reports several recent outbreaks of diarrhea in the daycare over the last 6 months. Lately he has been complaining of unusual fatigue, generalized malaise, minimal appetite, nausea, and is unable to eat without vomiting. Since he had the same illness a month ago, his mother brings him to the primary care provider after 2 days' illness. He denies sexual activity, drug use, or getting tattoos. He reports that his job is emptying garbage and mentions that the garbage contains diapers. He says, "Sometimes I have to push the diapers down in the bag for all of them to fit." He expressed disgust with the job, stating that he wants to go to college. His mother reports that the daycare infants have often had diarrhea since PM started to work there.

Clinical Assessment

Activity 5-1. Identifying Missing Subjective Information

Clinicians often use the acronym OLDCARTS (Onset, Location, Duration, Character, Aggravating/relieving, Radiation, Timing, Severity) to identify the information necessary to continue with their assessment. For this activity, identify the missing OLDCARTS information.

____

Activity 5-2. Anatomical Identification

Correctly identify the anatomy of a patient (**Activity Figure 5-2**).

A. ____________________________________

B. ____________________________________

C. ____________________________________

D. ____________________________________

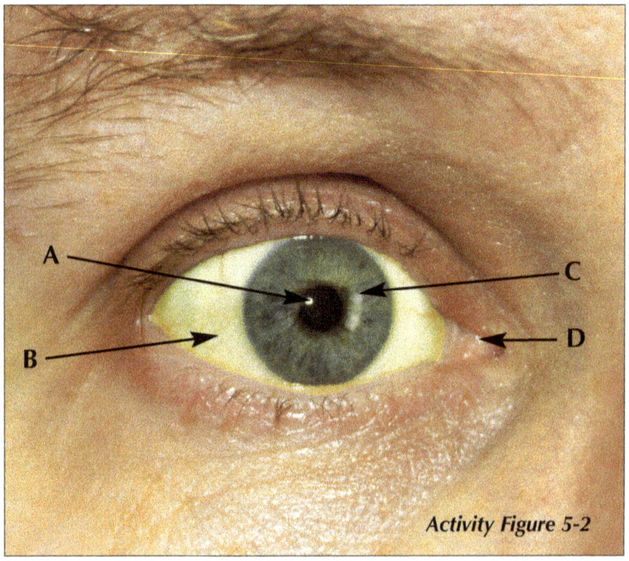

Activity Figure 5-2

Objective History

The patient's temperature is 101.5°F (38.6°C), pulse is 120 beats per minute, and blood pressure is 110/58 mm Hg. He appears healthy and slightly dehydrated, with mucous membranes that are pink and warm, and his skin is slightly clammy. The abdomen is soft with normal bowel sounds and without tenderness or hepatomegaly.

A complete blood cell count (CBC) and metabolic panel are within normal limits. Serological testing for anti-hepatitis A virus immunoglobulin M (anti-HAV IgM) and a hepatitis B panel are negative. Anti-HAV IgG is positive, which means that the patient was immunized or had hepatitis A at some point in the past.

Activity 5-3. Physical Examination Findings

Identify and document injuries, age-related normal variants, or medical conditions based on a review of the case photographs (**Activity Figure 5-3-a** through **b**).

____

____

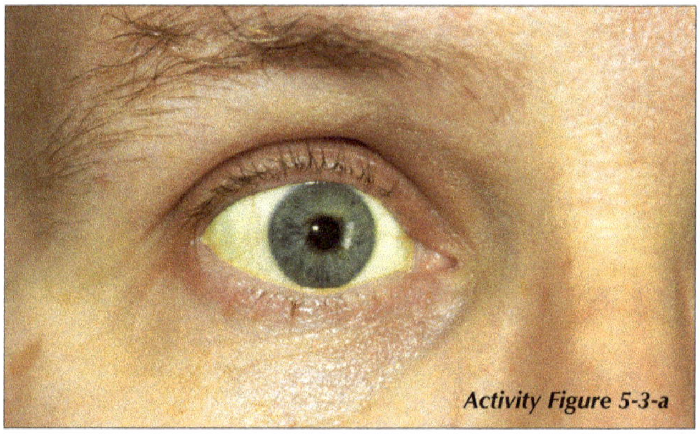
Activity Figure 5-3-a

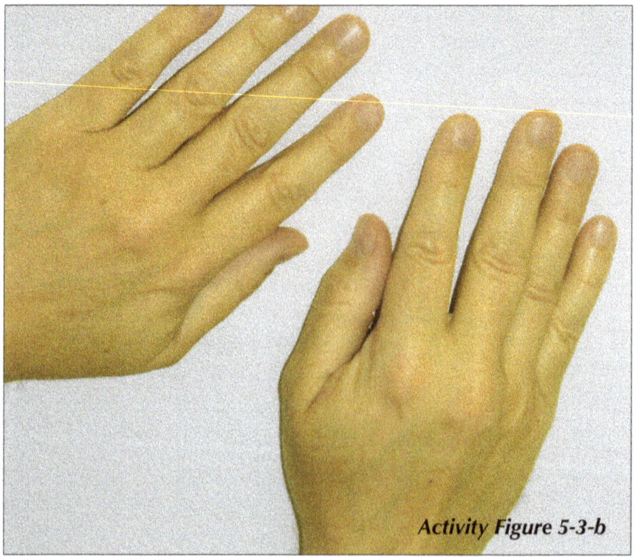
Activity Figure 5-3-b

Activity 5-4. Clinical Laboratory Improvement Amendments (CLIA) Laboratory Examination

Using the history and initial findings, list the items from the protocol that can be implemented to assist APPs and physicians in the clinical diagnosis.

Activity 5-5. Clinical Laboratory Testing

For APPs and physicians, using the history and initial findings, list the laboratory tests to assist in determining the definitive differential diagnosis.

Clinical Assessment

Activity 5-6. Forensic Evidence Collection

Determine whether or not the case history warrants medical forensic evidence collection. If so, list 3 items of evidence that should be collected, method for collection, and reason for collection.

Activity 5-7. Nursing Plan of Care Procedure

Assess and create a nursing diagnosis. Create a plan of care that includes a protocol for testing and demonstrates implementation of the plan of care and adherence to quality, with patient-centered and trauma-informed methods in the plan of care as needed.

Activity 5-8. APP and Physician Differential Diagnosis

For APPs and physicians, complete the previous activities and create a differential diagnosis based on the patient's history, laboratories, and clinical presentations. Of the possible differential diagnosis, what is the infection?

Treatment, Reporting, and Follow-Up Plan of Care

Activity 5-9. Treatment

Provide treatment options and prescribe medications to eradicate disease and provide comfort for the patient.

Activity 5-10. Reporting

Determine if the differential diagnosis of the disease is reportable. If yes, identify the entity in your community to which to report.

Activity 5-11. Follow-Up Recommendations in Plan of Care

Provide follow-up recommendations and patient education to include in the plan of care.

Case Study 6

Subjective

JT is a 14-year-old girl brought to her pediatrician's office by her mother for lesions around her mouth, on her hands, and on her lower abdomen and mons pubis. The lesions started approximately 1 month ago. JT denies discomfort, itching, fever, and redness to sites, but she does scratch the tops off, creating a scab. The child says when she scratches the tops off, they heal without a bump. The child is home-schooled, is up to date on immunizations, and has no chronic health conditions. The mother reports that JT was away at her grandparents' farm for the summer.

Activity 6-1. Identifying Missing Subjective Information

The acronym OLDCARTS (Onset, Location, Duration, Character, Aggravating/relieving, Radiation, Timing, Severity) is used to identify the information necessary to continue with your assessment. For the purposes of this activity, identify the absent OLDCARTS information.

____

Activity 6-2. Physical Examination Findings

Identify and document injuries, age-related normal variants, or medical conditions based on a review of the case photographs (**Activity Figure 6-2-a** through **b**).

A.______________________________________

B.______________________________________

C.______________________________________

D.______________________________________

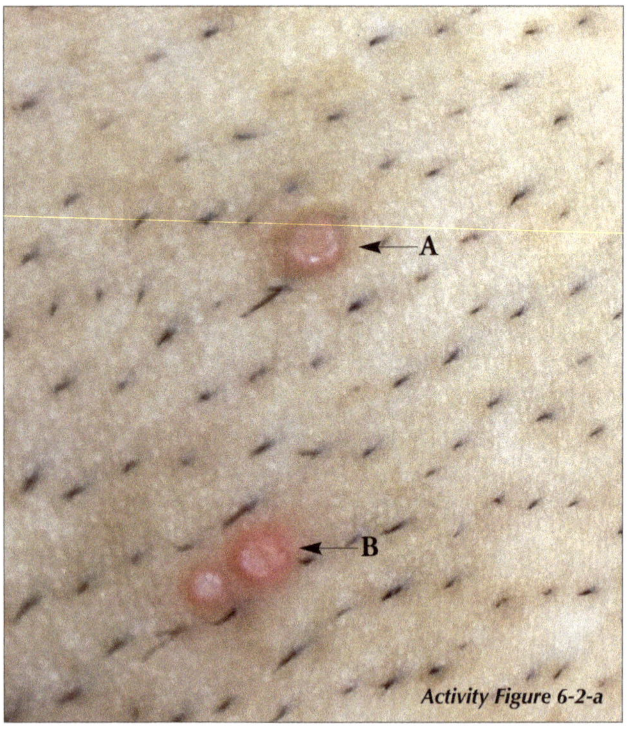

Activity Figure 6-2-a

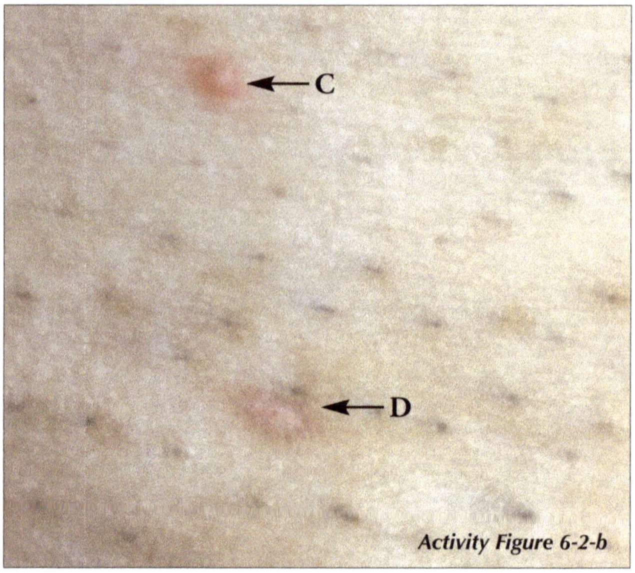

Activity Figure 6-2-b

Objective History and Findings

On examination, there are 3 raised, smooth, 2- to 3-mm round papules with white, depressed centers on the right cheek and 3 similar papules noted on the waistband area. JT has multiple lesions on her fingers. Papules are soft and nontender, and no ulceration, redness, or signs of infection are noted, except the lesions she scratched.

Viral herpes simplex virus (HSV) type-specific polymerase chain reaction (PCR) swab of lesion is negative for HSV-1 and HSV-2. The RN orders the office urine dipstick test, which shows a moderate increase in leukocytes, as well as trace blood. No other abnormalities are seen on the dipstick results. Based on clinical findings, a diagnosis of molluscum contagiosum is made.

Activity 6-3. Clinical Laboratory Improvement Amendments (CLIA) Laboratory Examination

Using the history and the initial urinary findings, list the items in the protocol to implement to assist APPs and physicians in the clinical diagnosis.

____

____

____

Activity 6-4. Clinical Laboratory Testing

For APPs and physicians, using the history and the initial urinary findings, list the laboratory tests to assist in the definitive differential diagnosis.

____

____

____

Clinical Assessment

Activity 6-5. Forensic Evidence Collection

Determine whether or not the case history warrants medical forensic evidence collection. If so, list 3 items of evidence that should be collected, method for collection, and reason for collection.

Activity 6-6. Nursing Plan of Care Procedure

Assess and create a nursing diagnosis. Create a plan of care that includes a protocol for testing, demonstrates implementation of the plan of care, and adheres to quality with patient-centered and trauma-informed methods in the plan of care.

Activity 6-7. APP and Physician Differential Diagnosis

For APPs and physicians, complete the previous activities and create a differential diagnosis based on the patient's history, laboratories, and clinical presentations. Of the possible differential diagnosis, what is the infection?

Treatment, Reporting, and Follow-Up Plan of Care

Activity 6-8. Treatment

Provide treatment options and prescribe medications to eradicate disease and provide comfort for the patient.

Activity 6-9. Reporting

Determine if the differential diagnosis of the disease is reportable. If yes, identify the entity in your community to which to report.

Activity 6-10. Follow-Up Recommendations in Plan of Care

Provide follow-up recommendations and patient education to include in the plan of care.

Case Study 7

Subjective History

An 18-year-old presents to a Title X STI clinic with a "sore" on his penis. Completing the subjective and objective assessments, the triage nurse and the primary care provider (PCP) record that the patient routinely has unprotected sexual intercourse and has since he was 15 years old. Before that, he reports being in foster care and says that he ran away because he was being abused. The patient states that he had multiple sexual experiences with different people, both male and female, in an effort to make enough money to pay for his drugs. He also works with a group of other men and women who sell sex. On questioning, he tells the PCP that he must turn his money over to his landlord. When asked about the lesion, the patient states that it "hurts a little."

Activity 7-1. Identifying Missing Subjective Information

Clinicians often use the acronym OLDCARTS (Onset, Location, Duration, Character, Aggravating/relieving, Radiation, Timing, Severity) to identify the information necessary to continue with their assessment. For this activity, identify the absent OLDCARTS information.

____

Activity 7-2. Anatomical Identification

Correctly identify the anogenital anatomy of a patient (**Activity Figure 7-2**).

A.____

B.____

C.____

D.____

E.____

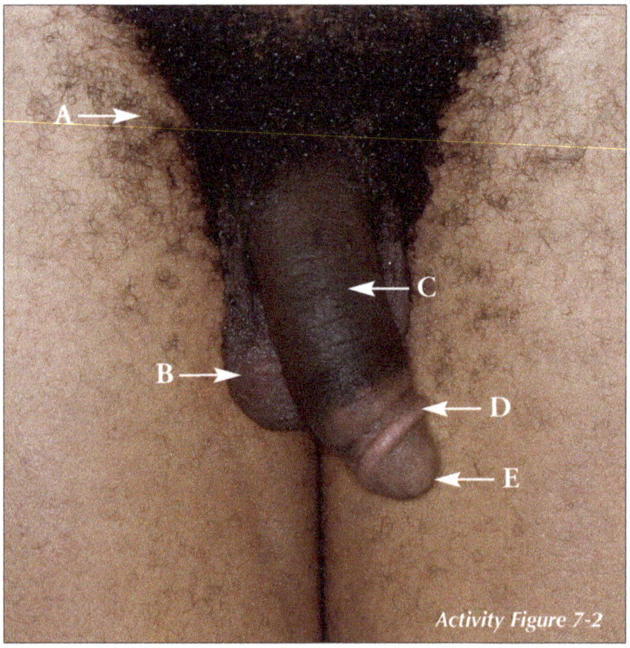

Activity Figure 7-2

Objective History

When a patient is infected with Donovan bodies, symptoms do not appear immediately. Symptoms can appear up to 12 weeks after infection, and many times the sores are not noticed because they are hidden in a fold and are not painful.

Activity 7-3. Physical Examination Findings

Identify and document injuries, age-related normal variants, or medical conditions based on a review of the case photographs (**Activity Figure 7-3**).

A.____

B.____

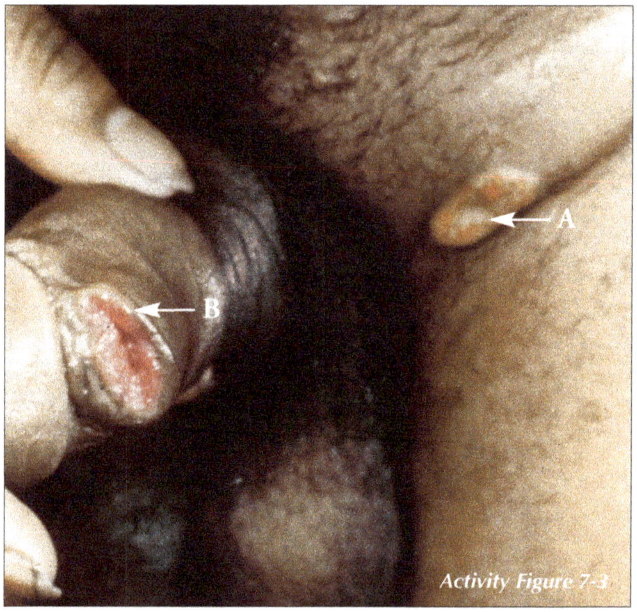

Activity Figure 7-3

Activity 7-4. Clinical Laboratory Improvement Amendments (CLIA) Laboratory Examination

Using the history and the initial findings, list the items in the protocol to implement to assist APPs and physicians in the clinical diagnosis.

____

____

____

____

____

____

____

____

____

Activity 7-5. Clinical Laboratory Testing

For APPs and physicians, using the history and initial findings, list the laboratory tests to assist in determining the definitive differential diagnosis.

Clinical Assessment

Activity 7-6. Forensic Evidence Collection

Determine whether or not the case history warrants medical forensic evidence collection. If so, list 3 items of evidence that should be collected, method for collection, and reason for collection.

Activity 7-7. Nursing Plan of Care Procedure

Assess and create a nursing diagnosis. Create a plan of care that includes a protocol for testing and demonstrates implementation of the plan of care and adherence to quality, with patient-centered and trauma-informed methods in the plan of care.

Activity 7-8. APP and Physician Differential Diagnosis

For APPs and physicians, complete the previous activities and create a differential diagnosis based on the patient's history, laboratories, and clinical presentations. Of the possible differential diagnosis, what is the infection?

Treatment, Reporting, and Follow-Up Plan of Care

Activity 7-9. Treatment

Provide treatment options and prescribe medications to eradicate disease and provide comfort for the patient.

Activity 7-10. Reporting

Determine if the differential diagnosis of the disease is reportable. If yes, identify the entity in your community to which to report.

Activity 7-11. Follow-Up Recommendations in Plan of Care

Provide follow-up recommendations and patient education to include in the plan of care.

Case Study 8

Subjective History

JD is a 21-year-old transgender man (born female) who presents to the primary care clinic for STI testing. He is sexually active with men and women and reports multiple partners in the last 12 months. He reports oral sex (fellatio and cunnilingus), receptive anal sex, and penile-vaginal sex. The last sexual contact was 3 days ago, and no protective barriers were used. A female partner from 1 month ago contacted him to tell him he should get tested for STIs. He denies any symptoms at this time. JD uses self-prescribed testosterone therapy, has no significant medical history, and has no known drug allergies.

Activity 8-1. Identifying Missing Subjective Information

Clinicians often use the acronym OLDCARTS (Onset, Location, Duration, Character, Aggravating/relieving, Radiation, Timing, Severity) to identify the information necessary to continue with their assessment. For this activity, identify the absent OLDCARTS information.

____

____

Activity 8-2. Anatomical Identification

Correctly identify the anogenital anatomy of a patient (**Activity Figure 8-2**).

A.____________________________________

B.____________________________________

C.____________________________________

D.____________________________________

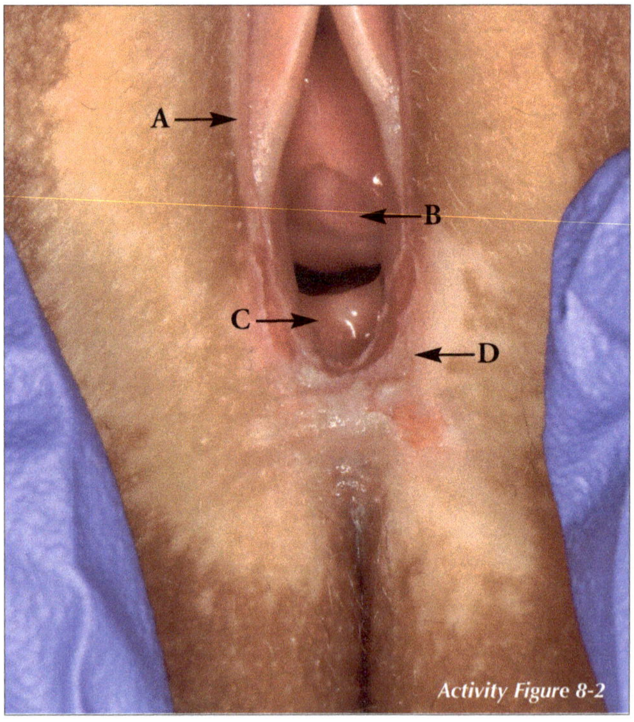

Activity Figure 8-2

Objective History

Physical and anogenital examination are normal.

Urine NAAT for *Chlamydia trachomatis* and *Neisseria gonorrhoeae* (CT/NG) is negative. Pharyngeal NAAT for CT/NG is positive for *C. trachomatis*. Rectal NAAT for CT/NG is positive. Dipstick urinalysis is normal. Human immunodeficiency virus (HIV) antibody test, *Treponema pallidum* total antibody screen, and acute hepatitis panel are negative.

Activity 8-3. Physical Examination Findings

Identify and document injuries, age-related normal variants, or medical conditions based on a review of the case photographs (**Activity Figure 8-3**).

____

____

____

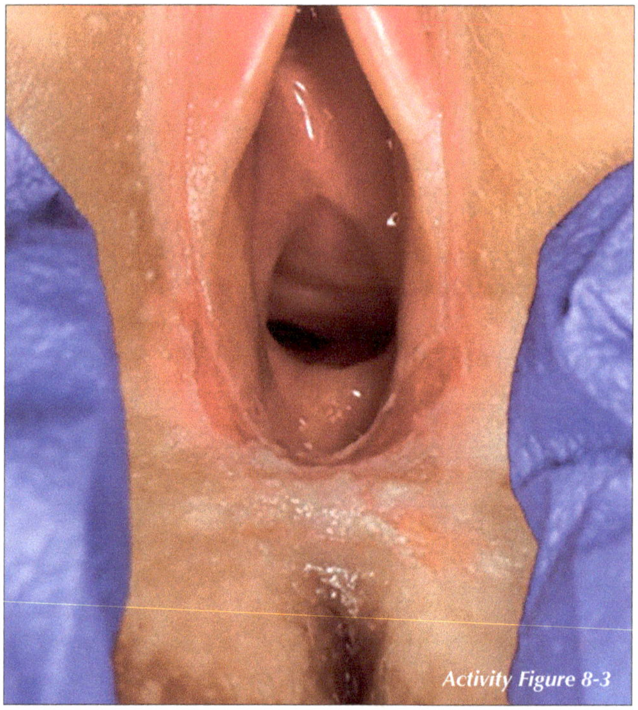
Activity Figure 8-3

Activity 8-4. Clinical Laboratory Improvement Amendments (CLIA) Laboratory Examination

Using the history and the initial urinary findings, list the items in the protocol to implement to assist APPs and physicians in the clinical diagnosis.

____

____

____

____

Activity 8-5. Clinical Laboratory Testing

For APPs and physicians, using the history and the initial urinary findings, list the laboratory tests to assist in the definitive differential diagnosis.

Clinical Assessment

Activity 8-6. Forensic Evidence Collection

Determine whether or not the case history warrants medical forensic evidence collection. If so, list 3 items of evidence that should be collected, method for collection, and reason for collection.

Activity 8-7. Nursing Plan of Care Procedure

Assess and create nursing diagnoses. Create a plan of care that includes a protocol for testing and demonstrates implementation of the plan of care and adherence to quality, with patient-centered and trauma-informed methods in the plan of care.

Activity 8-8. APP and Physician Differential Diagnosis

For APPs and physicians, complete the previous activities and create a differential diagnosis based on the patient's history, laboratories, and clinical presentations. Of the possible differential diagnosis, what is the infection?

Treatment, Reporting, and Follow-Up Plan of Care

Activity 8-9. Treatment

Provide treatment options and prescribe medications to eradicate disease and provide comfort for the patient.

Activity 8-10. Reporting

Determine if the disease is reportable. If yes, identify the entity in your community to which to report.

Activity 8-11. Follow-Up Recommendations in Plan of Care

Provide follow-up recommendations and patient education to include in the plan of care.

Case Study 9

Subjective History

The patient is a 62-year-old woman who presents to the emergency department (ED) for left knee pain secondary to a fall 5 weeks prior. Patient reports history of stage 2 chronic kidney disease, hypertension (reports that she has not taken her medication in about 3 months), obesity, tobacco use (45 pack-year history), and frequent use of marijuana. She also reports drinking alcohol approximately 5 times per week.

Risk factors include a history of intravenous drug use ("once or twice in the 1970s"), as well as a long-term sexual partner who is reportedly positive for hepatitis (type unknown). Her last medical care was a radiograph in the ED after her fall.

Activity 9-1. Identifying Missing Subjective Information
The acronym OLDCARTS (Onset, Location, Duration, Character, Aggravating/relieving, Radiation, Timing, Severity) is used to identify the information necessary to continue with your assessment. For the purposes of this activity, identify the absent OLDCARTS information.

____

____

Objective History and Findings

At her initial new patient sick visit, screening protocols were discussed and tests were ordered for cervical, breast, and colon cancer. Because of the birth cohort screen, the patient is checked for presence of anti–hepatitis C virus (HCV). The physical examination is unremarkable, including no hepatomegaly or abdominal tenderness.

Routine laboratory tests are ordered. Patient has elevated blood urea nitrogen level, a creatinine level of 1.6 mg/dL, a vitamin D level of 19.3 ng/mL, and elevated triglyceride levels at 335 mg/dL. Estimated glomerular filtration rate is 41 mL/min.

A CBC is within normal limits. Aspartate aminotransferase and alanine aminotransferase, alkaline phosphatase, and total bilirubin are all within normal limits. All screens are negative with the exception of anti-HCV.

The patient is contacted and asked to return to the clinic for HCV RNA testing by polymerase chain reaction and is found to have 1 570 000 IU/mL, genotype 1a. International normalized ratio is 1.1 and FibroSure score is F0-F1, indicating no to minimal fibrosis. Screening tests for hepatitis A, hepatitis B, and HIV are all negative.

Activity 9-2. Physical Examination Findings
Identify and document injuries, age-related normal variants, or medical conditions based on a review of the case photographs (**Activity Figure 9-2**).

____

____

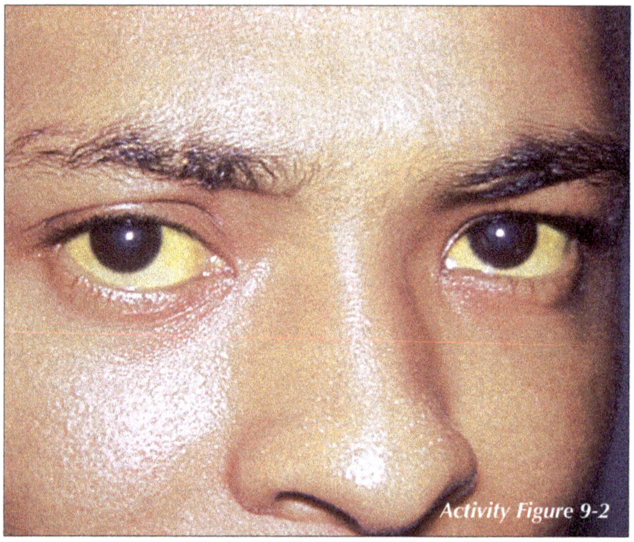

Activity Figure 9-2

Activity 9-3. Clinical Laboratory Improvement Amendments (CLIA) Laboratory Examination
Using the history and the initial urinary findings, list the items in the protocol to implement to assist APPs and physicians in the clinical diagnosis.

____

____

____

____

____

____

Activity 9-4. Clinical Laboratory Testing
For APPs and physicians, using the history and the initial urinary findings, list the laboratory tests to assist in the definitive differential diagnosis.

____

____

____

____

____

____

Clinical Assessment

Activity 9-5. Forensic Evidence Collection

Determine whether or not the case history warrants medical forensic evidence collection. If so, list 3 items of evidence that should be collected, method for collection, and reason for collection.

Activity 9-6. Nursing Plan of Care Procedure

Assess and create a nursing diagnosis. Create a plan of care that includes a protocol for testing and demonstrates implementation of the plan of care and adherence to quality, with patient-centered and trauma-informed methods in the plan of care.

Activity 9-7. APP and Physician Differential Diagnosis

For APPs and physicians, complete the previous activities and create a differential diagnosis based on the patient's history, laboratorics, and clinical presentations. Of the possible differential diagnosis, what is the infection?

Treatment, Reporting, and Follow-Up Plan of Care

Activity 9-8. Treatment

Provide treatment options and prescribe medications to eradicate disease and provide comfort for the patient.

Activity 9-9. Reporting

Determine if the differential diagnosis of the disease is reportable. If yes, identify the entity in your community to which to report.

Activity 9-10. Follow-Up Recommendations in Plan of Care

Provide follow-up recommendations and patient education to include in the plan of care.

Case Study 10

Subjective History

MB is a 23-year-old woman who presents to the clinic with a request for a vaginal examination. She reports yellowish discharge and pelvic pain during intercourse. She reports no new partners in the last 3 months.

Activity 10-1. Identifying Missing Subjective Information

The acronym OLDCARTS (Onset, Location, Duration, Character, Aggravating/relieving, Radiation, Timing, Severity) is used to identify the information necessary to continue with your assessment. For the purposes of this activity, identify the absent OLDCARTS information.

____

____

Activity 10-2. Anatomical Identification

Correctly identify the anogenital anatomy of a patient (**Activity Figure 10-2**).

A. ____________________________________

B. ____________________________________

C. ____________________________________

D. ____________________________________

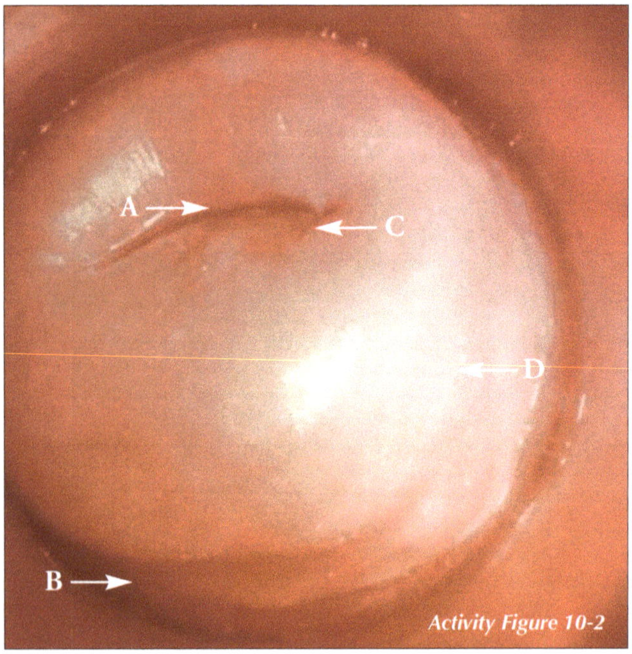

Activity Figure 10-2

Objective History and Findings

The patient is found to have cervical motion tenderness; copious yellow, thick discharge; and vaginal inflammation.

Routine cultures for *Chlamydia trachomatis* and *Neisseria gonorrhoeae* are obtained, and the patient is presumptively treated with 1 g azithromycin orally and 250 mg of ceftriaxone (Rocephin) via intermuscular injection. On follow-up, the patient continues to have pelvic pain and discharge. NAAT for *C. trachomatis* and *N. gonorrhoeae* is negative. NAAT for *Mycoplasma genitalium* is positive. (This NAAT was sent to a local research laboratory.)

Activity 10-3. Physical Examination Findings

Identify and document injuries, age-related normal variants, or medical conditions based on a review of the case photographs (**Activity Figure 10-3**).

A. ____________________________________

B. ____________________________________

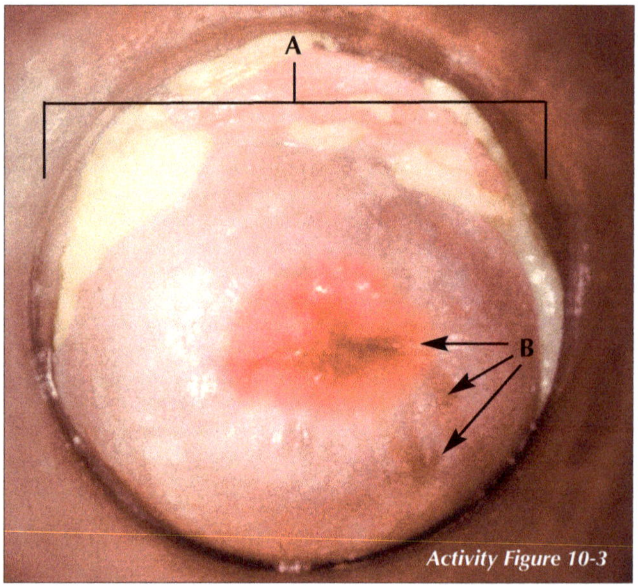

Activity Figure 10-3

Activity 10-4. Clinical Laboratory Improvement Amendments (CLIA) Laboratory Examination

Using the history and the initial urinary findings, list the items in the protocol to implement to assist APPs and physicians in the clinical diagnosis.

____

____

____

____

____

Activity 10-5. Clinical Laboratory Testing

For APPs and physicians, using the history and the initial urinary findings, list the laboratory tests to assist in the definitive differential diagnosis.

Clinical Assessment

Activity 10-6. Forensic Evidence Collection

Determine whether the case history warrants medical forensic evidence collection. If so, list 3 items of evidence that should be collected, method for collection, and reason for collection.

Activity 10-7. Nursing Plan of Care Procedure

Assess and create a nursing diagnosis. Create a plan of care that includes a protocol for testing and demonstrates implementation of the plan of care and adherence to quality, with patient-centered and trauma-informed methods in the plan of care.

Activity 10-8. APP and Physician Differential Diagnosis

For APPs and physicians, complete the previous activities and create a differential diagnosis based on the patient's history, laboratories, and clinical presentations. Of the possibilities included in the differential diagnosis, what is the infection?

Treatment, Reporting, and Follow-Up Plan of Care

Activity 10-9. Treatment

Provide treatment options and prescribe medications to eradicate disease and provide comfort for the patient.

Activity 10-10. Reporting

Determine if the differential diagnosis of the disease is reportable. If yes, identify the entity in your community to which to report.

Activity 10-11. Follow-Up Recommendations in Plan of Care

Provide follow-up recommendations and patient education to include in the plan of care.

Case Study 11

Subjective

EM is a 3-month-old girl whose mother brings her to the ED with complaints of lethargy, vomiting after feeding, and a rash. EM's mother states that she "won't stop crying, like she's hungry, but she won't eat. And she has this horrible diaper rash that's spreading. I don't know what's wrong with her!" The mother reports that when she does eat, EM seems to vomit much of what she is fed. For the last week EM has had copious nasal discharge and had a "bloody nose" the day before, according to her mother. "I thought it was a cold, but it seems like she just gets worse instead of better." Her mother reports no prenatal care before an uncomplicated delivery at a local hospital, although EM was diagnosed as having low birth weight.

Activity 11-1. Identifying Missing Subjective Information

The acronym OLDCARTS (Onset, Location, Duration, Character, Aggravating/relieving, Radiation, Timing, Severity) is used to identify the information necessary to continue with your assessment. For the purposes of this activity, identify the absent OLDCARTS information.

____

Activity 11-2. Anatomical Identification

Correctly identify the anogenital anatomy of the patient (**Activity Figure 11-2**).

A.______________________________________

B.______________________________________

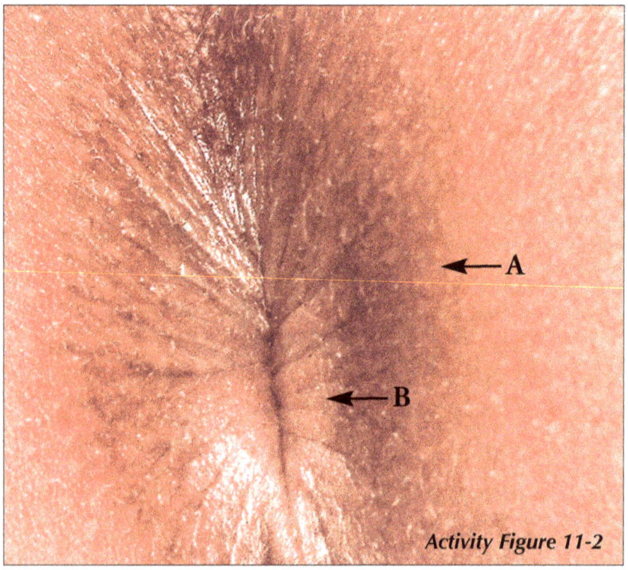

Activity Figure 11-2

Objective History and Findings

A complete physical and anogenital examination is performed. A papular rash is present around the mouth, as well as on the soles of the feet. Sores are noted in the groin area and buttocks. Hepatosplenomegaly is noted. Lumbar puncture and long-bone radiographs are completed, and the health care provider is waiting for the results.

Activity 11-3. Physical Examination Findings

Identify and document injuries, age-related normal variants, or medical conditions based on a review of the case photographs (**Activity Figure 11-3-a** through **c**).

A. ______________________________________

B. ______________________________________

C.______________________________________

D.______________________________________

E.______________________________________

F.______________________________________

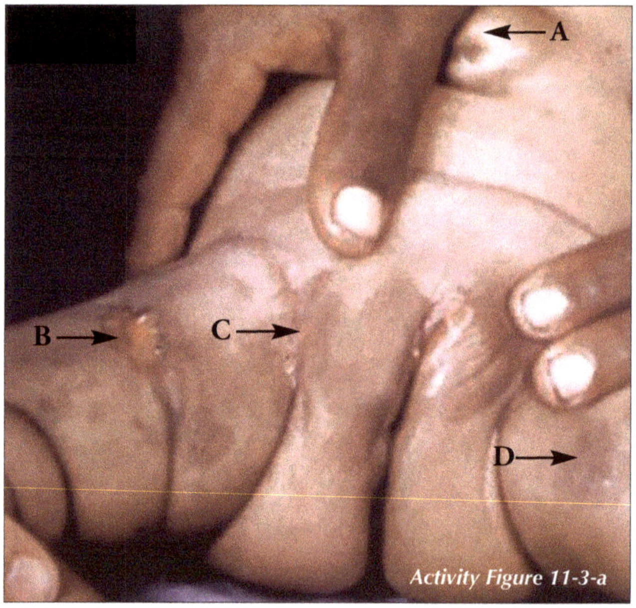

Activity Figure 11-3-a

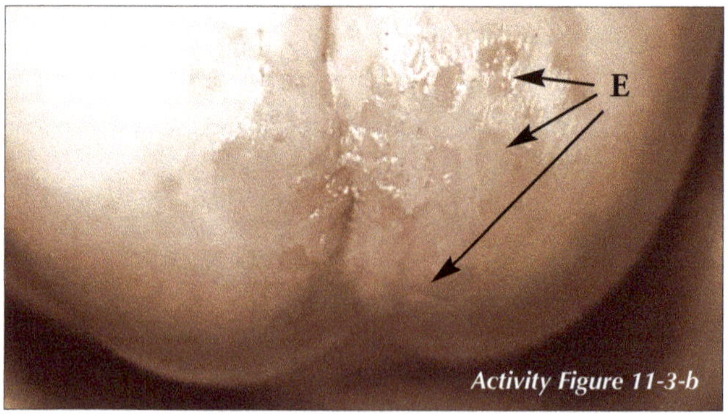

Activity Figure 11-3-b

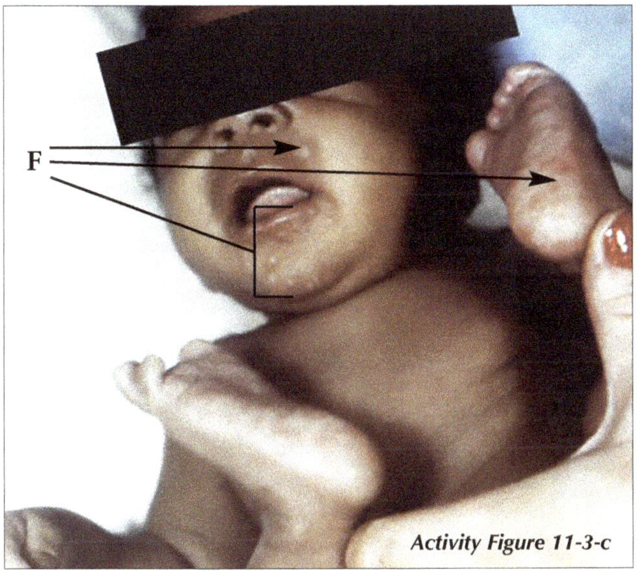

Activity Figure 11-3-c

Activity 11-4. Clinical Laboratory Improvement Amendments (CLIA) Laboratory Examination
Using the history and the initial urinary findings, list the items in the protocol to implement to assist APPs and physicians in the clinical diagnosis.

Activity 11-5. Clinical Laboratory Testing
For APPs and physicians, using the history and the initial urinary findings, list the laboratory tests to assist in the definitive differential diagnosis.

CLINICAL ASSESSMENT

Activity 11-6. Forensic Evidence Collection
Determine whether or not the case history warrants medical forensic evidence collection. If so, list 3 items of evidence that should be collected, method for collection, and reason for collection.

Activity 11-7. Nursing Plan of Care Procedure
Assess and create a nursing diagnosis. Create a plan of care that includes a protocol for testing and demonstrates implementation of the plan of care and adherence to quality, with patient-centered and trauma-informed methods in the plan of care.

Activity 11-8. APP and Physician Differential Diagnosis
For APPs and physicians, complete the previous activities and create a differential diagnosis based on the patient's history, laboratories, and clinical presentations. Of the possible differential diagnosis, what is the infection?

TREATMENT, REPORTING, AND FOLLOW-UP PLAN OF CARE

Activity 11-9. Treatment
Provide treatment options and prescribe medications to eradicate disease and provide comfort for the patient.

Activity 11-10. Reporting
Determine if the differential diagnosis of the disease is reportable. If yes, identify the entity in your community to which to report.

Activity 11-11. Follow-Up Recommendations in Plan of Care
Provide follow-up recommendations and patient education to include in the plan of care.

Case Study 12

Subjective History

JB is a 6-year-old girl whose mother brings her to the pediatric clinic after the patient complains of itching and bumps in her "underwear area." The child has made no claim of sexual assault or abuse to the mother or health care provider, and the mother expresses no immediate concern for sexual abuse. The patient is questioned without the mother present and denies anyone is harming her. Other household members include her father and 4-year-old brother.

Activity 12-1. Identifying Missing Subjective Information

The acronym OLDCARTS (Onset, Location, Duration, Character, Aggravating/relieving, Radiation, Timing, Severity) is used to identify the information necessary to continue with your assessment. For the purposes of this activity, identify the absent OLDCARTS information.

____

Activity 12-2. Anatomical Identification

Correctly identify the anogenital anatomy of a patient (**Activity Figure 12-2**).

A. ______________________________________

B. ______________________________________

C. ______________________________________

D. ______________________________________

E. ______________________________________

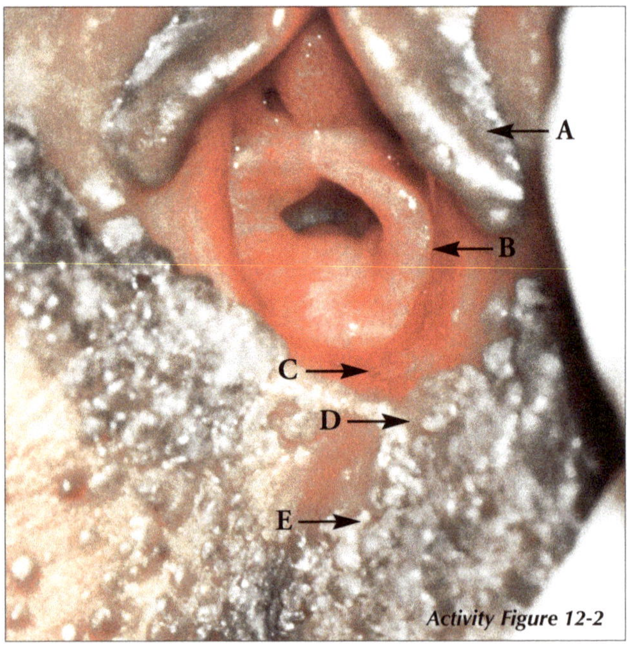

Activity Figure 12-2

Objective History and Findings

A physical examination identifies a 2.5 cm x 3 cm area of smooth papules on her perineum below and to the right of the posterior fourchette.

Human papillomavirus (HPV) testing is not indicated. STI testing for signs of sexual abuse includes urine NAAT for *Chlamydia trachomatis*, *Neisseria gonorrhoeae*, and *Trichomonas vaginalis*, which are all negative.

Activity 12-3. Physical Examination Findings

Identify and document injuries, age-related normal variants, or medical conditions based on a review of the case photographs (**Activity Figure 12-3**).

____

____

____

____

____

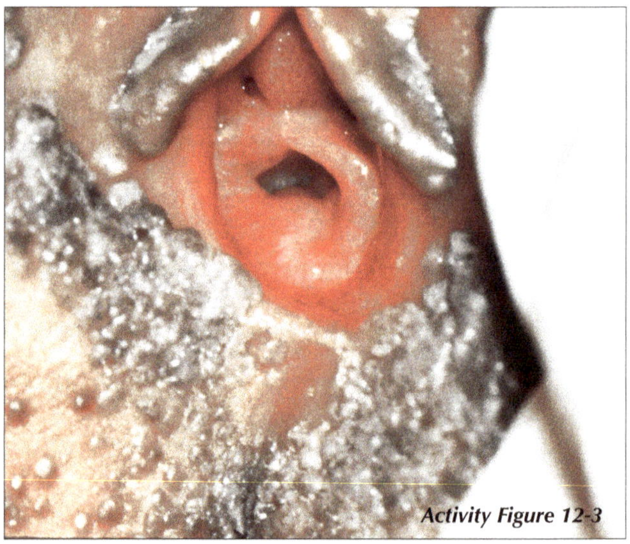
Activity Figure 12-3

Activity 12-4. Clinical Laboratory Improvement Amendments (CLIA) Laboratory Examination

Using the history and the initial urinary findings, list the items in the protocol to implement to assist APPs and physicians in the clinical diagnosis.

____

____

____

____

____

Activity 12-5. Clinical Laboratory Testing

For APPs and physicians, using the history and the initial urinary findings, list the laboratory tests to assist in the definitive differential diagnosis.

Clinical Assessment

Activity 12-6. Forensic Evidence Collection

Determine whether or not the case history warrants medical forensic evidence collection. If so, list 3 items of evidence that should be collected, method for collection, and reason for collection.

Activity 12-7. Nursing Plan of Care Procedure

Assess and create a nursing diagnosis. Create a plan of care that includes a protocol for testing and demonstrates implementation of the plan of care and adherence to quality, with patient-centered and trauma-informed methods in the plan of care.

Activity 12-8. APP and Physician Differential Diagnosis

For APPs and physicians, complete the previous activities and create a differential diagnosis based on the patient's history, laboratories, and clinical presentations. Of the possible differential diagnosis, what is the infection?

Treatment, Reporting, and Follow-Up Plan of Care

Activity 12-9. Treatment

Provide treatment options and prescribe medications to eradicate disease and provide comfort for the patient.

Activity 12-10. Reporting

Determine if the differential diagnosis of the disease is reportable. If yes, identify the entity in your community to which to report.

Activity 12-11. Follow-Up Recommendations in Plan of Care

Provide follow-up recommendations and patient education to include in the plan of care.

Case Study 13

Subjective History

DJ is a 42-year-old Caucasian man who presents to the ED with extreme fatigue and nausea and vomiting over the past 4 weeks as well as dark urine over the past few days. He reports a history of injection drug use, which escalated from prescription opioid use that began after a work-related injury. He states that he has been clean for 2 months. He identifies as heterosexual and reports having multiple female sexual partners. He lives with his brother. He reports smoking cigarettes at a rate of half a pack per day and denies use of alcohol or any illegal drugs. He denies any recent sick contacts and denies a family history of any chronic illnesses or infectious diseases. He denies having any other medical problems, including a history of HIV and hepatitis, and has no history of any surgical procedures. On review of symptoms, he reports mild abdominal pain as well as decreased appetite.

Activity 13-1. Identifying Missing Subjective Information

The acronym OLDCARTS (Onset, Location, Duration, Character, Aggravating/relieving, Radiation, Timing, Severity) is used to identify the information necessary to continue with your assessment. For the purposes of this activity, identify the absent OLDCARTS information.

____

Activity 13-2. Anatomical Identification

Correctly identify the anogenital anatomy of a patient (**Activity Figure 13-2-a** and **b**).

A.____

B.____

C. ____

D. ____

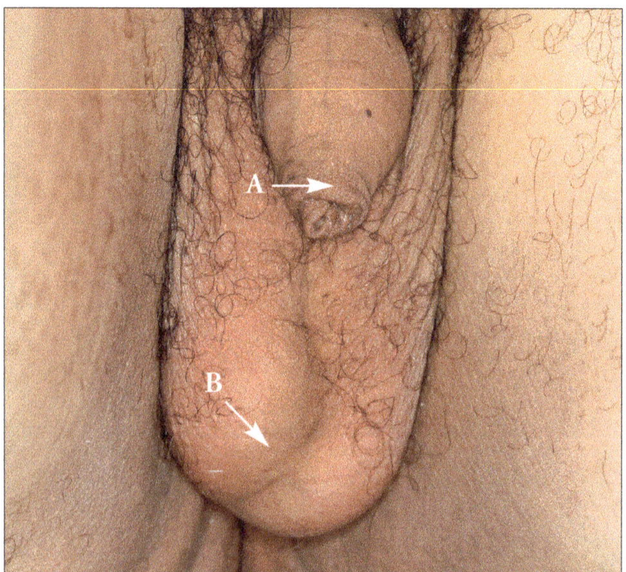

Activity Figure 13-2-a

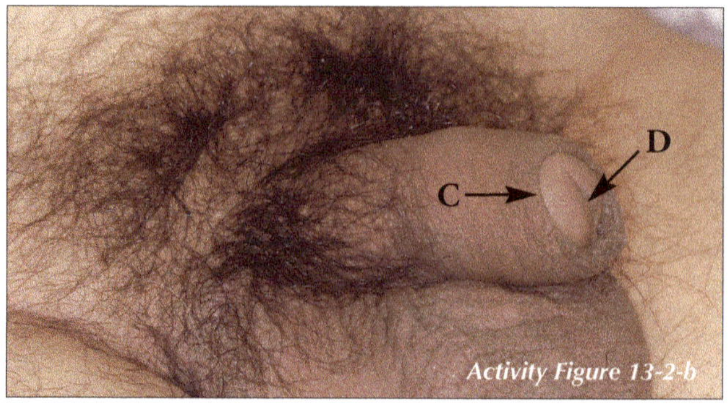

Activity Figure 13-2-b

Objective History and Findings

The patient has a temperature of 99.9°F. The sclera is slightly jaundice. There are no other skin changes. The abdomen is nontender; no hepatosplenomegaly is present.

Laboratory testing is ordered, and the results are as follows: alanine aminotransferase 1800 IU/mL, aspartate aminotransferase 1100 IU/mL, hepatitis A virus, hepatitis C virus, and hepatitis D virus antibody tests are negative. Hepatitis B surface antigen and immunoglobulin M antibody to core hepatitis B core antigen are positive. Hepatitis B virus DNA is undetectable.

Activity 13-3. Physical Examination Findings

Identify and document injuries, age-related normal variants, or medical conditions based on a review of the case photographs (**Activity Figure 13-3-a** and **b**).

A. ____

B. ____

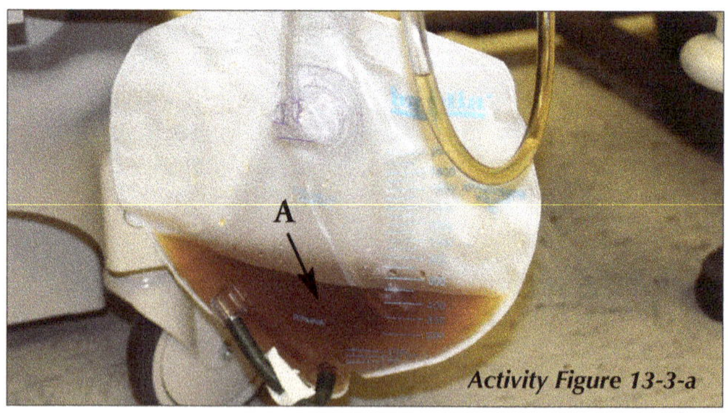

Activity Figure 13-3-a

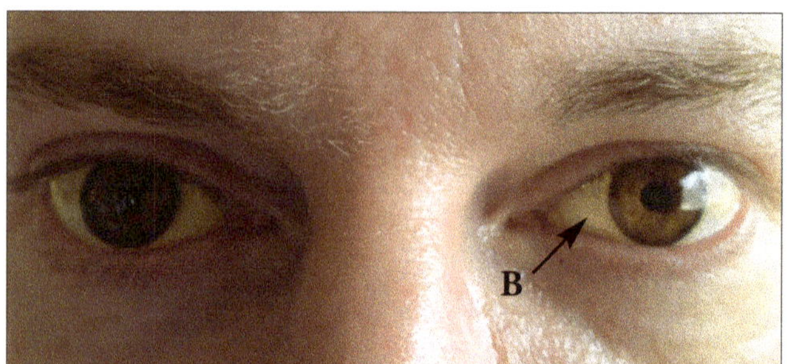

Activity Figure 13-3-b

Activity 13-4. Clinical Laboratory Improvement Amendments (CLIA) Laboratory Examination

Using the history and the initial urinary findings, list the items in the protocol to implement to assist APPs and physicians in the clinical diagnosis.

Activity 13-5. Clinical Laboratory Testing

For APPs and physicians, using the history and the initial urinary findings, list the laboratory tests to assist in the definitive differential diagnosis.

Clinical Assessment

Activity 13-6. Forensic Evidence Collection

Determine whether or not the case history warrants medical forensic evidence collection. If so, list 3 items of evidence that should be collected, method for collection, and reason for collection.

Activity 13-7. Nursing Plan of Care Procedure

Assess and create a nursing diagnosis. Create a plan of care that includes a protocol for testing and demonstrates implementation of the plan of care and adherence to quality, with patient-centered and trauma-informed methods in the plan of care.

Activity 13-8. APP and Physician Differential Diagnosis

For APPs and physicians, complete the previous activities and create a differential diagnosis based on the patient's history, laboratories, and clinical presentations. Of the possible differential diagnosis, what is the infection?

Treatment, Reporting, and Follow-Up Plan of Care

Activity 13-9. Treatment

Provide treatment options and prescribe medications to eradicate disease and provide comfort for the patient.

Activity 13-10. Reporting

Determine if the disease is reportable. If yes, identify the entity in your community to which to report.

Activity 13-11. Follow-Up Recommendations in Plan of Care

Provide follow-up recommendations and patient education to include in the plan of care.

Case Study 14

Subjective History

AJ, a 24-year-old Caucasian man who has recently returned from a Caribbean vacation with friends, presents to an outpatient STI testing clinic with reports of a 7-day history of a red, painful "sore" on his penis. He denies fever, chills, nausea, vomiting, dysuria, urethral discharge, or testicular pain. The patient reports that while on holiday, approximately 9 days before the onset of his symptoms, he had sexual contact with a woman he met in the hotel bar. He reports a regular female partner at home as well. He denies condom use with either partner.

Activity 14-1. Identifying Missing Subjective Information

The acronym OLDCARTS (Onset, Location, Duration, Character, Aggravating/relieving, Radiation, Timing, Severity) is used to identify the information necessary to continue with your assessment. For the purposes of this activity, identify the absent OLDCARTS information.

____

Activity 14-2. Anatomical Identification

Correctly identify the anogenital anatomy of a patient (**Activity Figure 14-2**).

A. ______________________________

B. ______________________________

C. ______________________________

D. ______________________________

E. ______________________________

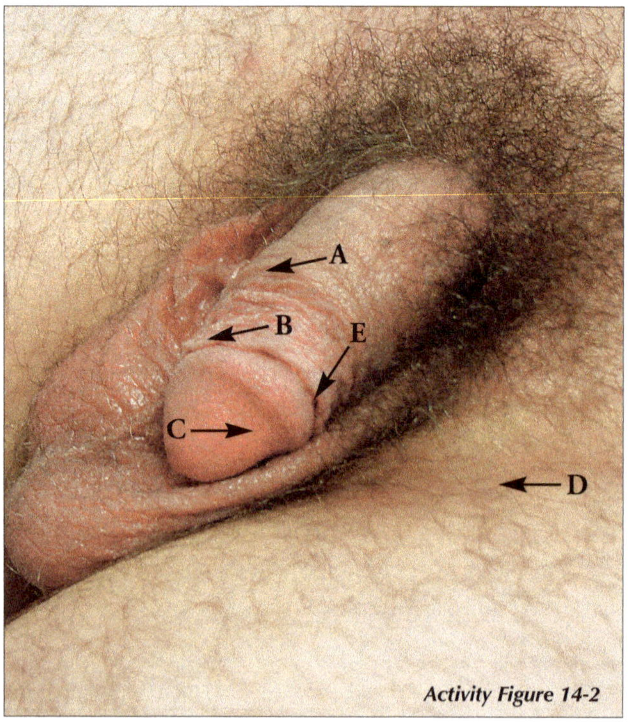

Activity Figure 14-2

Objective History and Findings

The patient has a 2-cm tender, erythematous, penile lesion on the shaft of his penis. On physical examination, 2 tender, palpable inguinal lymph nodes are noted. There is no urethral discharge, and the remainder of the genitourinary examination is unremarkable.

Activity 14-3. Physical Examination Findings

Identify and document injuries, age-related normal variants, or medical conditions based on a review of the case photograph (**Activity Figure 14-3**).

____

____

____

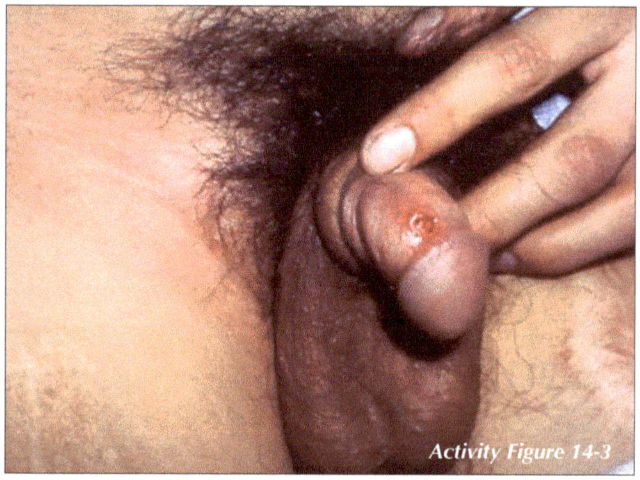
Activity Figure 14-3

Activity 14-4. Clinical Laboratory Improvement Amendments (CLIA) Laboratory Examination

Using the history and the initial urinary findings, list the items in the protocol to implement to assist APPs and physicians in the clinical diagnosis.

____

____

____

____

Activity 14-5. Clinical Laboratory Testing

For APPs and physicians, using the history and the initial urinary findings, list the laboratory tests to assist in the definitive differential diagnosis.

____

____

____

____

Clinical Assessment

Activity 14-6. Forensic Evidence Collection

Determine whether or not the case history warrants medical forensic evidence collection. If so, list 3 items of evidence that should be collected, method for collection, and reason for collection.

Activity 14-7. Nursing Plan of Care Procedure

Assess and create nursing diagnoses. Create a plan of care that includes a protocol for testing and demonstrates implementation of the plan of care and adherence to quality, with patient-centered and trauma-informed methods in the plan of care.

Activity 14-8. APP and Physician Differential Diagnosis

For APPs and physicians, complete the previous activities and create a differential diagnosis based on the patient's history, laboratories, and clinical presentations. Of the possible differential diagnosis, what is the infection?

Treatment, Reporting, and Follow-Up Plan of Care

Activity 14-9. Treatment

Provide treatment options and prescribe medications to eradicate disease and provide comfort for the patient.

Activity 14-10. Reporting

Determine if the differential diagnosis of the disease is reportable. If yes, identify the entity in your community to which to report.

Activity 14-11. Follow-Up Recommendations in Plan of Care

Provide follow-up recommendations and patient education to include in the plan of care.

Case Study 15

Subjective

A 20-year-old female university student presents to the student health center with a complaint of foul-smelling vaginal discharge after "lots of sex" over a 3-day beach vacation with her current boyfriend. She reports she had sex multiple times daily for the 3 days they were at the beach. She has been monogamous with this same sexual partner for the past 2 months but had multiple sexual partners, both male and female, over the past 2 years. She uses oral contraceptives to prevent pregnancy. She does not use any barrier protection because she "always forgets." She states she douches regularly. She denies dysuria, cloudy urine, frequent urination, pruritus, dyspareunia, burning sensation, or vaginal erythema or edema. When asked to describe the vaginal discharge, she states that it is a thin, white, fishy-smelling discharge that "seems like it's always there." She reports that she did not notice the discharge before her beach weekend, and now it is worrisome because of the amount of discharge and the odor, which is "so noticeable" that her boyfriend said something to her.

Activity 15-1. Identifying Missing Subjective Information

Clinicians can use the acronym OLDCARTS (Onset, Location, Duration, Character, Aggravating/relieving, Radiation, Timing, Severity) to identify the information necessary to complete a patient assessment. For this activity, identify the absent OLDCARTS information.

____

____

Activity 15-2. Anatomical Identification

Correctly identify the anogenital anatomy of a patient (**Activity Figure 15-2-a** and **b**).

A. ______________________________________

B. ______________________________________

C. ______________________________________

D. ______________________________________

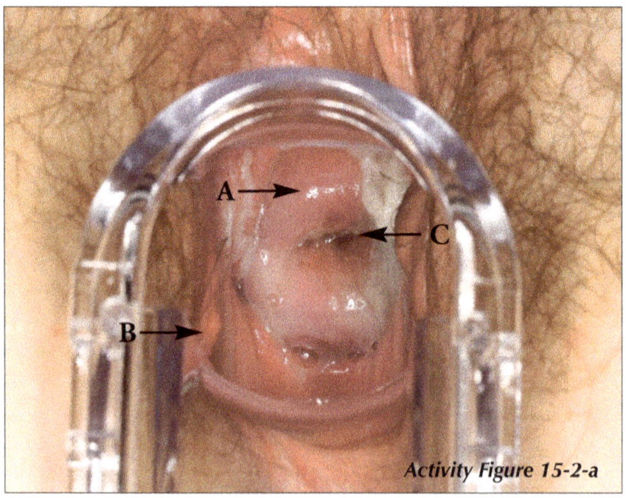

Activity Figure 15-2-a

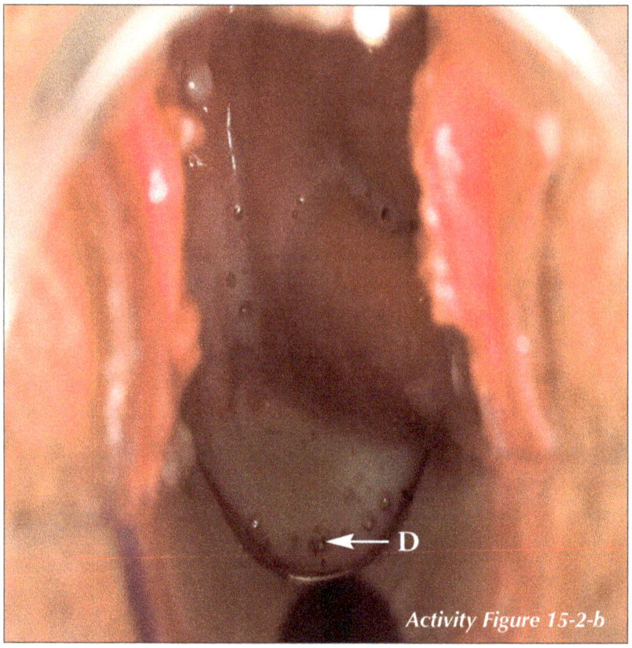

Activity Figure 15-2-b

Objective History and Findings

The vaginal discharge is off-white and thin, with bubbles and with a distinct "fishy" odor. The vaginal pH is 5.1 with a positive whiff test. The urine pregnancy test is negative.

Activity 15-3. Physical Examination Findings

Identify and document injuries, age-related normal variants, and medical conditions based on a review of the case photographs (**Activity Figure 15-3**).

____

____

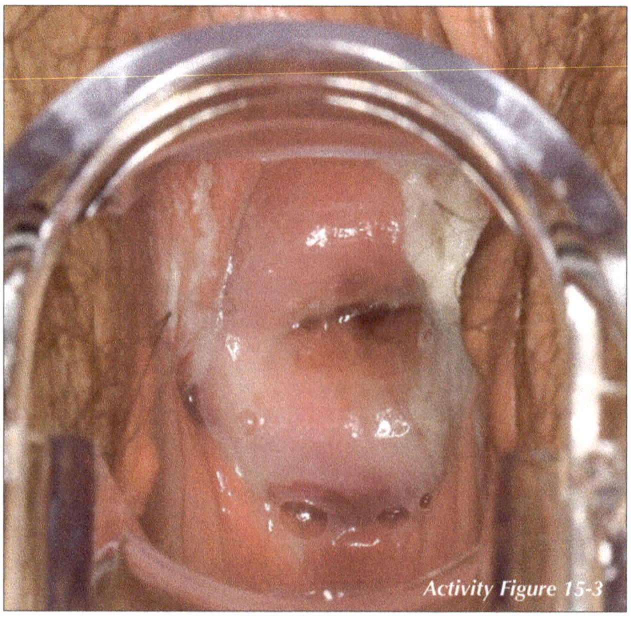

Activity Figure 15-3

Activity 15-4. Clinical Laboratory Improvement Amendments (CLIA) Laboratory Examination

Using the history and the initial findings, list the items in the protocol to implement to assist APPs and physicians in the clinical diagnosis.

Activity 15-5. Clinical Laboratory Testing

For APPs and physicians, using the history and the initial findings, list the laboratory tests to assist in the definitive differential diagnosis.

CLINICAL ASSESSMENT

Activity 15-6. Forensic Evidence Collection

Determine whether the case history warrants medical forensic evidence collection. If so, list 3 items of evidence that should be collected, the method for collection, and the reason for collection.

Activity 15-7. Nursing Plan of Care Procedure

Assess and create a nursing diagnosis. Create a plan of care that includes a protocol for testing and demonstrates the implementation of the plan of care and adherence to quality, with patient-centered and trauma-informed methods in the plan of care.

Activity 15-8. APP and Physician Differential Diagnosis

For APPs and physicians, complete the previous activities, and create a differential diagnosis based on the patient's history, diagnostics, and clinical presentation. Of the possible differential diagnoses, what is the priority differential?

TREATMENT, REPORTING, AND FOLLOW-UP PLAN OF CARE

Activity 15-9. Treatment

Provide treatment options and prescribe medications to eradicate disease and provide comfort for the patient.

Activity 15-10. Reporting

Determine if the differential diagnosis of the disease is reportable. If yes, identify the entity in your community to which to report.

Activity 15-11. Follow-Up Recommendations in Plan of Care

Provide follow-up recommendations and patient education to include in the plan of care.

Case Study 16

Subjective History

SD is a 25-year-old woman who presents to the primary care clinic for a required physical examination and meningitis immunization before starting a new job. In addition to the physical, she requests a birth control prescription refill, stating that she is a single mother of a 2-year-old, and she does not want more children at this time while she tries to get more economically secure. The HPV vaccination is offered, and patient education is provided about STI screening. SD states that she has never had an STI screening or the HPV vaccinations. She reports a sexual history of 6 different partners, with 1 male partner in the past 3 months. On further questioning, SD acknowledges that she has noticed increased vaginal discharge lately and some minor pain during intercourse. She also notes that she has had a "sore throat" and feels like she is "coming down with something." Exposure risks include fellatio, cunnilingus, penile vaginal intercourse, and inconsistent condom use. No significant medical history and no drug allergies are reported.

Activity 16-1. Identifying Missing Subjective Information

The acronym OLDCARTS (Onset, Location, Duration, Character, Aggravating/relieving, Radiation, Timing, Severity) is used to identify the information necessary to continue with your assessment. For the purposes of this activity, identify the absent OLDCARTS information.

____

Activity 16-2. Anatomical Identification

Correctly identify the anogenital anatomy of a patient (**Activity Figure 16-2**).

A. ____________________________________

B. ____________________________________

C. ____________________________________

D. ____________________________________

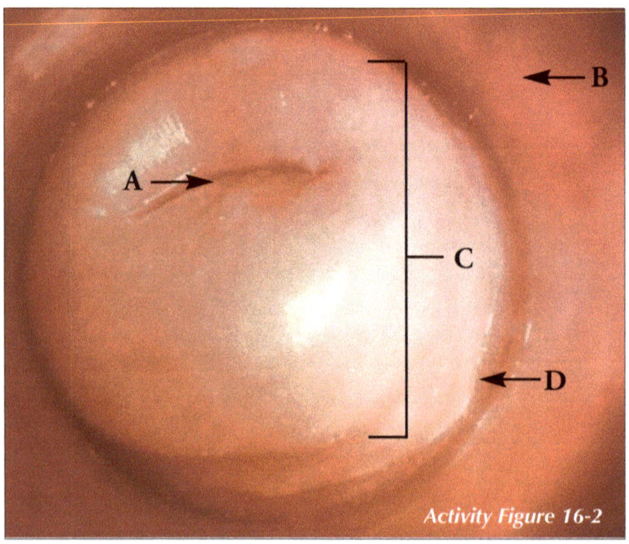

Activity Figure 16-2

Objective History and Findings

The patient has a temperature of 100.1°F (37.8°C). Blood pressure and pulse rate are normal. An oral examination reveals erythema of the soft palate and white spots on the tonsils. Enlarged lymph nodes are palpated under the jaw and on the neck.

Activity 16-3. Physical Examination Findings

Identify and document injuries, age-related normal variants, or medical conditions based on a review of the case photographs (**Activity Figure 16-3**).

____

____

____

____

____

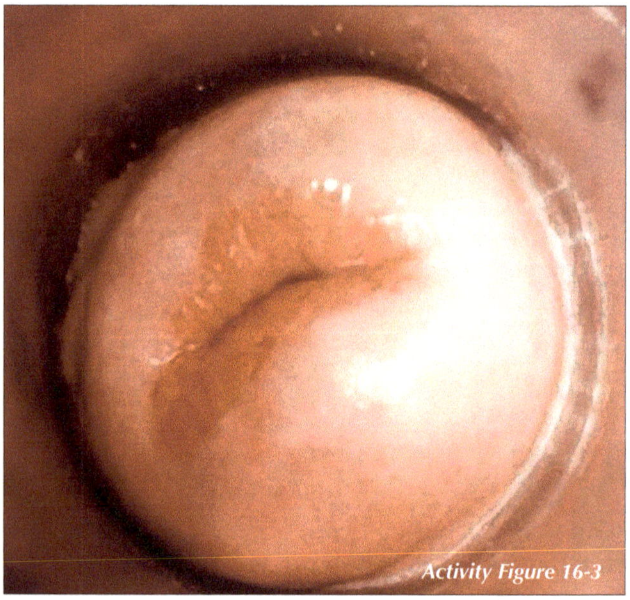
Activity Figure 16-3

Activity 16-4. Clinical Laboratory Improvement Amendments (CLIA) Laboratory Examination

Using the history and the initial urinary findings, list the items in the protocol to implement to assist APPs and physicians in the clinical diagnosis.

____

____

____

____

____

____

Activity 16-5. Clinical Laboratory Testing

For APPs and physicians, using the history and the initial urinary findings, list the laboratory tests to assist in the definitive differential diagnosis.

Clinical Assessment

Activity 16-6. Forensic Evidence Collection

Determine whether the case history warrants medical forensic evidence collection. If so, list 3 items of evidence that should be collected, method for collection, and reason for collection.

Activity 16-7. Nursing Plan of Care Procedure

Assess and create nursing diagnoses. Create a plan of care that includes a protocol for testing and demonstrates implementation of the plan of care and adherence to quality, with patient-centered and trauma-informed methods in the plan of care.

Activity 16-8. APP and Physician Differential Diagnosis

For APPs and physicians, complete the previous activities and create a differential diagnosis based on the patient's history, laboratories, and clinical presentations. Of the possible differential diagnosis, what is the infection?

Treatment, Reporting, and Follow-Up Plan of Care

Activity 16-9. Treatment

Provide treatment options and prescribe medications to eradicate disease and provide comfort for the patient.

Activity 16-10. Reporting

Determine if the differential diagnosis of the disease is reportable. If yes, identify the entity in your community to which to report.

Activity 16-11. Follow-Up Recommendations in Plan of Care

Provide follow-up recommendations and patient education to include in the plan of care.

Case Study 17

Subjective History

A teen boy was brought to the primary care clinic with a rash on his lower body and "bugs in his eyes." The "bugs" appeared 12 days ago, and the boy was unable to get transportation to the clinic. His distress is fairly constant, but he complains that the symptoms do seem to intensify at night. He is worried about the other children in his house. He denies others in the household having "bugs" and says that they are in other rooms and do not sleep with him.

Activity 17-1. Identifying Missing Subjective Information

The acronym OLDCARTS (Onset, Location, Duration, Character, Aggravating/relieving, Radiation, Timing, Severity) is used to identify the information necessary to continue with your assessment. For the purposes of this activity, identify the absent OLDCARTS information.

____

____

Activity 17-2. Anatomical Identification

Correctly identify the anogenital anatomy of a patient (**Activity Figure 17-2**).

A. ______________________________________

B. ______________________________________

C. ______________________________________

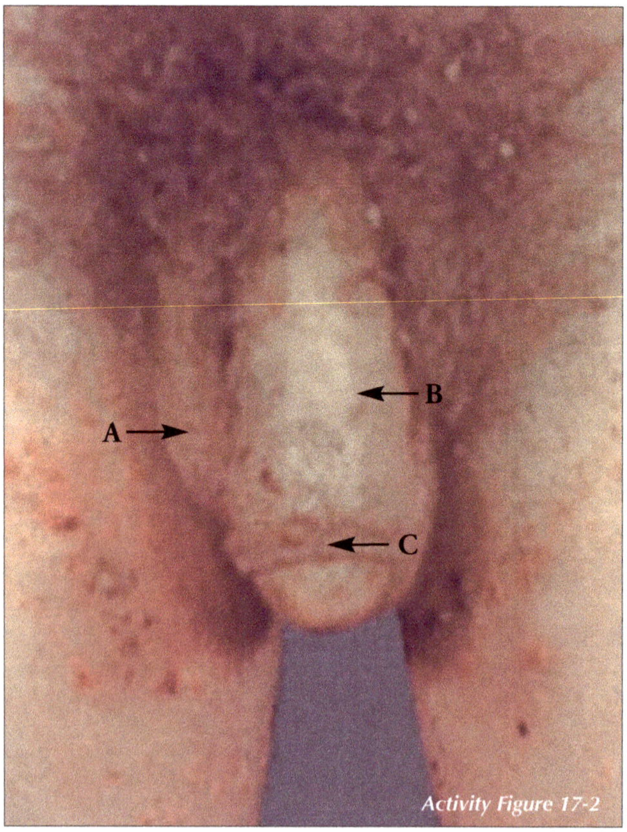

Activity Figure 17-2

Objective History and Findings

On inspection and application of clear tape to the eyelashes, the microscopic evaluation reveals scabies.

Activity 17-3. Physical Examination Findings

Identify and document injuries, age-related normal variants, or medical conditions based on a review of the case photographs (**Activity Figure 17-3**).

____

____

____

____

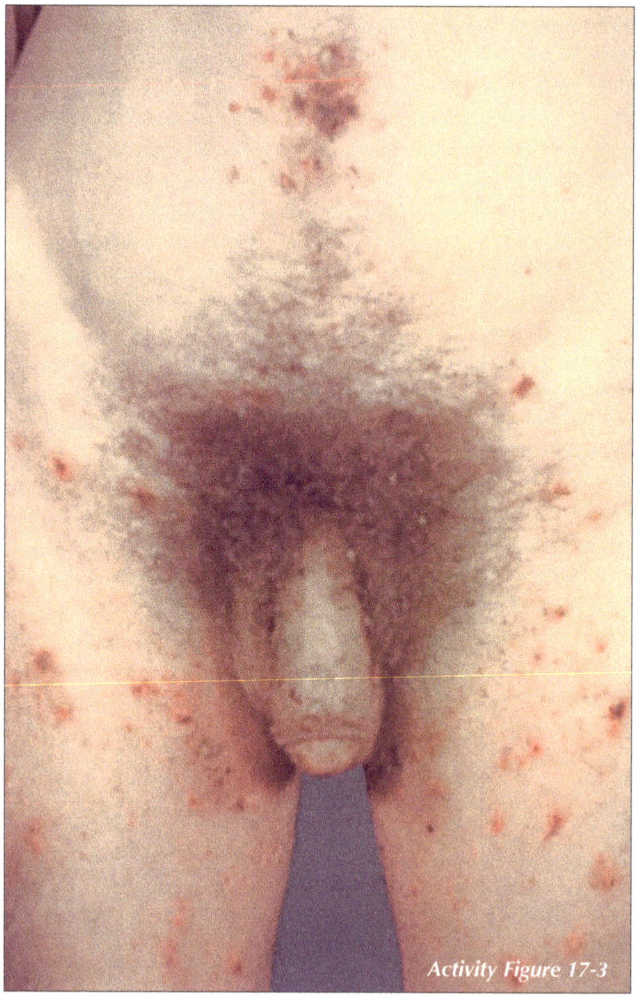
Activity Figure 17-3

Activity 17-4. Clinical Laboratory Improvement Amendments (CLIA) Laboratory Examination
Using the history and the initial urinary findings, list the items in the protocol to implement to assist APPs and physicians in the clinical diagnosis.

Activity 17-5. Clinical Laboratory Testing
For APPs and physicians, using the history and the initial urinary findings, list the laboratory tests to assist in the definitive differential diagnosis.

Clinical Assessment

Activity 17-6. Forensic Evidence Collection
Determine whether or not the case history warrants medical forensic evidence collection. If so, list 3 items of evidence that should be collected, method for collection, and reason for collection.

Activity 17-7. Nursing Plan of Care Procedure
Assess for and create a nursing diagnosis. Create a plan of care that includes a protocol for testing, demonstrates implementation of the plan of care, and adheres to quality with patient-centered and trauma-informed methods in the plan of care.

Activity 17-8. APP and Physician Differential Diagnosis
For APPs and physicians, complete the previous activities and create a differential diagnosis based on the patient's history, laboratories, and clinical presentations. Of the possible differential diagnosis, what is the infection?

Treatment, Reporting, and Follow-Up Plan of Care

Activity 17-9. Treatment
Provide treatment options and prescribe medications to eradicate disease and provide comfort for the patient.

Activity 17-10. Reporting
Determine if the differential diagnosis of the disease is reportable. If yes, identify the entity in your community to which to report.

Activity 17-11. Follow-Up Recommendations in Plan of Care
Provide follow-up recommendations and patient education to include in the plan of care.

Case Study 18

Subjective History

A 31-year-old man presents to an outpatient STI testing clinic. He reports a 2-week history of a painful, red, swollen ulcer on his penis. He denies fever, chills, night sweats, rashes, genital lesions, dysuria, urethral discharge, testicular pain, proctitis, rectal discharge, tenesmus, and diarrhea. He reports previous unprotected receptive and penetrative oral and anal sexual contacts with male partners.

Activity 18-1. Identifying Missing Subjective Information

The acronym OLDCARTS (Onset, Location, Duration, Character, Aggravating/relieving, Radiation, Timing, Severity) is used to identify the information necessary to continue with your assessment. For the purposes of this activity, identify the absent OLDCARTS information.

____

Activity 18-2. Anatomical Identification

Correctly identify the anogenital anatomy of a patient (**Activity Figure 18-2-a** and **b**).

A. ____________________________________

B. ____________________________________

C. ____________________________________

D. ____________________________________

E. ____________________________________

F. ____________________________________

G. ____________________________________

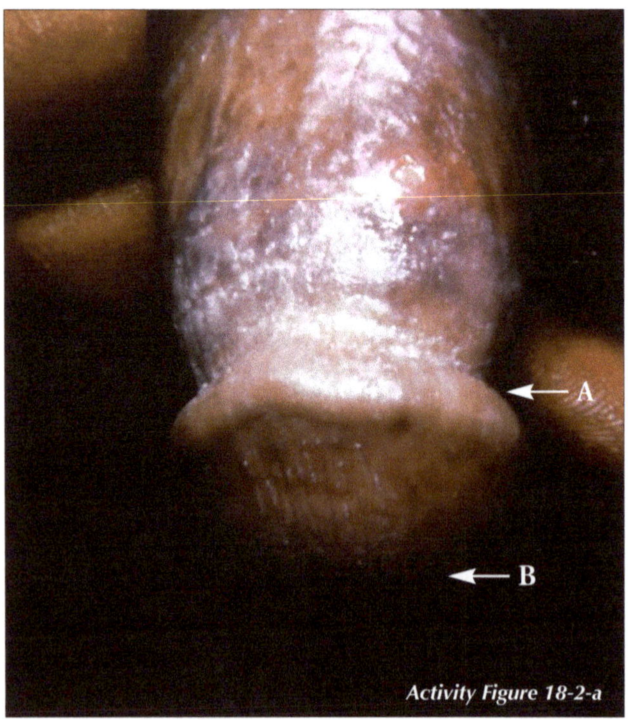

Activity Figure 18-2-a

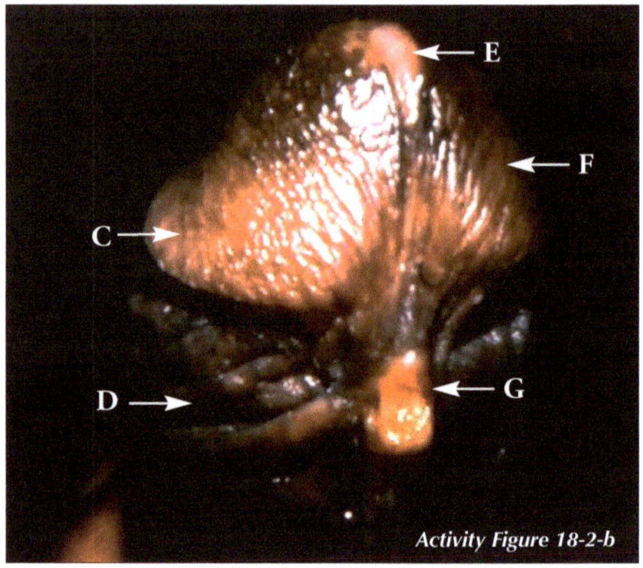

Activity Figure 18-2-b

Objective History

Examination reveals a 3-cm, tender, erythematous penile lesion free of discharge and ulceration. There is no visible groove sign (ie, inflammation of the inguinal nodes above and femoral nodes below the inguinal ligament). The genitourinary examination is otherwise unremarkable, as is the examination of his cervical lymph nodes and oropharynx.

Specimens are collected to test for gonorrhea and *Chlamydia*, including first-void urine for NAAT and pharyngeal and rectal swabs for culture. Lymphogranuloma venereum genotyping is requested for all specimens that have positive test results for *Chlamydia*. Samples for serological testing for syphilis, HIV, and *Chlamydia* serovar L are also sent.

Activity 18-3. Physical Examination Findings

Identify and document injuries, age-related normal variants, and medical conditions based on a review of the case photographs (**Activity Figure 18-3-a** through **b**).

A. ____________________________________

B. ____________________________________

Activity 18-4. Clinical Laboratory Improvement Amendments (CLIA) Laboratory Examination

Using the history and the initial urinary findings, list the items in the protocol to implement to assist APPs and physicians in the clinical diagnosis.

____

____

____

____

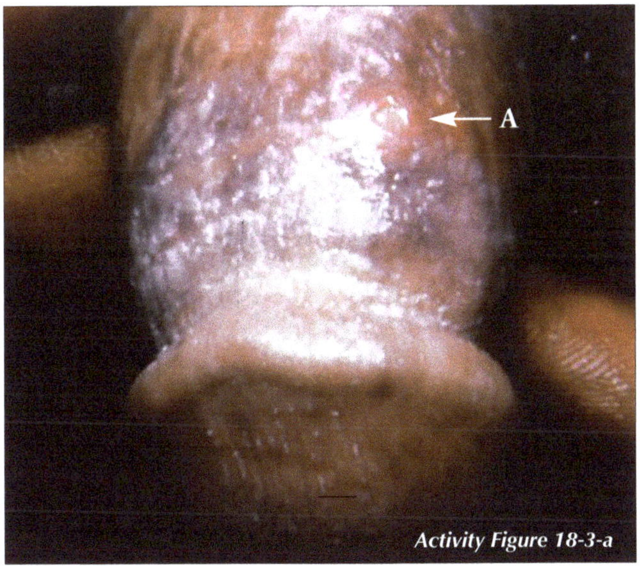

Activity Figure 18-3-a

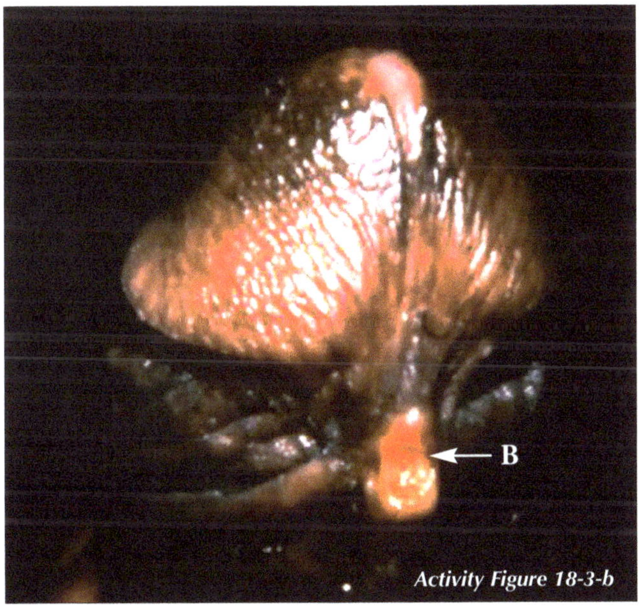

Activity Figure 18-3-b

Activity 18-5. Clinical Laboratory Testing

For APPs and physicians: Using the history and the initial urinary findings, list the laboratory tests to assist in the definitive differential diagnosis.

CLINICAL ASSESSMENT

Activity 18-6. Forensic Evidence Collection

Determine whether the case history warrants medical forensic evidence collection. If so, list 3 items of evidence that should be collected, method for collection, and reason for collection.

Activity 18-7. Nursing Plan of Care Procedure

Assess and create a nursing diagnosis. Create a plan of care that includes a protocol for testing, demonstrates implementation of the plan of care, and adheres to quality with patient-centered and trauma-informed methods in the plan of care.

Activity 18-8. APP and Physician Differential Diagnosis

For APPs and physicians: Complete the previous activities and create a differential diagnosis based on the patient's history, laboratories, and clinical presentations. Of the possible differential diagnosis, what is the infection?

TREATMENT, REPORTING, AND FOLLOW-UP PLAN OF CARE

Activity 18-9. Treatment

Provide treatment options and prescribe medications to eradicate disease and provide comfort for the patient.

Activity 18-10. Reporting

Determine if the differential diagnosis of the disease is reportable. If yes, identify the entity in your community to which to report.

Activity 18-11. Follow-Up Recommendations in Plan of Care

Provide follow-up recommendations and patient education to include in the plan of care.

Case Study 19

Subjective History

A 44-year-old male construction worker presents to the ED. He reports frequent upper respiratory infections and mouth sores. The patient is concerned because he has no energy, feels lethargic and sick, and is unable to work a full day. The symptoms have been present for several months. He reports he does not have a health care provider but uses the ED for his injuries on the job. He smokes and reports that he used to use crack. He also reports that several years ago, while he was in jail, he was raped by another inmate. When given the option, he prefers to not tell law enforcement about the rape. The APP begins the medical history interview and workup for symptoms.

Activity 19-1. Identifying Missing Subjective Information

The acronym OLDCARTS (Onset, Location, Duration, Character, Aggravating/relieving, Radiation, Timing, Severity) is used to identify the information necessary to continue with your assessment. For the purposes of this activity, identify the absent OLDCARTS information.

____

Activity 19-2. Anatomical Identification

Correctly identify the oral anatomy of a patient (**Activity Figure 19-2-a** through **c**).

A. ______________________________________

B. ______________________________________

C. ______________________________________

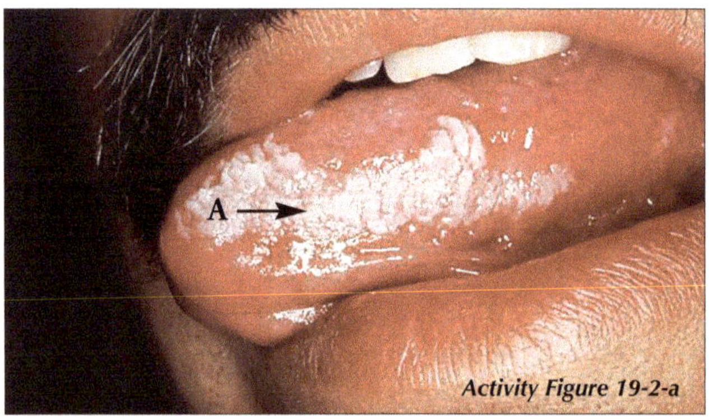

Activity Figure 19-2-a

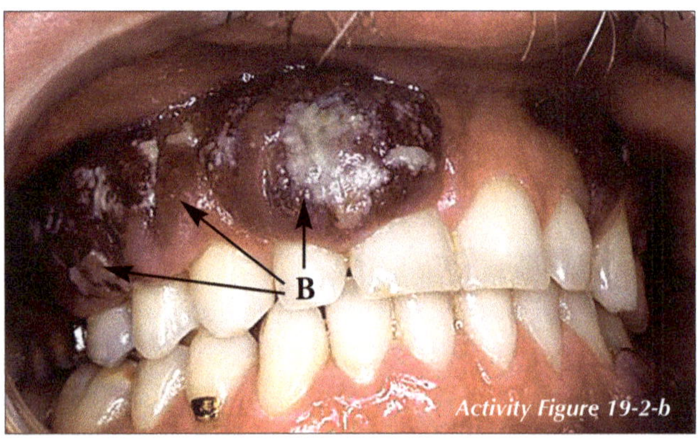

Activity Figure 19-2-b

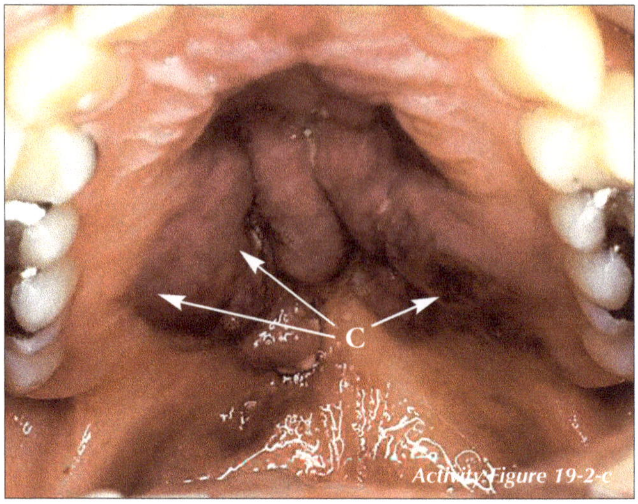

Activity Figure 19-2-c

Objective History

The evaluation found that the patient is without acute or previous injury in the anogenital area, but there are significant white patches over anal tissue. In the mouth there are a number of lesions on the lateral left tongue and soft palate, making it painful for the patient to swallow.

All laboratory tests are completed after the medical forensic evaluation. Tests include urinalysis; CBC; cultures for all orifices; drug screen; STI screening with NAAT for *Chlamydia*, gonorrhea, and HIV; and bloodwork plus chest radiographs.

The NAATs for *Chlamydia* and gonorrhea are negative, and the NAAT for HIV is positive. Further testing for CD4 count, HIV type, tuberculosis skin test, and other opportunistic infections are ordered.

Activity 19-3. Physical Examination Findings

Identify and document injuries, age-related normal variants, and medical conditions based on a review of the case photographs (**Activity Figure 19-3-a** through **c**).

A. ______________________________________

B. ______________________________________

C. ______________________________________

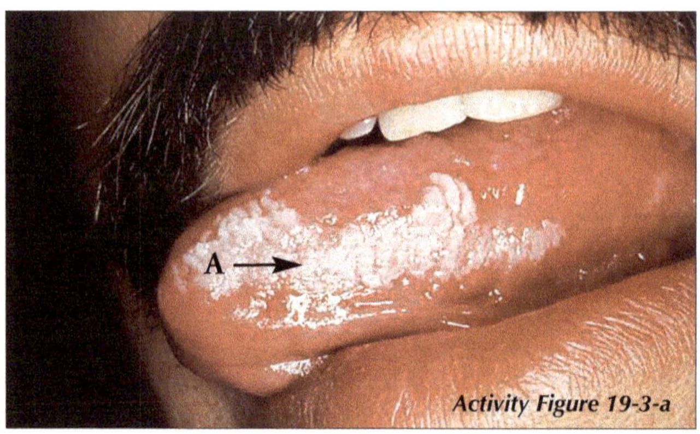

Activity Figure 19-3-a

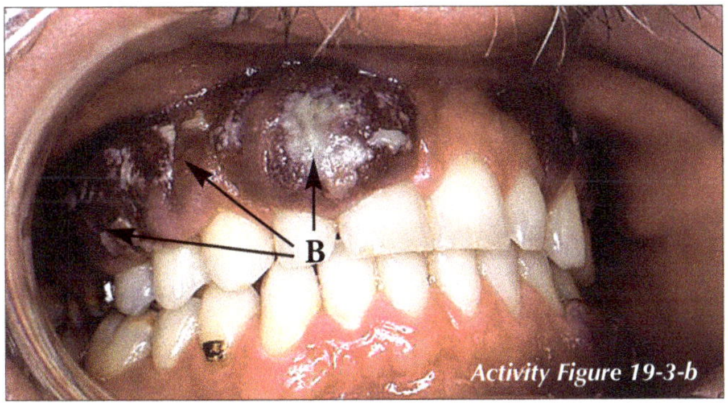

Activity Figure 19-3-b

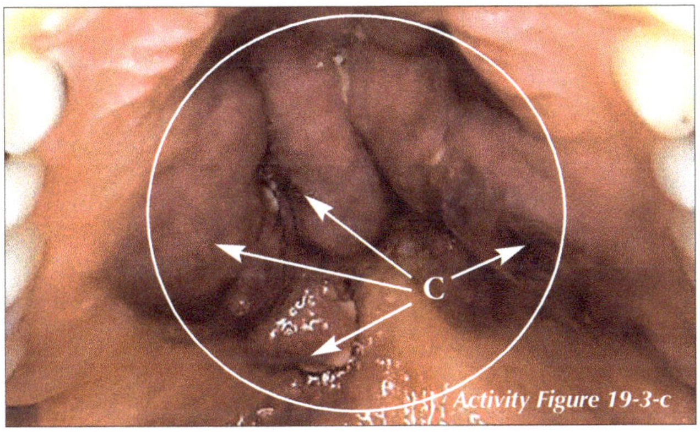

Activity Figure 19-3-c

Activity 19-4. Clinical Laboratory Improvement Amendments (CLIA) Laboratory Examination

Using the history and the initial laboratory findings, list the items in the protocol to implement to assist APPs and physicians in the clinical diagnosis.

Activity 19-5. Clinical Laboratory Testing

For APPs and physicians: Using the history and the initial NAAT findings, list the laboratory tests to assist in the definitive differential diagnosis.

Clinical Assessment

Activity 19-6. Forensic Evidence Collection

Determine whether or not the case history warrants medical forensic evidence collection. If so, list 3 items of evidence that should be collected, method for collection, and reason for collection.

Activity 19-7. Nursing Plan of Care Procedure

Assess and create a nursing diagnosis. Create a plan of care that includes a protocol for testing, demonstrates implementation of the plan of care, and adheres to quality with patient-centered and trauma-informed methods in the plan of care.

Activity 19-8. APP and Physician Differential Diagnosis

For APPs and physicians: Complete the previous activities and create a differential diagnosis based on the patient's history, laboratories, and clinical presentations. Of the possible differential diagnosis, what is the infection?

Treatment, Reporting, and Follow-Up Plan of Care

Activity 19-9. Treatment

Provide treatment options and prescribe medications to eradicate disease and provide comfort for the patient.

Activity 19-10. Reporting

Determine if the differential diagnosis of the disease is reportable. If yes, identify the entity in your community to which to report.

Activity 19-11. Follow-Up Recommendations in Plan of Care

Provide follow-up recommendations and patient education to include in the plan of care.

Section VIII

Answer Key

Note to Students

Community standards and agency protocols for evidence collection, prophylactic treatment, patient referrals, and follow-up vary across the United States and internationally. It is the student's responsibility to know his or her community standards, agency protocols, and the rationale surrounding any variations where national or international standards or recommendations exist.

When documenting findings in the medical forensic record, documentation should include approximate length, width, shape, and color of injuries. This level of documentation is not possible when reviewing photodocumentation as presented in these case studies. Limitations to assessment of injury via photodocumentation are related to several variables, including scale, angle, lighting, equipment settings, picture quality, and provider technique (eg, separation, traction).

The case studies in this book are brief summaries of complex patient encounters. The figures provided with each case study represent a sample of the photodocumentation collected during the medical forensic examination. Please note the detail and extent of evidence collection, prophylactic treatment, patient referrals, and recommended follow-up are based on these brief summaries, not on the additional details that would be available during an actual patient encounter. Also, the authors purposefully created the answer key for a broad audience to reflect the diversity and scope of practice of individuals completing this book. In doing so, it is recognized that the answer key may often reflect those roles that have a more limited scope of practice (eg, registered nurse [RN] versus advanced practice registered nurse [APRN] or doctor of medicine).

Case Study 1

Activity 1-1. Identifying Missing Subjective Information

Radiation, Severity, Aggravating/relieving factors

Activity 1-2. Anatomical Identification

A. Cervix

B. Cervical os

C. Squamocolumnar junction

Activity 1-3. Physical Examination Findings

The cervix is erythematous with punctate hemorrhages resembling a "strawberry cervix." Otherwise, the examination is normal.

Activity 1-4. Clinical Laboratory Improvement Amendments (CLIA) Laboratory Examination

— The RN orders the office urine dipstick, which shows moderate increase in leukocytes, as well as trace blood. No other abnormalities are seen in dipstick results.

— Implement the protocol for testing.

Activity 1-5. Clinical Laboratory Testing

— Nucleic acid amplification testing (NAAT) for *Trichomonas* on a vaginal swab or urine sample is the preferred method. If this is not possible, an immediate wet mount of the sample could suffice as a backup option if CLIA-provider approved.

— APTIMA *T. vaginalis* assay, if available, using a sample of urine, vaginal swab, or endocervical swab.

— Wet mount.

— Culture.

— Consider testing for other sexually transmitted infections (STIs), including human immunodeficiency virus (HIV) and syphilis.

Activity 1-6. Forensic Evidence Collection

This case does not warrant a medical forensic evaluation with evidence collection.

Activity 1-7. Nursing Plan of Care Procedure

Nursing diagnosis:

- — Damage to tissue integrity: Mucosal lesion in the cornea, the integument, or subcutaneous tissues.
- — Violation of the integrity of the oral mucosa: Out of the tissue layers of the oral cavity.
- — Violation of the integrity of the skin: Skin lesion; break in the integument, the largest multifunctional organ of the body.
- — Acute pain: Itching, distress, or malaise experienced and reported by the person.
- — Chronic pain: Pain lasting for more than 6 months.

Plan of care:

- — Adherence to quality, psychomotor activities in testing
- — Patient-centered collaborative activities
- — Trauma-informed collaboration and support with implementation of plan of care

Activity 1-8. Advanced Practice Provider (APP) and Physician Differential Diagnosis

— The differential diagnosis includes bacterial vaginosis (BV), group B *Streptococcus* infection, trichomoniasis, cancer, iatrogenic injury, scarring, and recent semen deposit.

— The infection is trichomoniasis.

Activity 1-9. Treatment

— Metronidazole 2 g orally (PO) once ***OR***

— Tinidazole 2 g PO once ***OR***

— Metronidazole 500 mg PO twice a day for 7 to 14 days, depending on compliance and chronicity

Activity 1-10. Reporting

— Trichomoniasis is not a reportable disease.

— *Note: Children exposed to well (bathing) water or lake water (swimming) may have an infection from normal activities. Call local public health epidemiologist for further investigation of the community's water quality.*

Activity 1-11. Follow-Up Recommendations in Plan of Care

— Avoid alcohol for 24 hours after treatment with metronidazole and 72 hours after treatment with tinidazole.

— Avoid sexual intercourse until the treatment of the patient and all partners is completed and the patient is no longer exhibiting symptoms.

— Immediately discontinue douching permanently, because douching increases the risk for STIs.

— Additionally, all sexual partners should be seen at the clinic for examination and treatment. Condom use is recommended and is essential in preventing STIs.

— Follow-up recommendations: Patient follow-up should include retesting 3 months after completion of treatment for a test of cure. Avoid NAAT testing because DNA remains for months, even if the organism is dead, particularly in the nonestrogenized genital environment of children and elders.

Case Study 2

Activity 2-1. Identifying Missing Subjective Information

Aggravating/relieving, Radiation, Timing, Severity

Activity 2-2. Anatomical Identification

Arrow A: Clitoral Hood

Arrow B: Labia Major

Arrow C: Labia Minor

Arrow D: Uretha

Arrow E: Hymen

Arrow F: Posterior Forchette

Activity 2-3. Physical Examination Findings

The examination reveals multiple red lesions (approximately 8 to 12) with white centers covering labia majora, labia minora, urethra, and vestibule. Kissing lesions present adjacent to urethra majora adjacent to urethra, and vaginal orifice at 3 o'clock. One cluster coalesced on labia majora at mons. Discharge is clear, caking in slight glossy film.

Arrow A: Blisters/vesicles

Arrow B: Ulcers on mucous membrane

Arrow C: Ulcers on skin

Activity 2-4. Clinical Laboratory Improvement Amendments (CLIA) Laboratory Examination

— The RN ordered the office urine dipstick, and child was unable to void because of pain.

— Implement the protocol for testing.

— Laboratory testing:

  — NAAT Results: Laboratory loses NAAT, never logged into custody. Not reported to provider.

  — Culture Results: Scraping of lesions completed for culture, which was sent to another laboratory.

  — Positive for herpes simplex virus 2 (HSV-2).

Activity 2-5. Clinical Laboratory Testing

— Urine NAAT for *Chlamydia* and gonorrhea

— Urine analysis (UA)

— Epstein-Barr virus and cytomegalovirus

— NAAT culture, rectal and oral

Activity 2-6. Forensic Evidence Collection

This case does warrant a medical forensic evaluation, but evidence collection may not be possible because of levels of pain. Alternate items worn before symptoms may be collected for analysis (eg, undergarments).

Activity 2-7. Nursing Plan of Care Procedure

Nursing Diagnosis:

- — Damage to tissue integrity: Mucosal lesion on urethra or surrounding integument or subcutaneous tissues
- — Violation of the integrity of the genital mucosa: Out of the tissue layers of the anogenital areas
- — Violation of the integrity of the skin: Skin lesion; break in the integument, the largest multifunctional organ of the body
- — Acute pain: Distress or malaise experienced and reported by the person
- — Chronic pain: Pain severity associated with neuralgia

Plan of care:

- — Adherence to quality evidence-based interventions to manage disease and pain syndromes
- — Patient-centered collaborative activities (eg, knowledge and treatment of disease), including diminished spread
- — Trauma-informed collaboration and support with implementation of plan of care
- — Identification of source, reporting to authorities

Activity 2-8. APP and Physician Differential Diagnosis

- — Herpes simplex virus (HSV), self-injury, vesicular eczema, tinea cruris, Epstein-Barr virus and cytomegalovirus, impetigo or cellulitis.
- — The infection is HSV-2.

Activity 2-9. Treatment

Medical treatment:

- — Discharged home with acyclovir (75 mg/kg per day orally divided 5 times each day, for a maximum 1000/day for 7 days, to be started immediately) and told to return in 72 to 96 hours for reevaluation.

Follow-up plan of care:

- — Follow-up instructions include scheduling the next visit anytime symptoms worsen or in 72 to 96 hours.
- — No further testing ordered.
- — Transmission may occur from routine touch of an infected person, where auto-transfer occurs with children sucking on their fingers and transferring the virus to the genitals in their sleep. There is no definitive test that determines the source, other than a prodromal disease from others with description of symptoms.
- — The link between anogenital herpes and sexual abuse requires an understanding of viral transmission and typing to properly interpret its significance, including that asymptomatic adults spread the virus without outbreak of symptoms.
- — Anogenital herpes in children require primary care providers to have an understanding of the appearance and mode of transmission of anogenital herpes, as well as techniques for diagnosis.

— Centers for Disease Control and Prevention (CDC) guidelines for diagnosing, evaluating, and medically managing anogenital herpes in children is clear; however, the social ramifications related to reporting to child protective services (CPS) is not. Due to the nature of the genital infection, current recommendations include reporting to CPS for a medical forensic examination and forensic interview.

Activity 2-10. Reporting

HSV infection is suspicious of child sexual abuse, requiring a report to CPS, with knowledge that the HSV virus is subject to self-inoculation (oral-genital contact) and adults with HSV do not often know if or when they shed the virus.

Activity 2-11. Follow-Up Recommendations in Plan of Care

— Call the mother within 48 hours to remind her of the follow-up appointment and evaluate for medication initiation and tolerance. If not started, instruct to start medication as soon as possible.

— Follow-up recommendations: The patient should be followed-up with and managed by a pediatric health care provider familiar with HSV treatment and management in childhood. There is no test of cure because, once exposed, the virus is detectable and erupts frequently, requiring continuous monitoring.

— Infection symptoms testing HSV: This infection is suspicious of child sexual abuse. Self-inoculation (a child with oral herpes may self-inoculate genitalia) or inoculation by an adult with oral or genital herpes during caretaking contact such as diaper changes must be ruled out.

— Dysuria, genital or perianal vesicles/ulcers. Primary infection often results in a high fever and may be accompanied by malaise and fatigue. Obtain specimens from all mucocutaneous lesions and send for viral culture or polymerase chain reaction (PCR) testing. Note that culture is rapidly being replaced by PCR in many laboratories because of cost and improved performance.

— Serology: Serologic testing in the absence of lesions will detect HSV antibody 2 to 3 weeks after infection. Providers should request type-specific HSV-2 and/or HSV-1 serologic assays.

Activity 2-12. Identifying Missing Subjective Information

Aggravating/relieving, Radiation, Timing, Severity

Activity 2-13. Physical Examination Findings

The examination reveals multiple red lesions (approximately 8 to 12) with white centers covering labia majora, labia minora, urethra, and vestibule. Kissing lesions present adjacent to urethra majora and vaginal orifice at 3 o'clock. One cluster coalesced on labia majora at mons. Discharge is clear, caking in slight glossy film.

Arrows A. Hyperpigmented circular lesions on skin.

Arrows B. Hyperpigmented circular lesions on skin.

Arrows C. Mucous membrane lesions healed without distinction. *Note: May respond to alternate light source to detect neovascularization; may not match specifically as disease progresses for days, yielding different stages of healing not evident in this photograph.*

Arrows D. Hymen is normal in appearance without evidence of acute injury.

Activity 2-14. Clinical Laboratory Improvement Amendments (CLIA) Laboratory Examination

— Positive laboratory for HSV-2.

— Lesions continue to heal on antiviral medication. No dysuria noted at return visit; UA without leukocytes or blood.

Activity 2-15. Clinical Laboratory Testing

UA for white blood cells

Activity 2-16. Forensic Evidence Collection

This case was referred for a medical forensic evaluation with evidence collection at the previous visit; therefore, no referral is necessary at the follow-up visit. In the event another STI occurs, another referral is necessary.

Activity 2-17. Nursing Plan of Care Procedure

Nursing diagnosis:

- — Damage to tissue integrity
- — Violation of the integrity of the skin: Skin lesion; break in the integument, the largest multifunctional organ of the body
- — Acute pain: Distress or malaise experienced and reported by the patient

Plan of care:

- — Adherence to plan of care, vigilant for new lesions or symptoms of returning disease
- — Patient-centered collaborative activities
- — Trauma-informed collaboration and support with implementation of plan of care

Activity 2-18. APP and Physician Differential Diagnosis

- — HSV, self-injury, insect bites, impetigo, cellulitis, Epstein-Barr virus and cytomegalovirus, vesicular eczema, tinea cruris
- — The infection is HSV-2

Activity 2-19. Treatment

Medical treatment:

- — Discharged home with acyclovir (75mg/kg per day orally, divided 5 times each day for a maximum 1000/day for 7 days, to be started immediately). Told to return as needed for reevaluation in the event of another eruption.

Follow-up plan of care:

- — Follow-up instructions include scheduling the next visit.
- — No further testing ordered.
- — Transmission may occur from routine touch of an infected person, and auto-transfer occurs with children sucking on their fingers and transferring the virus to the genitals in their sleep. There is no definitive test that determines the source, other than a prodromal disease from others with description of symptoms.
- — The link between anogenital herpes and sexual abuse requires an understanding of viral transmission and typing to properly interpret its significance.
- — Anogenital herpes in children creates serious medical, social, and legal implications. It is important that primary care providers have an understanding of the appearance, mode of transmission, and diagnostic technique of anogenital herpes.
- — CDC guidelines for diagnosing, evaluating, and medically managing anogenital herpes in children is clear; however, the social ramifications related to reporting to CPS is not. Due to the nature of the genital infection, current recommendations include reporting to CPS for a medical forensic examination and forensic interview.

Activity 2-20. Reporting

This infection is suspicious of child sexual abuse, requiring report to CPS, with knowledge that the HSV virus is subject to self-inoculation. In this case, the second visit is not reportable.

Activity 2-21. Follow-Up Recommendations in Plan of Care

— Call the mother to remind her of the next routine visit, or if symptoms erupt, discuss a plan to address the symptoms before the appointment. It is recommended that the child return with the mother if symptoms erupt for a sick child visit, available routinely to all children.

— Follow-up recommendations: The patient should be followed-up with and managed by a pediatric health care provider familiar with HSV treatments. There is no test of cure because once exposed, the virus is detectable.

Infection symptoms testing:

— This infection is suspicious of child sexual abuse.

— Dysuria, genital or perianal vesicles/ulcers. Primary infection may be accompanied by malaise and fatigue.

— Obtain specimens from all mucocutaneous lesions, and send for viral culture or PCR testing. Note that culture is rapidly being replaced by PCR in many laboratories because of cost and improved performance.

— Serology: Serologic testing in the absence of lesions will detect HSV antibody 2 to 3 weeks after infection.

— Providers should request type-specific HSV-2 and/or HSV-1 serologic assays.

Activity 2-22. Identifying Missing Subjective Information

Aggravating/relieving, Radiation, Timing, Severity

Activity 2-23. Physical Examination Findings

No lesions noted.

Activity 2-24. Clinical Laboratory Improvement Amendments (CLIA) Laboratory Examination

None, as there are no clinical symptoms to distinguish differential diagnosis.

Activity 2-25. Clinical Laboratory Testing

No testing necessary at the visit.

Activity 2-26. Forensic Evidence Collection

This case does not meet the criteria for the medical forensic evaluation with evidence collection.

Activity 2-27. Nursing Plan of Care Procedure

Nursing diagnosis: Normal examination

Activity 2-28. APP and Physician Differential Diagnosis

History of HSV-2; no evidence of acute HSV-2

Activity 2-29. Treatment

Medical treatment:

— Discharged home with Acyclovir refills, to be started when any symptoms of itching, burning, or pain return.

Follow-up plan of care:

— No further testing warranted.

— Follow-up instructions include scheduling the next visit with symptoms or developments.

— The child is referred for counseling with the following education information:

— The link between anogenital herpes and sexual abuse requires an understanding of viral transmission and typing to properly interpret its significance.

— Anogenital herpes in children creates serious medical, social, and legal implications. It is important that primary care providers have an understanding of the appearance, mode of transmission, and diagnostic technique of anogenital herpes.

— Implications for practice will provide guidelines for diagnosing, evaluating, and properly managing anogenital herpes in children.

— CDC guidelines for diagnosing, evaluating, and medically managing anogenital herpes in children is clear; however, the social ramifications related to reporting to CPS is not. Due to the nature of the genital infection, current recommendations include reporting to CPS for a medical forensic examination and forensic interview.

Activity 2-30. Reporting

This infection is suspicious of child sexual abuse, requiring a report to CPS, with knowledge that the HSV virus is subject to self-inoculation. In this case, the follow-up visit is not reportable.

Activity 2-31. Follow-Up Recommendations in Plan of Care

— Follow-up recommendations: The patient should be followed-up with and managed by a pediatric health care provider familiar with HSV treatments. There is no test of cure, because once exposed, the virus is detectable.

— Infection symptoms testing HSV:

— This infection is suspicious of child sexual abuse.

— Dysuria, genital or perianal vesicles/ulcers. Primary infection may be accompanied by malaise and fatigue.

— Obtain specimens from all mucocutaneous lesions, and send for viral culture or PCR testing. Note that culture is rapidly being replaced by PCR in many laboratories because of cost and improved performance.

— Serology: Serologic testing in the absence of lesions will detect HSV antibody 2 to 3 weeks after infection.

— Providers should request type-specific HSV-2 and/or HSV-1 serologic assays.

Case Study 3

Activity 3-1. Identifying Missing Subjective Information

Radiation, Severity, Aggravating/relieving factors

Activity 3-2. Anatomical Identification

A. Foreskin

B. Meatus/urethral opening

C. Scrotum

Activity 3-3. Physical Examination Findings

A. Follicular injury

B. White nit

Activity 3-4. Clinical Laboratory Improvement Amendments (CLIA) Laboratory Examination

— Implement the protocol for testing.

— Prepare a saline slide with the louse for analysis by the laboratory.

Activity 3-5. Clinical Laboratory Testing

— Diagnosis is made by the naked eye and can be confirmed by using a hands lens or microscope to identify the eggs (nits) and louse.

— If you do not have a louse, distinguish between yeast and various dermatitises (including seborrhea and eczema conditions).

Activity 3-6. Forensic Evidence Collection

This case does not warrant a medical forensic evaluation with evidence collection.

Activity 3-7. Nursing Plan of Care Procedure

Nursing diagnoses:

— Damage to tissue integrity: Follicular lesion, damage to the capillaries in the integument or subcutaneous tissues

— Violation of the integrity of the skin: Skin lesion; break in the integument, the largest multifunctional organ of the body

— Acute pain: Itching distress experienced and reported by the person

Plan of care:

— Adherence to quality, psychomotor activities in testing for louse

— Patient-centered collaborative activities related to topical treatments

— Trauma-informed collaboration and support with implementation of plan of care

Activity 3-8. APP and Physician Differential Diagnosis

— The differential diagnosis includes scabies, pediculosis pubis, yeast or fungus, and streptococcal or staphylococcal infection.

— The infection is pediculosis pubis, resulting in tissue injury from infestation.

Activity 3-9. Treatment

Medical treatment:

— Both over-the-counter and prescription medications are available for treatment of pubic lice infestations. A lice-killing lotion containing 1% permethrin or a mousse containing pyrethrins and piperonyl butoxide can be used to treat pubic ("crab") lice.

— Treatment should include using Permethrin 1% cream applied to affected areas and washed off after 10 minutes.

— Nits can be removed with fingernails, a nit comb, or tweezers.

Activity 3-10. Reporting

Pediculosis pubis is not a reportable disease.

Activity 3-11. Follow-Up Recommendations in Plan of Care

— Tell the family that clean underwear and clothing should be put on after treatment.

— More than 1 application may be necessary to get rid of the infestation.

— Evaluation may be necessary after 1 week if symptoms persist.

— Retreatment also may be necessary if lice are found or if eggs are seen at the hair–skin junction.

— Sexual partners should be informed so that they may be examined and treated.

— Shaving is not necessary.

— Condoms should be used but do not prevent transmission of the pediculosis pubis louse.

— Bedding and clothing used by the infested person should be machine washed in hot water or dry cleaned as soon as possible, but within the following 2 to 3 days.

Case Study 4

Activity 4-1. Identifying Missing Subjective Information

Radiation, Severity, any Relieving self-treatment

Activity 4-2. Anatomical Identification

A. Edematous labia minora

B. Erythematous vestibular tissue

C. Clitoral hood

Activity 4-3. Physical Examination Findings

The cervix and vaginal walls are erythematous, with thick, white, "chunky," adherent discharge noted. Otherwise, the examination is normal.

Activity 4-4. Clinical Laboratory Improvement Amendments (CLIA) Laboratory Examination

— The RN orders an in-office urine dipstick test, which shows a moderate increase in leukocytes, as well as trace blood. No other abnormalities are seen in dipstick results.

— Implement the protocol for testing.

Activity 4-5. Clinical Laboratory Testing

Wet mount is used to identify the presence of yeast pseudohyphae and yeast buds and to rule out the presence of clue cells and *Trichomonas vaginalis*; pH testing is often found to be within normal limits (3.8 to 4.2), and there will be no amine odor change to the solution.

Activity 4-6. Forensic Evidence Collection

This case does not warrant a medical forensic evaluation with evidence collection.

Activity 4-7. Nursing Plan of Care Procedure

Nursing diagnosis:

— Acute pain: Distress or malaise experienced and reported by the person

Plan of care:

— Adherence to quality, psychomotor activities in testing

— Patient-centered collaborative activities

— Trauma-informed collaboration and support with implementation of plan of care

Activity 4-8. APP and Physician Differential Diagnosis

— The differential diagnosis includes BV, *Chlamydia*, trichomoniasis, cancer, iatrogenic injury, and recent semen deposit.

— The infection is candidiasis.

Activity 4-9. Treatment

AD is prescribed fluconazole 150 mg, 1 tablet by mouth today, and repeat in 72 hours. Often, pediatric patients are uncomfortable or unable to use an intravaginal treatment.

Activity 4-10. Reporting

Candidiasis is not a reportable disease.

Activity 4-11. Follow-Up Recommendations in Plan of Care

— Tell the family that clean underwear and clothing should be put on after treatment.

— Evaluation may be necessary after 2 weeks, if symptoms persist.

Case Study 5

Activity 5-1. Identifying Missing Subjective Information
Radiation, Timing, Severity

Activity 5-2. Anatomical Identification
A. Pupil

B. Sclera

C. Iris

D. Inner canthus

Activity 5-3. Physical Examination Findings
Jaundice of the sclera and skin

Activity 5-4. Clinical Laboratory Improvement Amendments (CLIA) Laboratory Examination
Objective documentation of the physical assessment and findings, which should include constitutional findings (height, weight, temperature, heart rate, respiratory rate, skin condition [eg, turgor]); assessment of the integument for signs and symptoms of hydration and color; assessment of the head, ears, eyes, nose, and throat and of the chest, abdomen, and extremities. The RN may have protocol to order a urine analysis dip.

Activity 5-5. Clinical Laboratory Testing
— Urinalysis

— Complete blood cell count (CBC) with differential

— Liver panel (minimally including alanine aminotransferase [ALT], previously known as serum glutamic pyruvic transaminase [SGPT]; aspartate aminotransferase [AST], also known as serum glutamic-oxaloacetic transaminase [SGOT]; albumin/globulin; alkaline phosphatase [ALP]; and bilirubin [total/direct])

— IgM antibodies

— IgG antibodies

Activity 5-6. Forensic Evidence Collection
This case does not warrant a medical forensic evaluation with evidence collection.

Activity 5-7. Nursing Plan of Care Procedure
Nursing diagnosis:

— Imbalanced nutrition: Less than body requirements related to nausea/vomiting as evidenced by patient reports of nausea and vomiting

— Fatigue related to nausea/vomiting

— Evidence of the patient's diagnosis of hepatitis

— Knowledge deficit related to hygiene (fecal/oral transmission)

Plan of care:

— Minimize progressive degeneration/necrosis of the liver (no consumption of alcohol or other liver toxic medications (eg, acetaminophen [Tylenol]).

— Improve lifestyle habits: More frequent hand washing (fecal/oral transmission) and adoption of standard and contact precautions for diapered or incontinent patients.

— Ensure optimal nutrition for liver function.

Activity 5-8. APP and Physician Differential Diagnosis

— The differential diagnosis includes acute hepatitis A, B, C, D, and E virus infection; cytomegalovirus; Epstein-Barr virus; systemic lupus erythematosus; cancer; cirrhosis; and fatty liver disease.

— Acute hepatitis A virus exposure with recurrent infection is the diagnosis.

Activity 5-9. Treatment

In this case, PM has recurrent symptoms, so instructions for supportive care are given with minimal restrictions on activity and diet, although the patient is instructed to avoid alcohol and acetaminophen or other liver-toxic medications, until laboratory results return to normal. The patient is also instructed to return if the fever, nausea, and vomiting continue for 3 days. Additional symptoms to watch for include dark-colored urine and pale-colored stools. The patient receives a combined hepatitis A and B vaccine to boost immunity and prevent recurrence of hepatitis A. If improving, the patient is instructed to return to the clinic for laboratory monitoring in 1 month to 6 weeks. If symptoms worsen, return to the clinic after calling for additional assessments.

Activity 5-10. Reporting

This is not a reportable disease. Although not reportable, it is possible that the local health department would want to conduct an epidemiological investigation, which is necessary to find the sentinel case of hepatitis A and immunize the community of families using the daycare center to improve herd immunity, preventing spread to others.

Activity 5-11. Follow-Up Recommendations in Plan of Care

There is an increased risk of bleeding because of liver function challenge (determined by laboratory tests) and if abnormal, the patient requires specific instructions to avoid bleeding:

— Do not use straight razors. Do use soft toothbrushes, engage in good oral hygiene, and use stool softeners to avoid straining.

— Avoid medications that stress the liver, including acetaminophen. Hydrate and monitor electrolytes if vomiting persists.

— Avoid alcohol and illicit drugs, exposure to dirty needles, and contact with semen, blood, stool, and vomit.

Case Study 6

Activity 6-1. Identifying Missing Subjective Information

Character, Aggravating/relieving, Radiation, Severity

Activity 6-2. Physical Examination Findings

There are 3 raised, smooth, 2- to 3-mm round papules with white, depressed centers on the right cheek and 3 similar papules noted on the waistband area. Papules are soft and nontender, and no ulceration, redness, or signs of infection are noted.

A. Molluscum lesion

B. Molluscum lesion

C. Acute lesion

D. Healed lesion – note does not involve the follicle

Activity 6-3. Clinical Laboratory Improvement Amendments (CLIA) Laboratory Examination

— The RN orders the office urine dipstick test, which shows a moderate increase in leukocytes, as well as trace blood. No other abnormalities are seen on the dipstick results.

— Implement the protocol for testing.

Activity 6-4. Clinical Laboratory Testing

— There are not any tests to run for molluscum contagiosum.

— Diagnosis is made by the naked eye and can be confirmed by using a hands lens to identify the lesions(s).

Activity 6-5. Forensic Evidence Collection

This case does not warrant a medical forensic evaluation with evidence collection.

Activity 6-6. Nursing Plan of Care Procedure

Nursing diagnosis:

— Damage to tissue integrity: Mucosal lesion in the integument or subcutaneous tissues.

— Violation of the integrity of the skin: Skin lesion; break in the integument, the largest multifunctional organ of the body.

Plan of care:

— Patient-centered collaborative activities related to skin integrity and spread of the disease via scratching.

— Trauma-informed collaboration and support with implementation of plan of care.

Activity 6-7. APP and Physician Differential Diagnosis

— The differential diagnosis includes human papillomavirus (HPV), pediculosis pedis, condyloma acuminata, and basal cell carcinoma.

— The infection is molluscum contagiosum.

Activity 6-8. Treatment

— A discussion regarding treatment options includes (1) no treatment because molluscum contagiosum often will self-resolve; (2) in-office procedures to physically remove or destroy the lesions (curettage, cryotherapy, laser podophyllin resin, trichloroacetic acid, and cantharidin); and (3) at-home treatment options including topical creams or oral therapy.

— Parent opted to complete at-home topical treatment with podophyllotoxin cream (0.5%) applied twice daily to papules for 3 days per week and repeated weekly for 1 month. Parent is directed to the potential for integument burn, and APP demonstrated application of petroleum jelly around the lesion to avoid spread to normal skin.

— Patient is to return to the clinic for reevaluation at 1 month. Parent is directed to aid child in avoiding self-inoculation by scratching and nail hygiene.

Activity 6-9. Reporting

Molluscum contagiosum is not a reportable disease.

Activity 6-10. Follow-Up Recommendations in Plan of Care

— Tell the family that clean underwear and clothing should be put on after treatment.

— Evaluation may be necessary after 1 week if symptoms persist after treatment.

— Shaving is not necessary.

— Bedding and clothing used by the infected person should be machine washed in hot water or dry cleaned.

Case Study 7

Activity 7-1. Identifying Missing Subjective Information

Radiation, Severity

Activity 7-2. Anatomical Identification

A. Right inguinal area

B. Scrotum

C. Shaft

D. Corona

E. Glans

Activity 7-3. Physical Examination Findings

A. Left inguinal chancre eroded

B. Lateral left penis shaft, adjacent to penile corona, chancre eroded; bleeds easily

The primary care provider assesses the penis lesion, noting a 2 cm × 2 cm, beefy-red, velvety, raised ulcer with irregular margins that has gradually increased in size.

Activity 7-4. Clinical Laboratory Improvement Amendments (CLIA) Laboratory Examination

Identify and document any of the following:

— Lumpy red bumps in groin, genital, and anal regions

— Sores around genital or anal region

— Bleeding from the sores

— Skin discoloration scarring

— Foul-smelling ulcers with granulation around margins

— Fever

Activity 7-5. Clinical Laboratory Testing

Scraping or biopsy of the lesion is confirmatory for granuloma inguinale. Inject a local anesthetic and take a tissue sample.

Activity 7-6. Forensic Evidence Collection

This case does warrant a medical forensic evaluation with evidence collection. Because the patient's history includes multiple sex partners as a minor and working with a group to provide sex for money, human sex trafficking and child sexual abuse should be suspected. Under Title X, once human sex trafficking is suspected, the provider is a mandated reporter because the crimes occurred when the patient was a child, and many states have no statute of limitation on child sexual abuse or human sex trafficking.

The items collected should include the patient's underwear. Look for injuries and inspect anal folds first, then collect and package samples using 2 cotton-tipped applicators. Evidence should also be collected from the genitalia, including the penis and scrotum, as indicated by the patient history. Penile swabbing should include the shaft and scrotum. If the suspect is uncircumcised, the clinician should swab beneath the foreskin. Dry, package, and secure in evidence collection kit, making ready for transfer.

Activity 7-7. Nursing Plan of Care Procedure

Nursing diagnosis:

- Violation of the integrity of the skin: Skin lesion; break in the integument, the largest multifunctional organ of the body.

— Acute pain: Distress or malaise experienced and reported by the person, particularly after the biopsy.

Plan of care:

— Adherence to quality, psychomotor activities in testing

— Patient-centered collaborative activities

— Trauma-informed collaboration and support with implementation of plan of care

Activity 7-8. APP and Physician Differential Diagnosis

— The differential diagnosis includes primary syphilis, secondary syphilis (condylomata lata), chancroid, lymphogranuloma venereum (LGV), genital herpes, neoplasm, and amoebiasis.

— The infection is granuloma inguinale.

Activity 7-9. Treatment

Oral antibiotics, such as the following, are most effectively used to treat granuloma inguinale:

— Azithromycin 1 g orally once per week or 500 mg daily for at least 3 weeks and until all lesions have completely healed.

Alternative Regimens:

— Doxycycline 100 mg orally twice a day for at least 3 weeks and until all lesions have completely healed ***OR***

— Ciprofloxacin 750 mg orally twice a day for at least 3 weeks and until all lesions have completely healed ***OR***

— Erythromycin base 500 mg orally 4 times a day for at least 3 weeks and until all lesions have completely healed ***OR***

— Trimethoprim-sulfamethoxazole 1 double-strength (160 mg/800 mg) tablet orally twice daily for at least 3 weeks and until all lesions have completely healed

The antibiotics are typically prescribed for a duration of 3 to 4 weeks. The antibiotic course should be completed as prescribed by the health care professional, even if the visible signs and symptoms of the condition disappear. The nurse educates the patient on how to protect himself to avoid STIs. This includes the use of condoms and abstinence.

Activity 7-10. Reporting

This is a reportable disease. First, although rare, in a patient who reports multiple partners for years, the sentinel case must be identified to prevent the spread of the disease in the population. Second, under Title X, once human sex trafficking is suspected, the provider is a mandated reporter because the crimes occurred when the patient was a child, and many states have no statute of limitation on child sexual abuse or human sex trafficking.

Activity 7-11. Follow-Up Recommendations in Plan of Care

— Evaluation may be necessary after 2 weeks if symptoms persist.

— In this case, the patient is informed that the public health department will attempt to find all partners for medical treatment and that child protective services will be notified under the state's legislation on child sexual abuse and human sex trafficking. The use of trauma-informed, patient-centered care is important, encouraging collaboration to facilitate the safe rescue of other victims.

Case Study 8

Activity 8-1. Identifying Missing Subjective Information

Onset, Location, Duration, Character, Aggravating/relieving, Radiation, Timing, Severity

Activity 8-2. Anatomical Identification

A. Labium minus

B. Vaginal introitus

C. Hymen

D. Fossa navicularis

Activity 8-3. Physical Examination Findings

Hypopigmentation is present circumferentially with healing lesions. The hymen is normal, as is the visible vaginal vault.

Activity 8-4. Clinical Laboratory Improvement Amendments (CLIA) Laboratory Examination

— The nurse orders the office urine dipstick test, which indicates a moderate increase in leukocytes, as well as trace blood. No other abnormalities are seen in dipstick results.

— Implement the protocol for testing.

Activity 8-5. Clinical Laboratory Testing

A full STI panel of the oral and anogenital areas is warranted because of the history of multiple partners.

Activity 8-6. Forensic Evidence Collection

This case does not warrant a medical forensic evaluation with evidence collection.

Activity 8-7. Nursing Plan of Care Procedure

Nursing diagnosis:

— Damage to tissue integrity: Mucosal lesion in the cornea, the integument, or subcutaneous tissues

— Violation of the integrity of the skin: Skin lesion; break in the integument, the largest multifunctional organ of the body

— Acute pain: Distress or malaise experienced and reported by the person

Plan of care:

— Adherence to quality, psychomotor activities in testing

— Patient-centered collaborative activities

— Trauma-informed collaboration and support with implementation of plan of care

Activity 8-8. APP and Physician Differential Diagnosis

— The differential diagnosis includes urinary tract infection, oral pharyngitis, beta *Streptococcus* infection, trichomoniasis, cancer, iatrogenic injury, and recent semen deposit.

— The infection is *Chlamydia trachomatis.* Persons who receive a diagnosis of *Chlamydia* should be tested for HIV, gonorrhea, and syphilis.

Activity 8-9. Treatment

Diagnosis of *C. trachomatis* urethral infection can be made by testing a urethral swab or first-catch urine specimen. NAATs are the most sensitive tests for these specimens and therefore are recommended for detecting *C. trachomatis* infection. Rectal and oropharyngeal *C. trachomatis* infection in persons engaging in receptive anal or oral intercourse can be diagnosed by testing at the anatomic site of exposure. NAATs are not approved by the Food and Drug Administration for use with rectal or oropharyngeal swab specimens. However, NAATs have been found to have improved sensitivity and specificity compared with culture for the detection of *C. trachomatis* at rectal sites and at oropharyngeal sites among men.

The medication regimen includes the following:

— Azithromycin 1 g orally in a single dose ***OR***

— Doxycycline 100 mg orally twice daily for 7 days

Alternative Regimens:

— Erythromycin base 500 mg orally 4 times a day for 7 days ***OR***

— Erythromycin ethylsuccinate 800 mg orally 4 times a day for 7 days ***OR***

— Levofloxacin 500 mg orally once daily for 7 days ***OR***

— Ofloxacin 300 mg orally twice daily for 7 days

Note: Detection of *C. trachomatis* from an oropharyngeal specimen should be treated with azithromycin or doxycycline. The efficacy of alternative antimicrobial regimens in resolving oropharyngeal *Chlamydia* remains unknown.

Activity 8-10. Reporting

Chlamydia is not a reportable disease. However, because of the testing method (NAAT polymerase chain reaction detection of organism in fluid sample), if symptoms persist, culture the area to determine if there is persistent infection or reinfection of the area. If treatment fails, notify the CDC for further analysis of resistant strains.

Activity 8-11. Follow-Up Recommendations in Plan of Care

— Evaluation may be necessary after 1 week if symptoms persist.

— Sexual partners should be informed so that they may be examined and treated.

— Condoms should be used to prevent reinfection.

Case Study 9

Activity 9-1. Identifying Missing Subjective Information

Aggravating/relieving, Radiation, Timing, Severity

Activity 9-2. Physical Examination Findings

Icterus, or jaundice, of the conjunctivae and facial skin

Activity 9-3. Clinical Laboratory Improvement Amendments (CLIA) Laboratory Examination

— Implement universal precautions

— Gather height, weight, temperature, blood pressure, O2 saturation, respirations, and heart rates/minute

— Complete head-to-toe integument assessment, including ocular, hair, nails, and coloring

— Collect urine for analysis and draw blood for liver panel

— Implement the existing protocol to assist with the differential diagnosis

Activity 9-4. Clinical Laboratory Testing

To assess liver damage in chronic hepatitis C, consider:

1. Magnetic resonance elastography. The test is a noninvasive alternative to a liver biopsy, detecting active liver disease and scarring (fibrosis).

2. Transient elastography. A noninvasive ultrasound test, transmitting vibrations into the liver measuring stiffness.
3. Liver biopsy. Tissue is taken from the liver, guided by an ultrasound to cirrhotic tissues, and used for differential diagnosis with cancer.
4. Blood tests, drawn under the existing protocol, to measure the function of the liver, contributing to the differential diagnosis.

Activity 9-5. Forensic Evidence Collection

This case does not warrant a medical forensic evaluation with evidence collection.

Activity 9-6. Nursing Plan of Care Procedure

Nursing diagnosis:

— Impaired skin integrity related to pruritis: Skin lesion or icteric changes of skin or conjunctiva; break in the integument, the largest multifunctional organ of the body.

— Acute pain related to the tender, enlarged liver: Distress, malaise or focal upper right quadrant pain experienced and reported by the person.

— Chronic pain: Pain lasting for more than 6 months.

— Imbalanced nutrition: Less than body requirements related to anorexia, nausea and vomiting.

— Activity intolerance related to fatigue and generalized malaise.

— Hyperthermia related to the body's defensive reaction to invading organisms.

— Risk for infection related to diminished immune function.

Plan of care:

— Adherence to quality, psychomotor activities in testing

— Patient-centered collaborative activities

— Trauma-informed collaboration and support with implementation of plan of care

Activity 9-7. APP and Physician Differential Diagnosis

— The differential diagnosis includes hepatitis B, cirrhosis, cancer.

— The infection is hepatitis C.

Activity 9-8. Treatment

The choice of medications and length of treatment depend on the hepatitis C genotype, presence of existing liver damage, other medical conditions, and prior treatments. The recommended medical treatment consists of an 8 to 12-week regimen of ledipasvir/sofosbuvir (Harvoni).

The patient must stop drinking alcohol and taking illicit drugs 6 months before treatment. Alcohol speeds the progression of liver disease.

Activity 9-9. Reporting

Hepatitis C is a reportable disease. Local laws may vary, but in most cases, providers are required to report hepatitis to their state department of health.

Activity 9-10. Follow-Up Recommendations in Plan of Care

— Monthly clinic visits should be arranged for this patient to monitor for readiness for therapy.

— Avoid any medications that cause liver damage and review your medications with the health care provider, including over-the-counter medications, herbal preparations, and dietary supplements.

— Avoid contact with your blood by covering wounds. Do not share razors or tooth brushes. Do not donate blood, body organs, or semen.

— Advise health care workers and your sex partner that you have the virus, and always use condoms during intercourse.

Case Study 10

Activity 10-1. Identifying Missing Subjective Information

Duration, Aggravating/relieving, Radiation, Severity

Activity 10-2. Anatomical Identification

A. Slit-like cervical opening

B. Posterior fornix

C. Endocervical transition

D. Cervical neck

Activity 10-3. Physical Examination Findings

A. Discharge is circumferentially visible around superior cervical neck.

B. Erosion noted on cervix at 4, 5, and 12 o'clock.

The cervix is erythematous, and there is copious yellow, thick discharge.

Activity 10-4. Clinical Laboratory Improvement Amendments (CLIA) Laboratory Examination

— The nurse ordered the office urine dipstick test, which showed a moderate increase in leukocytes, as well as trace blood. No other abnormalities were identified in the dipstick results.

— Implement the protocol for testing.

Activity 10-5. Clinical Laboratory Testing

— Wet mount testing is completed with a finding of cervicitis (pH normal, whiff negative, numerous white blood cells and lack of clue cells, negative for yeast and *Trichomonas vaginalis* on microscopy).

— NAAT is ideal for identification of Mycoplasma genitalium (Mgen). However, diagnosis of Mgen is often made based on persistent/recurrent cervicitis and/or the presence of pelvic inflammatory disease.

— Consider testing for *Trichomonas vaginalis* via NAAT.

Activity 10-6. Forensic Evidence Collection

This case does not warrant a medical forensic evaluation with evidence collection.

Activity 10-7. Nursing Plan of Care Procedure

Nursing diagnosis:

— Acute pain: Distress or malaise experienced and reported by the person

— Chronic pain: Pain lasting for more than 6 months

Plan of care:

— Adherence to quality, psychomotor activities in testing

— Patient-centered collaborative activities

— Trauma-informed collaboration and support with implementation of plan of care

Activity 10-8. APP and Physician Differential Diagnosis

— The differential diagnosis includes *Chlamydia trachomatis*, *Neisseria gonorrhoeae*, BV, group B *Streptococcus*, trichomoniasis, cancer, iatrogenic injury, and recent semen deposit.

— The infection is Mgen.

Activity 10-9. Treatment
The patient and her partner were treated with a 14-day course of moxifloxacin 400 mg daily, which resolved the infection.

Activity 10-10. Reporting
Mgen is not a reportable disease.

Activity 10-11. Follow-Up Recommendations in Plan of Care
— Evaluation may be necessary after 2 weeks if symptoms persist.

— Sexual partners should be informed so that they may be examined and treated.

— Educate the patient on safe-sex practices including using condoms.

Case Study 11

Activity 11-1. Identifying Missing Subjective Information
Aggravating/relieving, Radiation

Activity 11-2. Anatomical Identification
A. Perianal skin

B. Anal folds

Hyperpigmented perianal skin, as shown in **Activity Figure 11-2**, is a normal finding in children of color.

Activity 11-3. Physical Examination Findings
A. Umbilical hernia. These typically disappear by age 5 years; if not, surgery is performed to correct it.

B. Primary chancre

C. Early cutaneous condyloma lata

D. Cutaneous hyperpigmentation from diaper rash

E. Cutaneous syphilids (chancre) of primary congenital syphilis

F. Papular rash of primary syphilis. The systemic distribution of the rash indicates congenital syphilis.

Activity 11-4. Clinical Laboratory Improvement Amendments (CLIA) Laboratory Examination
— The nurse orders the office urine dipstick test, which shows a moderate increase in leukocytes, as well as trace blood. No other abnormalities are seen in dipstick results.

— Implement the protocol for testing.

Activity 11-5. Clinical Laboratory Testing
— CBC differential

— Cerebrospinal fluid analysis for Venereal Disease Research Laboratory (VDRL) test, cell count, and protein

— HIV antibody testing

— VDRL *Treponema pallidum* particle agglutination assay

— Rapid plasma reagin

— Liver function tests

Activity 11-6. Forensic Evidence Collection
This case does not warrant a medical forensic evaluation with evidence collection.

Activity 11-7. Nursing Plan of Care Procedure

Nursing diagnosis:

- — Damage to tissue integrity: Mucosal lesion in the cornea, the integument, or subcutaneous tissues.
- — Violation of the integrity of the oral mucosa: Out of the tissue layers of the oral cavity.
- — Violation of the integrity of the skin: Skin lesion; break in the integument, the largest multifunctional organ of the body.
- — Acute pain: Distress or malaise experienced and reported by the person.

Plan of care:

— Adherence to quality, psychomotor activities in testing

— Patient-centered collaborative activities

— Trauma-informed collaboration and support with implementation of plan of care

Activity 11-8. APP and Physician Differential Diagnosis

— The differential diagnosis includes TORCH infections (**to**xoplasmosis, **r**ubella, **c**ytomegalovirus, HSV), neonatal hepatitis, and HIV.

— The infection is congenitally acquired syphilis.

Activity 11-9. Treatment

EM is admitted to the pediatric unit and administered aqueous crystalline penicillin G 100 000 to 150 000 units/kg per day, administered as 50 000 units/kg/dose intravenously every 12 hours during the first 7 days of life and every 8 hours after for a total of 10 days. Because this infection was congenitally acquired, EM's mother is also tested. If the mother's results are positive for syphilis, and she should begin treatment as well.

Activity 11-10. Reporting

Syphilis is a reportable disease. The local public health district should be notified.

Activity 11-11. Follow-Up Recommendations in Plan of Care

— Evaluation may be necessary after 1 week if symptoms persist.

— Teach that it is important to keep all follow-up appointments for the mother and baby so that providers can ensure that the treatment is effective.

— The mother should use condoms for all sexual activity.

— The mother should alert all sexual partners to get tested and treated if necessary.

— Inform the mother that reinfection is possible if the partner is not treated and condoms are not used.

Case Study 12

Activity 12-1. Identifying Missing Subjective Information

Onset, Duration, Character, Aggravating/relieving, Radiation, Timing, Severity

Activity 12-2. Anatomical Identification

A. Left labia minora

B. Hymen

C. Fossa navicularis

D. Posterior fourchette

E. Perineum

Activity 12-3. Physical Examination Findings

The area surrounding the hymen from 1 to 11 o'clock is reddened. This can be a normal finding in prepubescent children because of increased vascularization of the tissue; it could also be consistent with irritation and the child scratching the area. Erythema by itself is not diagnostic of sexual abuse. There are no acute injuries noted to the hymen and no notches or clefts present that could be indicative of past trauma. Inspect the anal area during the physical examination.

Activity 12-4. Clinical Laboratory Improvement Amendments (CLIA) Laboratory Examination

Urine testing for STIs is indicated in children if sexual abuse is possible. Urine NAAT STI testing is the least invasive option for children and easier to collect because the child does not need to clean the anogenital area before collection. A positive STI test in a prepubescent child is diagnostic of sexual abuse if it is not related to perinatal transmission. In the present case, urine STI tests were all negative.

Activity 12-5. Clinical Laboratory Testing

Testing for HPV is not warranted. Diagnosis is made by visual examination. Most anogenital warts are caused by HPV strains that are not high-risk cancer strains, and most cases of anogenital warts in children will resolve spontaneously or with treatment.

Activity 12-6. Forensic Evidence Collection

Discuss concerns for sexual abuse with the mother. If the mother identifies a potential perpetrator, and the potential perpetrator had contact with the child within the timeframe for evidence collection in your facility, collect evidence if the child consents. Contact child protective services and law enforcement. The child will be referred for a forensic interview at a child advocacy center. Contact your child advocacy center or pediatric SANE if your facility has one to conduct the examination. If you are the provider conducting the medical forensic examination, use your facility or state standardized sexual assault medical forensic examination protocols and evidence collection document forms or the documentation in the sexual assault evidence collection kit, if applicable.

Evidence collected should include photographic documentation if possible. Underwear should be retained. Look for injuries and inspect anal folds first, then collect and package samples using 2 cotton-tipped applicators per collection site. Moisten swabs with a small amount of sterile, normal saline or water. Change gloves and look for injuries in the vulva area, including the hymen. Inspect the vulva, and then collect and package samples using 2 new swabs to sample vulva. Avoid touching the hymen, as hymens are very sensitive to touch in prepubescent individuals. Do not insert swabs into the vagina or anus or use a speculum on a prepubescent child (unless medically necessary and under anesthesia). Follow your program policy regarding swab drying, and package swabs and secure in a kit, making ready for transfer.

Activity 12-7. Nursing Plan of Care Procedure

Nursing diagnosis:

- — Impaired skin integrity: Multiple papules on perineum.
- — Acute pain: Complaint of itching and discomfort in underwear area.
- — Risk for sexually transmitted infection: HPV was potentially sexually transmitted; the child is at risk for other STIs.
- — Risk for rape trauma syndrome: If the patient was sexually abused, the patient is at risk to experience a traumatic stress response.

Plan of care:

- — Refer to a pediatric dermatologist to treat anogenital warts; recommend warm baths for comfort; change underwear frequently; use distraction to prevent child from scratching the area.

- — Initial STI tests were negative; instruct the caregiver to the monitor for symptoms, and retest if needed.
- — Refer to a child advocacy center for forensic interview and counseling if sexual abuse is suspected or identified.
- — Ensure trauma-informed collaboration and support with implementation of plan of care.

Activity 12-8. APP and Physician Differential Diagnosis

— The differential diagnosis includes condylomata lata, condylomata acuminata, herpes simplex, lichen planus, psoriasis, and molluscum contagiosum.

— The infection is HPV.

Activity 12-9. Treatment

JB is referred to a pediatric dermatologist for appropriate treatment of anogenital warts. She is advised to take warm baths without soap or bubble bath for relief from itching and is instructed not to scratch herself. JB is referred to a child advocacy center for a forensic interview and follow-up medical forensic examination, if indicated and available at the child advocacy center. Law enforcement and child protective services are notified. HPV vaccine will be started at age 9. Consider examination of patient's 4-year-old brother, and inform child protective services that another child resides in the household.

Activity 12-10. Reporting

HPV is not a reportable disease in some states. Contact your state health department for reporting requirements in your area.

Activity 12-11. Follow-Up Recommendations in Plan of Care

— Refer the patient to pediatric dermatology for treatment.

— Inform the mother and patient that more than 1 treatment might be necessary, and warts may return.

— Instruct the patient to wear clean underwear and avoid scratching her underwear area and to take warm baths for comfort.

— Advised the patient's mother to keep all appointments with the child advocacy center.

Case Study 13

Activity 13-1. Identifying Missing Subjective Information

Aggravating/relieving, Radiation

Activity 13-2. Anatomical Identification

A. Foreskin

B. Testes

C. Foreskin

D. Urethra/glans

Activity 13-3. Physical Examination Findings

A. Dark urine, symptomatic of hepatitis B infection

B. Scleral jaundice

Activity 13-4. Clinical Laboratory Improvement Amendments (CLIA) Laboratory Examination

— Implement universal precautions

- — Gather height, weight, temperature, blood pressure, O2 saturation, respirations, and heart rates/minute
- — Complete head-to-toe integument assessment, including ocular, hair, nails, and coloring
- — Collect urine for analysis and draw blood for liver panel

Activity 13-5. Clinical Laboratory Testing

- — Hepatitis B virus (HBV) has several serological markers that are known to be present or absent in varying combinations depending on the chronicity and timing of infection. These markers include HBsAg, anti-HBs, HBeAg (hepatitis B e antigen), anti-HBe (hepatitis B e antibody), and anti-HBc, anti-HBc IgM (IgM antibody to hepatitis B core antigen), and anti-HBc IgG (IgG antibody to hepatitis B core antigen). Serological markers follow predictable patterns throughout the progression of both acute and chronic infections. Accurate clinical interpretation of the markers is essential for proper diagnosis and treatment.
- — HBV DNA can be used to directly measure the viral load and can help the provider assess the activity of the virus as well as monitor response to treatment when taken into consideration with other laboratory values.

Activity 13-6. Forensic Evidence Collection

This case does warrant a medical forensic evaluation with evidence collection.

Activity 13-7. Nursing Plan of Care Procedure

Nursing diagnosis:

- — Impaired skin integrity related to pruritis: Skin lesion or icteric changes of skin or conjunctiva; break in the integument, the largest multifunctional organ of the body.
- — Acute pain related to the tender, enlarged liver: Distress, malaise or focal upper right quadrant pain experienced and reported by the person.
- — Chronic pain: Pain lasting for more than 6 months.
- — Imbalanced nutrition: Less than body requirements related to anorexia, nausea and vomiting.
- — Activity intolerance related to fatigue and generalized malaise.
- — Hyperthermia related to the body's defensive reaction to invading organisms.
- — Risk for infection related to diminished immune function.

Plan of care:

- — Adherence to quality, psychomotor activities in testing
- — Patient-centered collaborative activities
- — Trauma-informed collaboration and support with implementation of plan of care

Activity 13-8. APP and Physician Differential Diagnosis

- — The differential diagnoses include hepatitis A, C, D, and E; alcoholic hepatitis; autoimmune hepatitis; drug-induced liver injury; and cirrhosis.
- — Based on the test results, the infection is hepatitis B.

Activity 13-9. Treatment

DJ is told to avoid alcohol and acetaminophen and to increase fluid intake to replace volume lost. He is educated on transmission of HBV and the possible outcomes (eg, developing the core IgM antibodies, becoming a carrier) and the importance of following up with the gastroenterologist. In addition to encouraging testing of his sexual partners, he is told to use barrier protection during sexual intercourse and to not share toothbrushes, razors, needles, or any other injection equipment. He is told to cover open cuts and scratches and to clean any blood spills with bleach solution. He is advised to not donate blood, organs, or sperm. He is referred to a local liver/gastro-intestinal clinic and encouraged to keep his follow-up appointment because he will need extended monitoring.

Activity 13-10. Reporting

— This is a reportable disease for acute or chronic infections.

— Exposure that results in development of the core antibodies is reportable for data, but not for investigation.

— The purpose of disease surveillance is to (1) identify contacts of case-patients who require postexposure prophylaxis; (2) detect outbreaks; (3) identify infected persons who need counseling and referral for medical management; (4) monitor disease incidence and prevalence; and (5) determine the epidemiologic characteristics of infected persons, including the source of their infection, to assess and reduce missed opportunities for vaccination.

Activity 13-11. Follow-Up Recommendations in Plan of Care

— The patient is encouraged to alert sexual partners, who should be informed so that they may be examined and treated. Prophylaxis is available if risk of a new infection is discovered before infection is confirmed.

— Patient education is critical to ensure that infected individuals understand the need for lifelong monitoring, transmission prevention, and the appropriate lifestyle changes.

— Lifestyle changes should include limiting or abstaining from alcohol and drug intake.

— Education about nutrition and maintenance of gastrointestinal symptoms that may be controlled with diet, exercise, and supplements, maintaining hydration and controlling pain.

— Caution should be exercised when taking drugs that are metabolized by the liver, such as acetaminophen.

— Those with HBsAg positivity should be counseled on transmission prevention.

— Patient should be monitored by a gastroenterologist until antibodies develop, and if antibodies do not develop, monitored for chronic infection.

— It is recommended that the patient follow up even if the disease symptoms improve.

Case Study 14

Activity 14-1. Identifying Missing Subjective Information

Aggravating/relieving, Radiation, Severity

Activity 14-2. Anatomical Identification

A. Shaft of penis

B. Foreskin

C. Glans penis

D. Area of inguinal lymph nodes

E. Corona

Activity 14-3. Physical Examination Findings

A painful, deep, erythematous ulcer with well-demarcated margins is present on the shaft near the glans penis. Enlarged lymph nodes can be palpated in the groin. No discharge is present and the examination is otherwise unremarkable.

Activity 14-4. Clinical Laboratory Improvement Amendments (CLIA) Laboratory Examination

— First-catch urine specimens are collected for NAAT.

— Blood samples are collected for serological testing.

— The nurse orders the office urine dipstick test, which shows moderate increase in leukocytes. No other abnormalities are seen in the dipstick results.

— Implement the protocol for testing.

Activity 14-5. Clinical Laboratory Testing

— A specimen is taken from the base of the ulcer for dark-field examination to rule out syphilis.

— Serological tests should be ordered to identify syphilis and HSV, the 2 more prominent differential diagnoses, and HIV because risk of transmission of HIV increases significantly when chancroid is present.

— Urine NAAT for gonorrhea and *Chlamydia* is indicated.

Activity 14-6. Forensic Evidence Collection

This case does not warrant a medical forensic evaluation with evidence collection.

Activity 14-7. Nursing Plan of Care Procedure

Nursing diagnoses:

— Infection: Risk for infection transmission related to contact transmission exposure, multiple sexual partners, and unprotected sexual intercourse.

— Damage to tissue integrity: Mucosal lesion in the cornea, the integument, or subcutaneous tissues.

— Violation of the integrity of the skin: Skin lesion; break in the integument, the largest multifunctional organ of the body.

— Acute pain: Distress or malaise experienced and reported by the person.

Plan of care:

— Adherence to quality, psychomotor activities in testing

— Patient-centered collaborative activities

— Trauma-informed collaboration and support with implementation of plan of care

Activity 14-8. APP and Physician Differential Diagnosis

— The differential diagnosis includes syphilis and herpes simplex. Other infections are considered but are not part of the differential diagnosis and include *Chlamydia*, LGV, and *N. gonorrhoeae*.

— Test for HIV because the open wound of chancroid increases the transmission of HIV.

— The infection is chancroid.

Activity 14-9. Treatment

All tests came back negative, and the patient returned to the clinic 7 days later for reevaluation. On examination the lesion is ulcerated and remains painful. Fluctuant lymphadenopathy to the inguinal area remains. In 25% of all *H. ducreyi* cases, the lymph nodes become bulbous, breaking open. In 75% of all *H. ducreyi* cases, the disease spontaneously resolved in 3 months.

Based on the negative laboratory tests and clinical presentation, a probable diagnosis of *Haemophilus ducreyi* infection (chancroid) is made and the patient is given a stat dose of azithromycin 1 g. The patient's regular partner is notified and treated with azithromycin 1 g. The patient attempts to contact the woman he had sex with while on vacation to notify her that she might be infected, but he is unable to locate her.

Activity 14-10. Reporting

Chancroid is a reportable disease. Chancroid should be reported both to the CDC and, in most states, to the state Department of Health. Contact your local health department for instructions on how to report.

Activity 14-11. Follow-Up Recommendations in Plan of Care

— Anticipatory guidance about the subsequent epidemiologic investigation to identify partners with reportable diseases; use trauma-informed care principles, without judgement.

— Further reevaluation may be necessary if symptoms do not resolve. Inform the patient that lymphadenopathy may take longer to resolve than the lesion.

— Sexual partners should be informed so that they may be examined and treated. In women, chancroid can be painless, and women may not know they are infected. Therefore, all sexual partners should be tested, even if asymptomatic.

— Condoms should be used during every sexual encounter.

Case Study 15

Activity 15-1. Identifying Missing Subjective Information

The patient identifies aggravating factors; however, attempts to relieve the symptoms are not presented and could be pertinent to the assessment, diagnosis, and treatment. The history does not include radiation, although the patient denies dysuria, dyspareunia, or burning.

Activity 15-2. Anatomical Identification

A. Cervix

B. Hymen remnant

C. Cervical os

D. Frothy discharge

Activity 15-3. Physical Examination Findings

The cervix is erythematous and discharge is whitish-grey and thin. Otherwise, the examination is within normal limits.

Activity 15-4. Clinical Laboratory Improvement Amendments (CLIA) Laboratory Examination

— The RN orders an in-office urine dipstick test. The urine dipstick results indicate trace leukocytes and trace blood. No other abnormalities observed on the dipstick results.

— The APP performs a speculum examination and collects samples of vaginal discharge for a wet mount and to determine vaginal pH, as well as point-of-care testing for BV.

Activity 15-5. Clinical Laboratory Testing

— The pH of vaginal discharge/fluid is acidic.

— Wet mount of the vaginal discharge with 1 to 2 drops of 0.9% normal saline solution at room temperature on a glass slide. If microscopy is available, examine the sample for clue cells. If not, send slide to laboratory for Gram stain, which is 98% effective in the detection of clue cells.

— Amine or "whiff" test. Perform by adding 10% potassium hydroxide (KOH) to the wet mount slide and then smelling ("whiffing") the slide for the presence or absence of a fishy odor. Occasionally, the fishy odor is prominent but requires validation with the KOH test.

Activity 15-6. Forensic Evidence Collection

This case does not warrant a medical forensic evaluation with evidence collection.

Activity 15-7. Nursing Plan of Care Procedure

Nursing diagnosis:

— Risk for infection related to invasion or proliferation of microorganisms

— Readiness for enhanced knowledge

Plan of care:

— Adherence to quality, psychomotor activities in testing

— Patient-centered collaborative activities

— Trauma-informed collaboration and support with implementation of plan of care

Activity 15-8. APP and Physician Differential Diagnosis

— The differential diagnosis includes BV, vulvovaginal candidiasis, trichomoniasis, atrophic vaginitis, and desquamative inflammatory vaginitis.

— Based on the patient's description of the discharge (homogeneous, thin, white, fishy odor) and her lack of dysuria, cloudy urine, frequent urination, pruritus, dyspareunia, burning sensation, vaginal erythema, or edema, the priority differential is a diagnosis of BV.

Activity 15-9. Treatment

Medical treatment:

— Definitive diagnosis is made in this case by meeting 3 of the 4 Amsel criteria: (1) characteristic discharge; (2) positive whiff test; and (3) vaginal pH greater than 4.5.

— The patient receives a prescription for metronidazole 500 mg twice daily for 7 days, and instructions included reoccurrence. The patient is instructed to stop douching and is educated on the negative effects of douching, such as changes the vaginal environment that creates susceptibility to infection.

Activity 15-10. Reporting

BV is not a reportable disease.

Activity 15-11. Follow-Up Recommendations in Plan of Care

— Male sex partners do not need treatment. The patient should provide notification of the BV diagnosis to female sex partners.

— Follow-up with a health care provider after completion of treatment is essential to prevent a recurrence.

— It is essential to complete the entire course of treatment as prescribed.

— Advise patient to refrain from alcohol for 24 hours after completion of metronidazole.

— Some women have a recurrence of BV within 1 year and may require additional treatment.

— BV is a risk factor for HIV, HSV, gonorrhea, *Chlamydia*, and trichomoniasis.

— Condoms are the best way to lower the risk of BV or other sexually transmitted infections.

Case Study 16

Activity 16-1. Identifying Missing Subjective Information

Onset, Duration Radiation, Aggravating/relieving, Severity

Activity 16-2. Anatomical Identification

A. External os

B. Vaginal wall

C. Cervix

D. Fornix

Activity 16-3. Physical Examination Findings

The cervical os exposes the squamocolumnar junction (also known as transformation zone) and is erythematous, with early cervical erosion, tenderness, and scant discharge present. Otherwise, the anogenital examination is normal. The appearance of the transformation zone is affected by age, hormones, and exposure to disease.

Activity 16-4. Clinical Laboratory Improvement Amendments (CLIA) Laboratory Examination

— The nurse orders the office urine dipstick, which shows a moderate increase in leukocytes, as well as trace blood. No other abnormalities are seen in the dipstick results.

— Implement the protocol for testing.

Activity 16-5. Clinical Laboratory Testing

— Endocervical and pharyngeal specimens are collected using sterile swab techniques.

— A first-catch urine specimen is collected for NAAT for *Chlamydia trachomatis* and *Neisseria gonorrhoeae.*

— Sample testing with wet mount, potassium hydroxide.

Activity 16-6. Forensic Evidence Collection

This case does not warrant a medical forensic evaluation with evidence collection.

Activity 16-7. Nursing Plan of Care Procedure

Nursing diagnosis:

— Violation of the integrity of the oral mucosa: Out of the tissue layers of the oral cavity.

— Acute pain: Distress or malaise experienced and reported by the person.

Plan of care:

— Adherence to quality, psychomotor activities in testing

— Patient-centered collaborative activities

— Trauma-informed collaboration and support with implementation of plan of care

Activity 16-8. APP and Physician Differential Diagnosis

— The differential diagnosis includes *Chlamydia*, BV, gonorrhea, vaginitis (yeast), trichomoniasis, and recent semen deposit.

— The infection is *N. gonorrhoeae.*

Activity 16-9. Treatment

SD returns to the clinic for treatment and is administered ceftriaxone 250 mg intramuscularly and azithromycin 1 g orally taken with food offered in the clinic to avoid upset stomach and is advised of possible nausea/vomiting.

Activity 16-10. Reporting

This is a reportable disease. The local public health district should be notified per mandatory reporting requirements, and the patient should be notified regarding disease investigation follow-up procedures.

Activity 16-11. Follow-Up Recommendations in Plan of Care

— Trauma informed care, avoiding judgement

— Anticipatory guidance about the mandatory reporting of the disease and follow-up with local health department epidemiologist

— Advise on contact until test of cure (eg, the patient is advised to avoid all oral and genital contact for 7 days)

— Reevaluation may be necessary after 1 week if symptoms persist

— Explore comfort in talking to partner(s), and advise recent sexual partners should be informed so that they may be examined and treated

— Condoms are provided, and the patient is educated to use condoms for all sexual encounters

Case Study 17

Activity 17-1. Identifying Missing Subjective Information

Character, Aggravating/relieving, Radiation, Severity

Activity 17-2. Anatomical Identification

A. Scrotum

B. Shaft

C. Foreskin in uncircumcised male

Activity 17-3. Physical Examination Findings

Dermatologic condition that was differentially diagnosed as a case of human scabies caused an infestation of scabies.

Activity 17-4. Clinical Laboratory Improvement Amendments (CLIA) Laboratory Examination

CLIA-specific recommendations do not apply universally across the United States with a diagnosis of scabies. Consult with the public health department about the legal requirements in their jurisdictions. For guidance, consider reviewing the State Legal Requirements for Submission of Isolates and Other Clinical Materials by Clinical Laboratories: A Review of State Approaches.

Activity 17-5. Clinical Laboratory Testing

— A skin scraping sample is taken by placing a drop of mineral oil directly over multiple burrows on the patient's skin and scraping parallel and laterally across the skin gently with the side of a scalpel blade. The skin sample is examined under a light microscope, and the diagnosis of scabies is confirmed with the identification of mites and larvae present on the slide.

— Chronic infestation results in gross distribution of the live mites and may result in crusting around the lesions.

Activity 17-6. Forensic Evidence Collection

This case does not warrant a medical forensic evaluation with evidence collection.

Activity 17-7. Nursing Plan of Care Procedure

Nursing diagnoses:

— Impaired skin integrity: Infestation

— Acute pain: Distress or malaise experienced and reported by the person.

— Readiness for enhanced knowledge

Plan of care:

— Adherence to quality, psychomotor activities in testing

— Patient-centered collaborative activities

— Trauma-informed collaboration and support with implementation of plan of care

Activity 17-8. APP and Physician Differential Diagnosis

— The differential diagnoses include contact dermatitis, chickenpox, drug reaction, eczema, lice, herpes, psoriasis, and other skin conditions.

— Based on a positive tape test, the infection (infestation) is scabies.

Activity 17-9. Treatment

The adults in the household are provided with permethrin 5%, a topical lotion for the treatment of scabies. They are instructed to apply the lotion, leaving the medication on the skin for 8 to 14 hours and followed by a thorough rinse. At the end of that time, adults may reapply the lotion, particularly if live mites reappear.

The guardian/parent is also instructed to not apply the lotion to the children in the household. Any ocular involvement requires application of petroleum jelly to the brows and lashes for at least 7 days. As long as mites are visible, the adults should continue to apply petroleum jelly to the brows and eyelashes. If there were younger children in the household, infants and children aged 2 months to 10 years should be treated with a single application of permethrin 5% cream from head to toe and left on the skin for 8 to 14 hours and then rinsed off. Reapply in 7 days if mites reappear.

Activity 17-10. Reporting

Scabies is not a reportable disease, except when infestation is endemic or an epidemic in day cares or schools. Public health officials will partner with institutions where children congregate to provide information and treatment recommendations.

Activity 17-11. Follow-Up Recommendations in Plan of Care

— More than 1 application may be necessary to get rid of the infestation.

— Evaluation may be necessary after 1 week if symptoms persist.

— Retreatment also may be necessary if unresolved in 2 to 4 weeks.

— Bedding and clothing used by the infested person should be machine washed in hot water and dried in a hot dryer or dry cleaned within the preceding 2 to 3 days. Hot dryers kill the mites and eggs as well. Items that cannot be washed and dried or dry cleaned should be sealed in a plastic bag for at least 3 days, because the mite dies without a human blood meal within 72 hours.

— Clean and vacuum rooms, then empty the vacuum bag.

— It is recommended that people who have been in contact with the infected patient also be treated, especially if living in the household.

Case Study 18

Activity 18-1. Identifying Missing Subjective Information

Radiation, Severity

Activity 18-2. Anatomical Identification

A. Corona

B. Glans

C. Corona

D. Foreskin

E. Urethra

F. Glans

G. Frenulum

Activity 18-3. Physical Examination Findings

A. Cratered lesion, painful

B. Frenulum with red lesion

In this photograph, the ulcerative red painful lesion is located on the frenulum.

Activity 18-4. Clinical Laboratory Improvement Amendments (CLIA) Laboratory Examination

— The RN ordered the office urine dipstick, which showed moderate increase in leukocytes, as well as trace blood. No other abnormalities are seen in dipstick results.

— Implement the protocol for testing for other STIs.

Activity 18-5. Clinical Laboratory Testing

— Persons who receive a LGV diagnosis should be tested for other STIs, especially HIV, gonorrhea, *Chlamydia* and syphilis.

Activity 18-6. Forensic Evidence Collection

This case does not warrant a medical forensic evaluation with evidence collection.

Activity 18-7. Nursing Plan of Care Procedure

Nursing diagnosis:

— Damage to tissue integrity: Mucosal lesion in the corona, the integument, or subcutaneous tissues

— Violation of the integrity of the skin: Skin lesion; break in the integument, the largest multifunctional organ of the body

— Acute pain: Distress or malaise experienced and reported by the person

— Chronic pain: Pain lasting for more than 6 months with resolving lymph node

Plan of care:

— Adherence to quality, psychomotor activities in testing

— Patient-centered collaborative activities related to STI avoidance

— Trauma-informed collaboration and support with implementation of plan of care

Activity 18-8. APP and Physician Differential Diagnosis

— The differential diagnosis includes herpes simplex, syphilis, chancroid, and granuloma inguinale.

— The infection is LGV.

Activity 18-9. Treatment

— Patient is prescribed 100 mg doxycycline orally twice daily for 21 days ***OR*** Erythromycin 500 mg orally 4 times a day for 21 days. Although clinical data are lacking, azithromycin 1 g orally once weekly for 3 weeks is probably effective based on its chlamydial antimicrobial activity. Fluoroquinolone-based treatments also might be effective, but the optimal duration of treatment has not been evaluated.

— Buboes (as noted in first photograph of enlarged right inguinal lymph node) might require aspiration through intact skin or incision and drainage to prevent the formation of inguinal/femoral ulcerations.

Activity 18-10. Reporting

As required by state law, LGV cases should be reported to the health department.

Activity 18-11. Follow-Up Recommendations in Plan of Care

— Follow-up in 2 to 3 weeks is requested and after all symptoms resolve. Partners need referral for testing and treatment as soon as possible.

— The patient is encouraged to refrain from sexual activity until 7 days after he has completed his treatment and to inform all sexual partners from the previous 60 days to present for testing and empirical treatment.

Case Study 19

Activity 19-1. Identifying Missing Subjective Information

Onset, Duration, Aggravating/relieving factors, Radiation, Severity

Activity 19-2. Anatomical Identification

A. Lateral left tongue

B. Gingival tissue of the right upper maxilla

C. Soft palate

Activity 19-3. Physical Examination Findings

A. Area of white patches of fungal disease on lateral left tongue

B. Granulated tumors on the gingival tissue over the right upper maxilla imply tumor-type growths; referral to an HIV specialist and dental surgeon is necessary for treatment

C. Soft palate is distorted by tumor-like growths, potentially obstructing mastication, and crypts provide potential for food capture and further breakdown of the tissue; consider oral care instructions to avoid potential for infection

In this case, the man has a positive HIV NAAT, with oral changes reflecting a low CD4 count and tumor-like growths. At this stage of HIV disease, acquired immunodeficiency syndrome (AIDS) is evident and the viral load is high, making the patient highly infectious. Medication can reduce the viral load, but the HIV specialist will enlist the help of other specialists in the management of AIDS and the patient's failing immune system.

Activity 19-4. Clinical Laboratory Improvement Amendments (CLIA) Laboratory Examination

— Implement the protocol for testing for all STIs.

— Explain to the patient that he is highly infectious, and make recommendations to minimize spread of the virus to the patient's partners.

— Refer to the HIV specialist, helping the patient understand the severity of his disease.

— Reassure and provide recommendations to the patient about the following:

  — Preventing exposure to opportunistic pathogens

  — Preventing disease

  — Discontinuing primary prophylaxis after immune reconstitution

  — Treating disease

  — When to start antiretroviral therapy in the setting of an acute opportunistic infection

  — Monitoring for adverse effects (including immune reconstitution inflammatory syndrome)

  — Managing treatment failure

  — Preventing disease recurrence (secondary prophylaxis or chronic maintenance therapy)

  — Discontinuing secondary prophylaxis or chronic maintenance therapy after immune reconstitution

Activity 19-5. Clinical Laboratory Testing

— HIV

— HSV

— Syphilis

— Liver profile for hepatitis B and C

— NAAT for *Chlamydia* and gonorrhea

— Chest radiographs

Activity 19-6. Forensic Evidence Collection

This case does not warrant a medical forensic evaluation with evidence collection.

Activity 19-7. Nursing Plan of Care Procedure

Nursing diagnosis:

— Damage to tissue integrity: Mucosal lesion in the corona, the integument or subcutaneous tissues

— Violation of the integrity of the skin: Skin lesion; break in the integument, the largest multifunctional organ of the body

— Acute pain: Distress or malaise experienced and reported by the person

— Chronic pain: Pain lasting for more than 6 months with resolving lymph node

Plan of care:

— Adherence to quality, psychomotor activities in testing

— Patient-centered collaborative activities

— Trauma-informed collaboration and support with implementation of plan of care

Activity 19-8. APP and Physician Differential Diagnosis

— The differential diagnosis includes bacillary angiomatosis, pyogenic granuloma, oral nevus, lymphoma, oral hemangiomas or other benign vascular proliferations.

— The infection is HIV, and the lesions are associated with Kaposi sarcoma.

Activity 19-9. Treatment

— The CDC 2019 *Guidelines for the Use of Antiretroviral Agents in Adults and Adolescents with HIV* are available.

— Based on the results of 2 large, randomized controlled trials that showed that a 2-drug regimen of (dolutegravir [DTG]) plus lamivudine (DTG/3TC) was noninferior to DTG plus tenofovir disoproxil fumarate (TDF)/emtricitabine (FTC), the Panel has added DTG/3TC to the list of Recommended Initial Regimens for Most People with HIV, except for individuals:

— with pretreatment HIV RNA >500,000 copies/mL

— who are known to have active HBV coinfection

— who will initiate antiretroviral therapy before results of HIV genotype testing for reverse transcriptase or HBV testing are available

— The CDC guidelines have been updated with revised recommendations on the use of DTG in individuals of childbearing potential. Current data on the possible association between weight gain and the use of (integrase strand transfer inhibitors [INSTIs]) and tenofovir alafenamide (TAF) are reviewed in the sections on INSTIs and nucleoside reverse transcriptase inhibitors.

— The patient is referred to an HIV specialty clinic for management to begin antiretroviral therapy (ART). If the APP is skilled in HIV treatment, an antifungal treatment with a high barrier to drug resistance is often chosen. Inform the patient that missing just a few doses of his HIV treatment can cause HIV drug resistance, which means his current HIV medication may stop working. This could cause his viral load to go up and make his CD4+ cell count go down, weakening his immune system. His future treatment options may become limited, and his HIV drug resistance can also be passed on to others. There are new guidelines to guide HIV treatment and management in many populations.

Activity 19-10. Reporting

HIV is a reportable disease; the state health department can direct providers about their responsibility to protect the public. There is significant public health intervention when prevalence is high. Rural communities do not experience a similar level of support. Overall, 40% of persons with HIV do not have controlled disease.

Activity 19-11. Follow-Up Recommendations in Plan of Care

— ART is the approach recommended for all people living with HIV, regardless of how long they've had the virus or how healthy they are. ART must be taken every day.

— Taking HIV medication every day as prescribed helps control the HIV virus and may prevent the development of AIDS.

— Provide treatment options and prescribe medications to eradicate disease and provide comfort to the patient.

— In this case, if the APP is unfamiliar with HIV management, the patient should be sent to a special care center to continue the evaluation of disease progression and create a personalized plan of care.

— End-stage HIV infection requires skilled teams of providers to manage the disease and the symptoms.

www.ingramcontent.com/pod-product-compliance
Lightning Source LLC
LaVergne TN
LVHW070909210926
848482LV00017B/1026
* 9 7 8 1 9 3 6 5 9 0 8 5 8 *